Deep Learning for Smart Healthcare

Deep learning can provide more accurate results compared to machine learning. It uses layered algorithmic architecture to analyze data. It produces more accurate results since learning from previous results enhances its ability. The multi-layered nature of deep learning systems has the potential to classify subtle abnormalities in medical images, clustering patients with similar characteristics into risk-based cohorts, or highlighting relationships between symptoms and outcomes within vast quantities of unstructured data.

Exploring this potential, *Deep Learning for Smart Healthcare: Trends, Challenges and Applications* is a reference work for researchers and academicians who are seeking new ways to apply deep learning algorithms in healthcare, including medical imaging and healthcare data analytics. It covers how deep learning can analyze a patient's medical history efficiently to aid in recommending drugs and dosages. It discusses how deep learning can be applied to CT scans, MRI scans and ECGs to diagnose diseases. Other deep learning applications explored are extending the scope of patient record management, pain assessment, new drug design and managing the clinical trial process.

Bringing together a wide range of research domains, this book can help to develop breakthrough applications for improving healthcare management and patient outcomes.

Dr. K. Murugeswari is a Senior Assistant Professor in the School of Computing Science and Engineering at VIT Bhopal University, M.P, India.

Dr. B. Sundaravadivazhagan is a professor in the Department of Information Technology at the University of Technology and Applied Science-AL Mussanah in Oman.

Dr. S. Poonkuntran is a Professor and Dean of the School of Computing Science and Engineering at VIT Bhopal University, Madhya Pradesh, India.

Dr. Thendral Puyalnithi is an Assistant Professor Senior in the Mepco Schlenk Engineering College in the Department of Artificial Intelligence and Data Science, Tamil Nadu, India.

Deep Learning for Smart Healthcare
Trends, Challenges and Applications

Edited by
Dr. K. Murugeswari
Dr. B. Sundaravadivazhagan
Dr. S. Poonkuntran
Dr. Thendral Puyalnithi

CRC Press
Taylor & Francis Group
Boca Raton London New York

CRC Press is an imprint of the
Taylor & Francis Group, an **informa** business

AN AUERBACH BOOK

First edition published 2024
2385 NW Executive Center Drive, Suite 320, Boca Raton FL 33431

and by CRC Press
4 Park Square, Milton Park, Abingdon, Oxon, OX14 4RN

CRC Press is an imprint of Taylor & Francis Group, LLC

ISBN: 978-1-032-45581-5 (hbk)
ISBN: 978-1-032-74516-9 (pbk)
ISBN: 978-1-003-46960-5 (ebk)

DOI: 10.1201/9781003469605

Typeset in Times
by MPS Limited, Dehradun

Contents

Preface

Deep learning provides more accurate results compared to machine learning. It uses layered algorithmic architecture to analyze data. Each layer in artificial neural networks filters the data based on the feedback received from previous layers. It produces more accurate results since learning from previous results to enhance its ability. This multi-layered nature of deep learning models to classify subtle abnormalities in medical images, clustering patients with similar characteristics into risk-based cohorts, or highlight relationships between symptoms and outcomes within vast quantities of unstructured data. The specialty of deep learning is to make decisions without the involvement of humans.

Deep learning has the potential to identify any discomforts in our body faster than clinicians. The hospital setup is not sufficient to meet quality patient outcomes due to increasing population and diversifying diseases. Hence, it is important to shift from traditional approach to machine-level approach. Managing patient data is very critical and complex, but deep learning provides us a good solution to manage such complex and big data that are kept over the cloud. It assists medical professionals and researchers to analyze diseases accurately and helps them to treat in a better way.

Deep learning analyzes patients' medical history efficiently and helps to recommend drugs and their dosage. Medical imaging techniques such as CT scan, MRI scan, and ECG are used to diagnose diseases. Deep learning analyses these images in a faster and accurate way, which results in earlier diagnosis of the disease. Deep learning helps to classify healthcare data and optimize drug design. It extends the scope of patient record management, cervical pain assessment, and clinical trial process.

- The proposed book will be the baseline for the researchers and academicians who wish to explore applying deep learning algorithms in the healthcare sector. Here, medical imaging and healthcare data analytics are considered.
- Magnetic resonance (MR) and computed tomography (CT) are the commonly used medical imaging techniques for detecting disease and prediction. Deep learning models effectively interpret by combining the aspects of these imaging data such as tissue size, volume, and shape. Deep learning algorithms are used for early detection of Alzheimer's disease, diabetic retinopathy detection, and ultrasound detection of breast nodules.
- Nowadays smartphones and wearable devices are part of everyday life. They provide useful information about our lifestyle. Easy-to-monitor medical risk factors of patients using mobile apps will be analyzed by deep learning models. In 2019, the Food and Drug Administration (FDA) approved Current Health's AI wearable device as the first AI medical

monitoring wearables used at home. It is used to measure respiration, pulse, oxygen temperature, saturation, and mobility of patients.

This book is mainly for bringing all the related research in different fields under the single umbrella of deep learning in the healthcare domain. It has many path-breaking applications, such as patient data management, clinical trial process, disease diagnoses, medical imaging, and recent developments.

Contributors

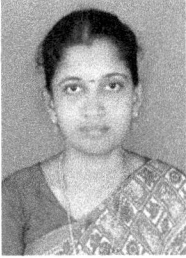

Dr. S. Angayarkanni Annamalai, M.E., Ph.D., is an assistant professor in the Department of Networking and Communication, with total teaching experience of 15.5 years. She obtained her B.Tech. (information technology) and M.E. (wireless technologies) from Anna University in 2005 and 2008. She scored 91.89 percentile in GATE – IT 2006 Examination. She completed her PhD in 2021 from Anna University. Her research domain is intelligent transportation systems. Her area of interest includes networking, wireless technologies, and intelligent road traffic system for Indian roads. She has published 4 papers in international journals and 5 papers in international conferences. She is a lifetime member of The Institution of Engineers (India) – IEI and Indian Society of Technical Education (ISTE).

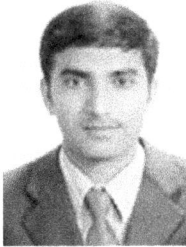

Dr. S.P. Balakannan received his Ph.D. degree from the Department of Electronics and Information Engineering at Chonbuk National University, South Korea (2010). He has received his master degree (5 years integrated) from the Department of Computer Science and Engineering, Bharathiar University, India, in the year 2003. He has worked as a project assistant in Indian Institute of Technology (IIT), Kharagpur, India from 2003 to 2006. Currently, he is working as senior associate professor in the Department of Information Technology, Kalasalingam University, Tamil Nadu, India. His areas of interest include wireless network, network coding, cloud & green computing, cryptography, and mobile communication.

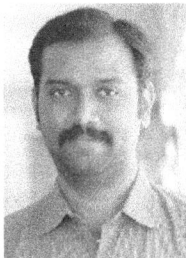

Dr. C. Balasubramanian received his bachelor of engineering in electronics and communication engineering from Anna University, Chennai by 2006. He received his master of engineering degree in applied electronics from Anna University, Chennai by 2008. He has completed Ph.D degree in the area of wireless sensor network in the Department of Information Technology under Kalasalingam Academy of Research and Education by 2020. He is currently working as an associate professor in the Department of Computer Science and Engineering, Kalasalingam Academy of Research and Education. He has 15 years of experience in teaching and research. He has published more than 25 papers in reputed international journals and conferences. His areas of interest are Internet of Things, image and signal processing, wireless sensor and ad hoc networks.

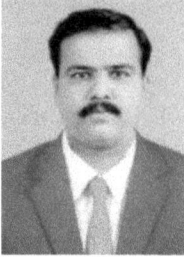

Dr. S. Balasubramaniam is Post-Doctoral researcher in the Department of Applied Data Science, Noroff University College, Kristiansand, Norway and He has a totally around 10+ years of experience in teaching, research and industry. Currently he is working as an Assistant Professor in School of Computer Science and Engineering, Kerala University of Digital Sciences, Innovation and Technology (Digital University of Kerala), Thiruvananthapuram, Kerala, India. He holds a Ph.D degree in Computer Science and Engineering from Anna University, Chennai, India. He has published nearly 20 research papers in reputed SCI/WoS/ Scopus indexed Journals. He has also granted with 1 Australian patent, 1 Indian Patent and published 3 Indian patents. He has presented papers at conferences, contributed chapters to the edited books and editor in few books published by international publishers. His research and publication interests include machine learning and deep learning-based disease diagnosis, cloud computing security, Generative AI and Electric Vehicles. EeanElElectric Vehicles.

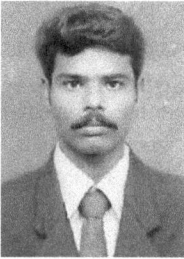

Dr. A. Chinnasamy obtained his bachelor degree (B.E.) in computer science and engineering from Anna University in 2005, his master's degree (M.E.) in computer science and engineering from Anna University in 2008, and his Ph.D. in information and communication engineering from Anna University, Chennai, 2017. He is currently working as assistant professor in the department of DSBS, SRMIST, Kattankulathur Chennai, (INDIA). He is having 15 years of teaching experience and published 21 articles in highly reputed international journals. He has an Anna University Guideship and is guiding 10 Ph.D. Research Scholars. His areas of interests include mobile ad hoc networks, VANET, and cloud computing. He is a member of the Computer Society of India (CSI), ISTE, IAENG and reviewer in *Measurement and Control Journal* and *Wireless Personal Communication.*

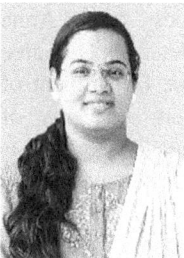

Dr. Bhumika Choksi received her Ph.D. from S. V. National Institute of Technology, Surat in the area of fluid flow through porous media. She has completed her M.Sc. & M.Phil. from VNSGU, Surat with top ranks and teaching engineering mathematics from the year 2009. Dr. Choksi has 9 research publications in ESCI, SCOPUS, UGC & other reputed peer-reviewed journals and has attended more than 30 national/ international conferences/seminars/workshops/STTPs. She is a life member of GAMS & Gujarat Ganit Mandal.

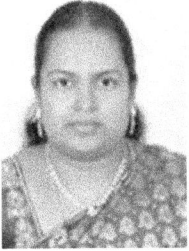

Dr. Beaulah David has completed her doctorate in the Department of Computer Science and Engineering and her master'a degree with a specialization of network and Internet engineering from Karunya Institute of Technology and Sciences, Coimbatore and her bachelor's degree in computer hardware and software engineering from Avinashilingam Institute for Home Science & Higher Education for Women, Coimbatore. At present she is working as an associate professor at Karpagam College of Engineering, Coimbatore. She has gained more than a decade of experience in teaching and her area of interest includes data sciences, pervasive computing, wireless sensor networks, and artificial intelligence. She has published many papers in refereed international journals, conference proceedings and also published patents.

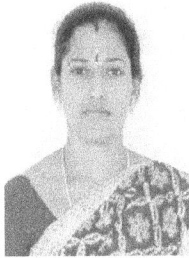

Dr. M. Renuka Devi completed her doctor of philosophy in 2012 in Bharathiar University, Coimbatore. She has nearly 21 years of post-graduate teaching experience in computer science. Currently working as an associate professor in the School of Information Science, Presidency University, Bangalore. There are 15 Ph.D. scholars and 13 MPhil scholars have completed their degree under her guidance. She has published 65 (30 Scopus + 30 UGC&WoS) papers in various international journals. She has organized various conferences and workshops. She has published 3 patents, 3 books, and 2 book chapters.

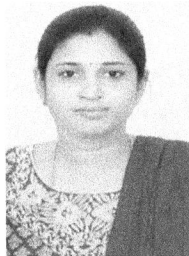

Ms. S. Devi is pursuing a Ph.D. from Presidency University, Bangalore and completed her M.Sc. (information technology) in 2006 in Bharathidasan University, Trichy and completed her M.Phil (computer science) in 2007 in Periyar University, Salem. She has nearly 8 years of industry and teaching experience in computer science & information science. Currently working as an assistant professor in School of Information Science, Presidency University, Bangalore. University, Bangalore. Research specializations include machine learning, natural language processing, and IOT. She has published over 10 research papers in reputed national and international conferences and journals, and attended and organized a number of seminars, workshops, FDP, etc.

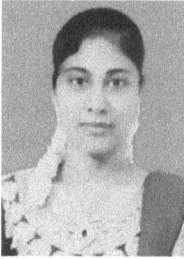

S. Aanjana Devi is a research scholar in the Department of Computer Application, Alagappa University, Karaikudi. She holds an M.Phil. degree in computer application from Alagappa University, Karaikudi. She is currently pursuing her Ph.D. degree. She has published papers in 2 national conferences, 4 international conferences, and 3 international journals in the area of bio metrics. Her research interests include network security, cloud computing, and deep learning.

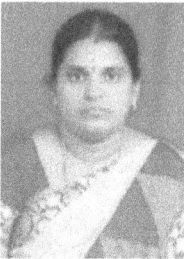

Dr. S. Dhanalakshmi is working as an associate professor, Department of Software Systems, Sri Krishna Arts and Science College, Coimbatore. She has nearly 19 years' experience. She has published more than 25 papers in international journals, and she has presented 15 papers in international conferences. Her research interests include preserving privacy, data mining, and security issues in databases.

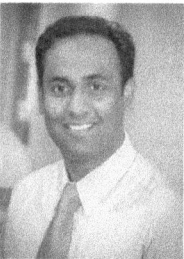

Robin Doss is the University's Strategic Research Centre (SRC) Director in Cyber Security Research and Innovation (CSRI). In addition, he leads Deakin University's participation in the Cyber Security Cooperative Research Centre (CSCRC). He is the theme leader for the CSCRC's research theme on "Development of Next Generation Authentication Technologies."

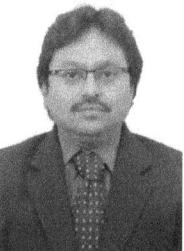

Dr. M. A. Saleem Durai, obtained his MCA from Bharathidasan University, Tiruchirappalli, M. Phil. from Madurai Kamaraj University, and completed his Ph.D. from VIT Vellore. He has served at VIT University since 2001 as a professor and associate dean in the School of Computer Sciences and Engineering VIT, Vellore, Tamil Nadu, India. He has authored many Scopus indexed journal papers. He is CO-PI for MHRD–SPARC Bilateral project with Deakin University, Australia: "Enabling Smart and Safe Cities Through IoT Technologies" with an overlay of 73 lakhs. His research interests include networking, data mining, machine learning, and IoT. He is closely associated with many professional bodies.

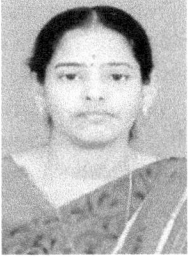

Dr. S. Vahini Ezhilraman, MCA., M.Phil., Ph.D., is presently working as an Assistant Professor in Shri Krishnaswamy College for Women, Chennai. She possesses good knowledge and experience in the field of computer application. She started her career in 2008, since then she has served as an assistant professor in the Computer Science Department in various reputed city colleges. She did her doctoral research on image processing and obtained her Ph.D. degree. She has attended various regional, national, and international conferences and presented research articles and published research papers in various reputed national and international journals.

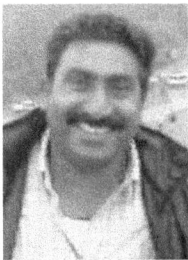

Mr. G. Ganesan is an assistant professor in the School of Computing Science and Engineering at VIT Bhopal University, M.P., India. He has 24+ years of experience in teaching and research and has published 15+ articles in various journals and conference proceedings and contributed chapters to the books. His research and publication interests include information security, machine learning, deep learning, cloud computing, network security, and cryptography.

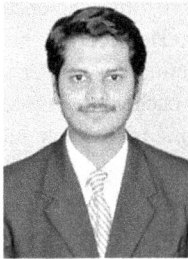

Dr. R. Gobinath is currently working as an Associate Professor at Christ university, Bangalore. He received his MCA Degree in Sri Ramakrishna Institute of Technology, Anna University, Coimbatore. He had Fourteen years of Excellence in teaching and twelve years in research experience. He started his teaching career as Assistant professor in the Department of Computer Application, Kovai Kalaimagal Arts and Science College, Coimbatore, Tamilnadu, Department of Computer Science, Nehru Arts and Science College, Coimbatore, Tamilnadu, Department of Information Technology, Dr. NGP Arts and Science College, Coimbatore, Tamilnadu and Associate professor Department of Computer Science, Vels University, Chennai, Tamilnadu. He obtained his Doctorate degree in the field of web mining and data mining in Karpagam University, Coimbatore, TamilNadu. He had published several papers in referred journals and conferences. His field of interest is Web Mining, Data Mining, Networking, wireless sensor networking, Image processing and Machine Learning. He acted as an editorial board member in several international journals and published many articles in Scopus indexed journals. He successfully guided Nine Ph.D research students and helped them in obtaining Ph.D degree, Vels University, Chennai. He obtained two awards for best research supervisor from SKCT, Thiruvanamalai, Tamil Nadu.

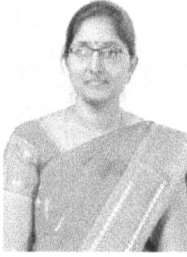

B. Gomathi is working as an associate professor in the Department of Computer Science and Engineering in PSG Institute of Technology and Applied Research at Coimbatore, India. She received her Ph.D. degree from Anna University Chennai in 2018. She is a life member of IEI. Her research areas include cloud computing, optimization techniques, and metric-driven development. Mail id: gomathi.babu@gmail.com.

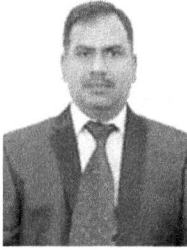

Dr. M. A. Mohammed Sahul Hameed is working as an Associate Professor at VIT Vellore, Tamil Nadu, India. His areas of interest and specialization are Language, Literature, Writing and Grammar. He has published more than 25 research papers, 3 books and has been training teachers and students on communication and writing skills. Delivered guest lectures on various topics in many colleges and universities.

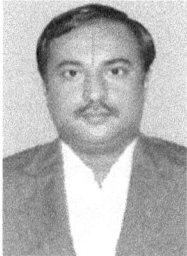

Dr. S. Hariharasitaraman is currently serving as senior assistant professor in the Division of Cyber Security and Digital Forensics, under the Faculty of Computing Science and Engineering, at VIT Bhopal University. He received his Ph.D. degree in computer science and engineering, his master's degree in computer science engineering, and bachelor's degree in computer science and engineering. He has more than 38 publications indexed in SCI/WoS/SCIE/Scopus databases, 4 book chapters, and authored four technical books with 1 national patent and 1 Australian patent granted. He is a recognized Ph.D. research supervisor and supervised 15 M.E/Mtech thesis. He is a known resource person, technical trainer, session chair, publication chair, and organiser for conducting technical workshops/webinars/industrial seminars/FDPs/conferences in technical, research, and quality domains targeted at various levels of audiences at national and international levels. He is the recipient of the Elsevier Publons Certified Journal Reviewer Award, and a reviewer for the Springer-Journal of Super Computing, MDPI, Wiley, Emerald, and IEEE publication house. He achieved a Grand Master position in Jedis rank towards generating open-sourced data to support speech and language technologies in Indian languages for "Crowdsourcing for Language Processing (CLAP)," a Project funded by MHRD and DST, Govt. of India under the IMPRINT 2 scheme, IIT Bombay, Synerg, Department of CSE. He is an active member of various technical national and international bodies like the Information Security Awareness Council-MeitY, GoI, ACM-Professional, IEEE-Student member, ISTE-Life Member, CSI, and IAEng-Life Member. His research area is security and machine learning.

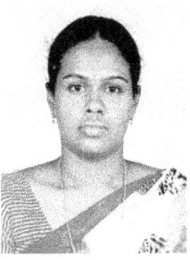

Mrs. K.E. Hemapriya is a research scholar. Her area of research is networking. With 10 years of teaching experience in the field of computer science, she is now working as assistant professor in the Department of Computer Technology at Sri Krishna Arts and Science College. She has presented and published her papers in the national and international conference and journals. She has also completed NPTEL course and has written a chapter "Cybertwin-Driven Resource Provisioning for IoE Applications at 6G-Enabled Edge Networks" in the book *New Approaches to Data Analytics and Internet of Things Through Digital Twin.*

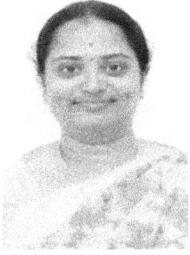

Mrs. S. Indhumathi has nearly 10 years' experience in teaching and working as an Assistant Professor, Department of Software Systems at Sri Krishna Arts and Science College, Coimbatore. She had published several papers in various International journals and presented several papers in national and international conferences.

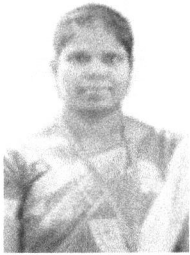

Dr. J. Joselin has nearly 17 years' experience in teaching and working as an Associate Professor at Sri Krishna Arts and Science College, Coimbatore. Had published 28 papers in various International journal and she has presented 21 papers in National and International conferences and her research broad area related to networking and security issues.

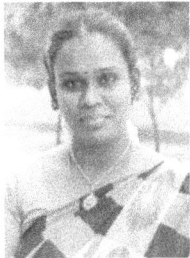

Dr. S. Karkuzhali received her B.E. degree in computer science and engineering from the Arulmigu Kalasalingam College of Engineering affiliated to Anna University, Chennai in 2008, and her M.E. degree in computer and communication engineering from the National Engineering College affiliated to Anna University of Technology Tirunelveli, in 2011. She secured first rank in her M.E. degree under those colleges, which are affiliated under Anna University of Technology Tirunelveli. She completed her PhD (Information and Communication Engineering) and the thesis entitled "Analysis of Retinal Images for Diagnosis of Eye Diseases using Feature Extraction" in Anna University, Chennai in the year 2018. She is currently working as assistant professor in Mepco Schlenk Engineering College, Sivakasi. Her research interests are in the areas of retinal image processing, computer vision, pattern recognition, and soft computing techniques. She has published more than 45 papers in national and international journals and conferences.

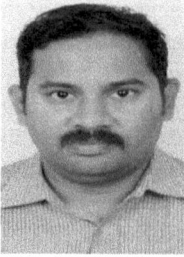

Dr. P. Karthikeyan earned his Ph.D. in Computer and Information Technology from Anna University, Chennai, India. He is having 15 plus years of experience in teaching/ research. Presently working as Associate professor and His research area of interest includes Image processing, artificial intelligence, and machine learning. He executed one funded research grants from the Research Organization, Government of India. He received two seminar grants from Anna University, Chennai, and the All-India Council for Technical Education-Indian Society for Technical Education. He has 2 patent publications and 40 plus technical paper publications. He has authored 6 books and 1 Chapter.

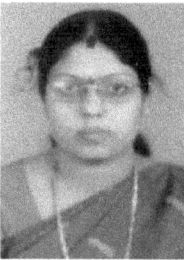

Dr. Kavitha V. obtained her B.E. degree in Computer Science and Engineering in 1996 from MS University and M.E. degree in Computer Science and Engineering in 2000 from Madurai Kamaraj University. She is the University Rank Holder received PhD degree in computer science and Engineering from Anna University Chennai in 2009. Presently she is working as a professor in the Department of CSE at University College of Engineering, Kanchipuram, Anna University, Chennai. In addition, she is the Dean of University College of Engineering, Kanchipuram campus. Currently, under her guidance research scholars are pursuing Ph.D. as full time and part time. Her research interests are wireless networks, mobile computing, network security, wireless sensor networks, image processing, and cloud computing. She has published many papers in national and international journal in areas such as network security, mobile computing, wireless network security, and cloud computing. She is a lifetime member of ISTE.

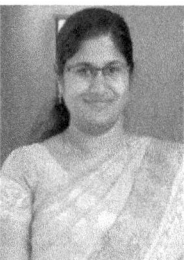

Mrs. S. Kowsalya is a research scholar with an aspiration to achieve new heights in the IT research sector and holds 9 years of teaching experience in computer science. She chooses her area of research as data mining so that to invade the maximum possibility of getting the mining techniques utilized for the present day's challenge faced by the people in medical field. Her desire is to make most of the mining techniques to impose in various health sector to make both medical officials and patients get benefit of it. Holding such a passion she serves as an assistant professor in the Department of Computer Applications at Sri Krishna Arts and Science College, India. Many of her papers have been published in national and international journals. She has also completed NPTEL courses and has written a chapter "Knowledge Discovery through Intelligent Data Analytics in Healthcare" in the book *New Approaches to Data Analytics and Internet of Things through Digital Twin.*

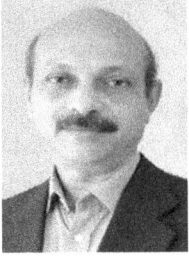

Dr. K. Satheesh Kumar is a professor and head of the Department of Futures Studies at the University of Kerala. Dr. Kumar graduated in mathematics and pursued his doctoral studies in suspension rheology at the CSIR Lab in Thiruvananthapuram. Later he worked as a post-doctoral research fellow at the Department of Chemical Engineering, Monash University, Melbourne, Australia and the Department of Physics POSTECH, Pohang, S. Korea. His research interests include suspension and polymer rheology, chaotic dynamics, nonlinear time series analysis, geo-physics, complex network analysis, and wind energy modelling and forecasting. Dr. Kumar has expertise in computational modelling and simulations, machine learning, parallel computing, and social network analysis. More information about Dr. Kumar can be found at https://keralauniversity.ac.in/dept/~kskumar.

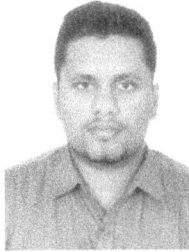

Dr. S. Aanjan Kumar received a B.Tech in information technology from Sudharsan Engineering College, Pudukkottai, Anna University, India in 2011; an M.E. in software engineering from Mount Zion College of Engineering and Technology, Pudukkottai, Anna University, India in 2013; and a Ph.D. from Anna University in 2022. He is now working as assistant professor grade 1 in VIT Bhopal University. He has 11 years of experience in teaching. He is a member of CSI, India and ISTE, India. He has published papers in 2 national conferences, 23 international conferences, 5 national journals and 19 international journals, 2 books and 2 book chapters for Springer and CRC Press on network security and image processing. He is a reviewer in 3 SCI and 1 Scopus journals. Presently he is working on computer vision for securing data and information security for government and public sector healthcare information systems. His areas of research interest include network security, software engineering, and healthcare in computer vision.

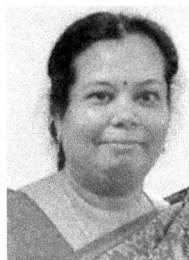

Dr. K. Maheswari, M.C.A., M.Phil., M.Ed., Ph.D., is currently employed in Anna Adarsh College for Women as an assistant professor in the Department of Computer Science. She has 19 years of extensive teaching expertise in the area of computer science. She earned her Ph.D. in data mining and big data analytics from Bharathiar University, India. She has 4 book chapters and 8 research papers published in international and national journals. Additionally, she has presented six papers at international conferences.

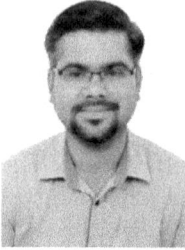

Dr. R. Manikandan is presently associated with CHRIST (Deemed to be University) in the capacity of associate professor in the School of Business and Management. He has obtained doctorate degree from Anna University, Chennai in the faculty of computer science. His area of expertise include data science, bio-inspired optimization techniques, and emerging technologies. He has published several research articles in reputed journals and has presented over 30 papers in international conferences. His has authored textbooks such as *Semantic Mining* and *Deep Learning*. This contribution is intended to make the readers understand the preliminary concepts and applications of emerging technology. The work is sincerely dedicated to his daughters Lakshitha and Yashvitha.

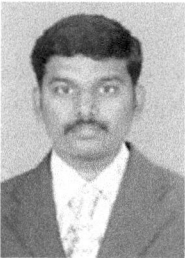

Dr. M. Maragatharajan received his bachelor's degree in electronics & communication engineering from Anna University by 2007. He has received his master's degree in information technology from Kalasalingam University, 2010. He has more than 13 years of teaching experience. Currently, he is working as an assistant professor in the School of Computing Science and Engineering, VIT Bhopal University, Kothirikalan, Madhya Pradesh, India. His areas of interest are wireless networks, machine learning, and deep learning.

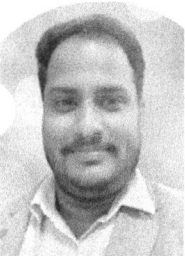

Dr. V. Muneeswaran holds a Ph.D. degree in electronics and communication engineering and has vast research experience in discipline of swarm intelligence, image/signal processing. He serves as a guest editor for *Applied Soft Computing,* a peer-reviewed journal published by Elsevier. As an author he has published several articles in reputed journals *Journal of Supercomputing, IEEE Access, Cognitive Systems Research* and also several works as book chapters in *Lecture Notes in Computer Science, Advances in Intelligent Systems and Computing, Lecture Notes in Electrical Engineering,* and *Smart Innovation, Systems and Technologies* published by Springer. The majority of the articles published were based on the application of swarm intelligence for engineering applications viz., medical image segmentation, optimization of neural networks, etc., On his credit, there are several awards including Publons Peer Review Awards 2018 for placing in the top 1% of reviewers in computer science. At present he is working on projects related to brain tumor segmentation using swarm intelligence techniques and key areas in medical image segmentation.

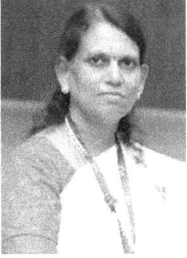

Dr. K. Murugeswari is a senior assistant professor in the School of Computing Science and Engineering at VIT Bhopal University, M.P., India. She holds a Ph.D. degree in information and communication engineering from the Anna University Chennai, India. She has 24+ years of experience in teaching and research, has published 15+ articles in various journals and conference proceedings and contributed chapters to the books. Her research and publication interests include information security, machine learning, deep learning, data analytics, network security, and cryptography.

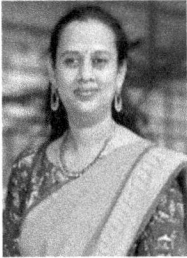

Dr. M. Mythily has completed her doctorate in software modeling from Anna Univeristy, Chennai, and her bachelor's and master's degrees with a specialization of computer science and engineering from Avinashilingam Deemed University and Government college of Technology, Coimbatore respectively. At present, working as an assistant professor at Karunya Institute of Technology and Sciences. As a whole, she gained more than a decade of experience in industry as well as in teaching. Her areas of interest include software engineering, design patterns and problem-solving techniques, secure software, and spring framework. She has published 15+ papers in refereed international journals and conference proceedings.

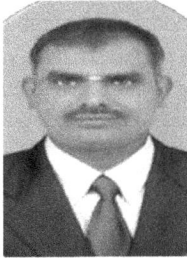

Dr. P. Nagaraj holds a Ph.D. degree in computer science and engineering and has vast research experience in the discipline of data science and analytics, computational intelligence. He has over 13 years of teaching and research experience. He serves as a guest editor for *Frontiers in Artificial Intelligence,* a peer-reviewed journal published by Frontiers Media S.A. As an author, he has published several articles in reputed journals like the *International Journal of Imaging Systems and Technology (IMA), Diabetes, Metabolic Syndrome and Obesity: Targets and Therapy, International Journal of Healthcare Information Systems and Informatics (IJHISI), IEEE Access,* and also several works as book chapters in *Lecture Notes on Data Engineering and Communications Technologies, Studies in Computational Intelligence, Communications in Computer and Information Science, Lecture Notes in Networks and Systems, Advances in Intelligent Systems and Computing* published by Springer and also works on Elsevier Book entitled *Cognitive and Soft Computing Techniques for the Analysis of Healthcare Data.* He has published more papers at IEEE Conference. Many of the articles published were based on the application of healthcare data analytics, health for engineering applications, diabetes healthcare management, optimization techniques, etc. He has participated in various events like webinars, workshops, and conferences and had been resource person in various seminars, faculty development program, and workshop. He also serves as a journal reviewer in top-listed journals like *IEEE Access, Applied Soft Computing,* etc.

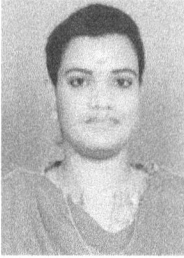

V. Navatharani is a PG-Research Scholar in the Department of Computer Science and Engineering, Anna University, Chennai. She is currently pursuing her M.E degree She has published papers in 1 national conference and 2 international conferences in the area of NETWORK SECURITY. Her research interests include network security, cloud computing, and deep learning.

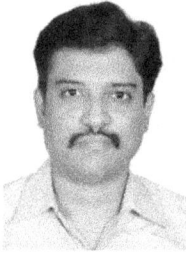

Dr. P. Naveen received B.E. in electronics and communication engineering from Arulmigu Kalasalingam College of Engineering in 2009. He obtained M.E. in power electronics and drives from Sri Sivasubramaniya Nadar College of Engineering in 2011. In 2022, he completed his Ph.D. in the field of image processing from Kalasalingam Academy of Research and Education. He has about 12 years of teaching experience at various levels and is presently holding the position of assistant professor in the Department of ECE, KPR Institute of Engineering and Technology, Coimbatore, India. Prior to KPR Institute of Engineering and Technology, he was associated as NIRF Co-ordinator in Sri Eshwar College of Engineering for 2 years and assistant director – Accreditation and Ranking in Kalasalingam Academy of Research and Education. His research interests include image processing and machine learning. He has published around 25 papers at international journals and international conferences. In addition to regular academic activities, he has played a vital role in various accreditation (ABET, NBA, NAAC, UGC, AICTE) and ranking activities, as well as placement cell activities, examination cell (Valuation Centre in-charge), and institution admission activities.

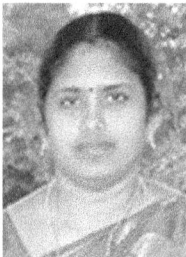

Ms. A. Nithya, is a research scholar in the Department of Computer Science and Applications, The Gandhigram Rural Institute (Deemed to be University), Dindigul, India. She received her Bachelor of Science (B.Sc) degree in physics in the year 2008 and M.Sc. (Information Technology) degree in the year 2010 from The Gandhigram Rural Institute (Deemed to be University) and M.Phil. (Computer Science) in the year 2012 from Bharathiar University. She is currently pursuing her Ph.D. degree at The Gandhigram Rural Institute (Deemed to be University). Her research focuses on breast cancer detection in mammograms, deep learning, and artificial intelligence.

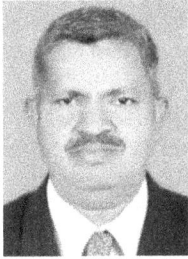

Prof V. Palanisamy earned his Ph.D. in computer science, India. He is having 35 plus years of experience in teaching/research. He is presently working as a professor, and his research area of interest includes image processing, artificial intelligence, and machine learning. He executed one funded research grants from the Research Organization, Government of India. He received two seminar grants from Anna University, Chennai, and the All-India Council for Technical Education-Indian Society for Technical Education. He has 2 patent publications and 121 plus technical paper publications. He has authored 2 books and 2 chapters.

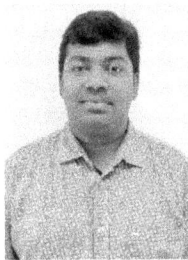

Dr. V. Pandimurugan working as has assistant professor in the Department of Networking and Communication, SRMIST, Kattankulathur, Chennai. He completed his B.E. (EEE) and M.E. (CSE) from Anna University in the years 2005 and 2008, respectively. He completed his Ph.D. (CSE) in 2019 from Manonmaniam Sundaranar University (MSU) Tirunelveli, Tamil Nadu. He has 15 years of teaching experience and has published 24 Scopus-indexed papers, which includes 8 SCI papers. His research interest includes health informatics, AI, and IoT. He has published, *Principles of Communication, Python,* and three Scopus-indexed book chapters. He has three granted and two published patents in his credit.

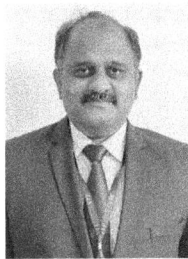

Dr. S. Poonkuntran is specialized in Computer and Information Technology with 18 years of experience in academia. He is presently associating with VIT Bhopal University, as a Professor and Dean for the School of Computing Science and Engineering. He has executed 3 funded research projects worth 1.10 crores from DRDO, ISRO & MNRE. He received 2 seminar grants worth 4 lacs from AICTE-ISTE and Anna University, Chennai. He has published more than 80+ technical publications, authored 7 books, 6 chapters, and holds 7 patents. He is a recipient of the Cognizant Best Faculty Award 2017-18 and served as a State Level Student Coordinator Position for Region VII, CSI, India in 2016-17. He is a lifetime member of IACSIT, Singapore, CSI, India, and ISTE, India. He has produced 2 PhD candidates. He has played a pivotal role in the development and implementation of innovative academic practices, setting up the state of art labs and office automation. His research areas of interest include information security, computer vision, artificial intelligence, and machine learning.

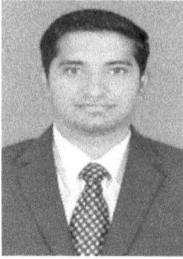

Dr. A. Prasanth received his B.E. degree in electronics and communication engineering from Anna University, Chennai and the M.E. degree in computer science and engineering (with specialization in Networks) from Anna University, Chennai and also received the Ph.D. degree in information and communication engineering from Anna University, Chennai, India. He served as a Recognized Anna University Ph.D. Supervisor. Four scholars doing their research under his guidance and one scholar completed the Ph.D. on March 2023. He is currently working as an assistant professor at Sri Venkateswara College of Engineering, Sriperumbudur, Tamil Nadu, India. He has published more than 35 research articles in reputed international journals among which 15 articles are indexed in SCI and 20 articles are indexed in Scopus. He has published 8 patents in IPR cell. Further, he has published more than 12 books under reputed publisher. He has served as resource person in 25 AICTE-sponsored STTP/FDP programs. Moreover, he has served as an editorial board member in various reputed SCI journals. His research interests include Internet of Things, blockchain, wireless sensor networks, medical image processing, and machine learning.

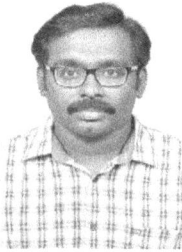

Dr. Thendral Puyalnithi is a vivid academician with 13+ years of experience in universities and colleges. He served as assistant professor senior in VIT University, Vellore for 9 years in the School of Computer Science and Engineering, then as associate professor in Kalasalingam Academy of Research and Education for 2 years in the Department of Computer Science and Engineering. Currently, he is serving as assistant professor senior in Mepco Schlenk Engineering College in the Department of Artificial Intelligence and Data Science for the past 2 years. He has published more than 10 research papers in reputed journals in the field of AI and ML. He has published 5 patents in the field of AI and healthcare. He has completed his undergraduate, bachelor of engineering (BE) in PSG College of Technology, Coimbatore, and post-graduation, master of engineering (M.E.) in BITS, Pilani. He has obtained his doctorate in VIT University, Vellore in the field of computational intelligence. His area of interest includes, AI, machine learning, deep learning, and big data.

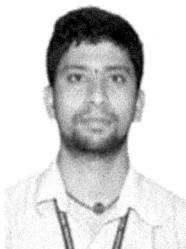

Dr. V. Rajaram is currently working as an assistant professor in the Department of Networking and Communication, School of Computing, SRM Institute of Science and Technology, Kattankulathur. He has completed his doctorate from Anna University, Chennai and has 13 years of teaching experience. He has published several research papers in international journals and international conferences. His research areas include wireless sensor networks and IoT. He has posted video lectures for the course Digital Logic, Microprocessors, and Computer Networks on YouTube.

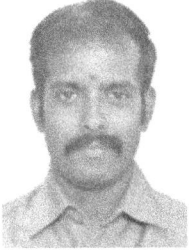

Dr. S. Ramkumar is currently working as an associate professor at Christ University, Bangalore. He received his MCA degree from Karunya University and his M.Phil. degree in Karpagam University. He had 12 years of excellence in teaching and 10 years in research. He had worked as an assistant professor in the PG Department of Computer Science at Subramanya College of Arts and Science, Palani, V.S.B. Engineering College, Karur, and Associate Professor at Kalasalingam Academy of Research and Education, Krishnan Koil in Tamil Nadu. He obtained his doctorate degree in computer science at Karpagam University, Coimbatore, Tamil Nadu. He had published several papers in referred journals and conferences. His field of interest is bio signal processing, artificial intelligence, human–computer interface, brain–computer interface, and machine vision. He is an editorial board member and reviewer of the several SCI, SCIE and Scopus-indexed journals, in India and all over the country. He had several articles in SCI and Scopus-indexed journals. He has conducted many conferences, faculty development programs, training program, seminars, and guest lecturers for faculty and students. He has acted as a chairperson and keynote speaker at several international conferences, and he has given hands-on training on Matlab for many students and research scholars in national seminars and also has gave many training programs for school teachers and students to update their knowledge in the latest technologies. He has received gold, silver, and bronze medals in national and international exhibitions for his research products on machine vision and human–computer interfaces. He had filed two patents. He got funded projects from funding agencies like DST and CSIR with a worth of 32 lakhs. He is the author of the textbooks *Java for Beginners, Magic Book for Quantitative Aptitude and Reasoning (Master the Tricks in 10 days), Problem Solving using C and C++, Basics of Internet with Web Design and Deep Learning.*

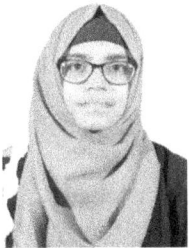

Syed Saba Raoof is pursuing Ph.D. from VIT Vellore at the School of Computer Science and Engineering. She received her master's degree in computer science engineering from Vardhaman College of Engineering in 2020 and a bachelor's degree in computer science engineering from Nizam College of Engineering in 2018. Her research interests include medical imaging, deep learning, machine learning, and IoT. Her current research interests include deep learning for medical imaging and deep learning and IoT for medical healthcare applications.

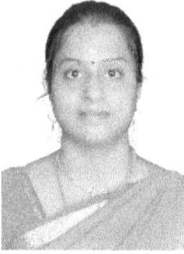

Dr. G. Saranya is working as an assistant professor in the Department of Networking and Communication, SRMIST, Kattankulathur, Chennai. She received her B.Tech degree in information technology from Sri Venkateswara College of Engineering, Sriperumbudur, Chennai, India in 2009 and her M.Tech degree in information technology from Vel Tech Multi Tech Dr.Rangarajan Dr.Sakunthala Engineering College, Avadi, Chennai, India in 2011. She completed her Ph.D. in computer science and engineering at Sathyabama Institute of Science and Technology, Chennai, India, in 2023. She has 10 years of teaching experience and 2 years of industry experience. Her research interests include big data analytics, machine learning, and deep learning.

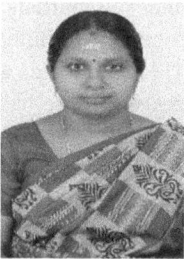

Dr. S. Saraswathi, MCA. M.Phil., Ph.D., Dean, Academic Affairs, has been associated with Nehru Arts and Science College as Dean Academic Affairs since 2022, prior to which she has 16 years of academic and administrative experience. In 2006, she started her career as lecturer in Sri Krishna College of Engineering and Technology, Coimbatore until 2013. In 2013, she joined as an assistant professor in the Department of Information Technology, Sri Krishna Arts and Science College until 2015 and promoted as the Head, Department of Computer Applications until 2022. She also visited the United States of America and got exposed to Western education provided by Clayton State University, Concordia University, Washington State University and Harvard University and learned the skill-based practices incorporated in the higher education system in 2019. Her expertise includes technology-based teaching process, effective mentoring, and curriculum formation with the objective of outcome-based education. She has held various responsibilities like head of the department, chairman board of studies in computer science, member academic council, institutional website, mal-practice committee, and other academic committees. Her area of interest is in the field of data mining, networking, and evolutionary computing. Her untiring effort and interest in research spans to present various research papers in national and international conferences. She has published her research work along with case studies at national and international conferences, and international journal and organized research conferences to the benefit of students and faculty community. She is OCJP-certified professional and completed various online courses like NPTEL, spoken tutorial that are integrated with the faculty development program.

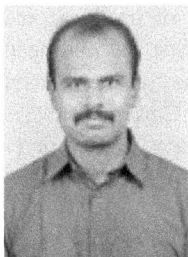

Dr. S. Senthilkumar holds B.Sc. (1997–2000), M.Sc. (2000–2002), M.Phil. (2002–2003), and Ph.D. (2004–2010) degree in chemistry from Madurai Kamaraj University, Madurai. He was awarded the Commonwealth Splite-site Doctoral Scholarship to visit (2005–2006) the University of Manchester, UK. He spent one year (2010–2011) as a postdoctoral fellow at the Hanyang University, Seoul, South Korea. He has published nearly 13 papers in reputed journals and presented more than 20 papers in various national/ international conferences. At present, he has been working as an assistant professor of chemistry in Ayya Nadar Janaki Ammal College (affiliated to Madurai Kamaraj University), Sivakasi.

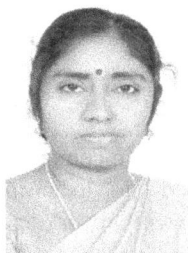

Dr. P. Shanmugavadivu serves as a professor of computer science and applications, at The Gandhigram Rural Institute (Deemed to be University), with 31 years of academic experience and 21 years of research experience. Her research areas include medical image & data vision, parallel computing, software engineering, content-based image retrieval and AI models. She holds a master's degree in computer applications (REC, Tiruchirapalli, 1990), Ph.D. in digital image restoration (GRI-DU, Gandhigram, 2008), MBA (IGNOU, New Delhi 2017), and M.Sc. (applied psychology) (Bharathiar University, Coimbatore, 2019), and M.Tech. (data science & engineering) (BITS Pilani, (2023). She is a recipient of funded research project from UGC, DST, ICMR and PMMMNMTT, of worth Rs. 2.39 Cr.

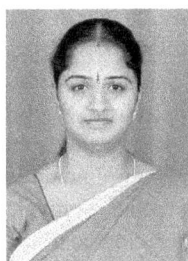

Dr. V. Sindhu completed her doctorate of philosophy in 2022 at Bharathiar University, Coimbatore. She has nearly 12 years of post-graduate teaching experience in the field of computer science. Currently working as an assistant professor in the Department of Computer Science, Christ University, Yeshwanthpur campus, Bangalore. She has published 12 (Scopus and WoS) papers in various international journals. She has acted as session chair and reviewer in various conferences. She has published 2 books and 1 book chapter.

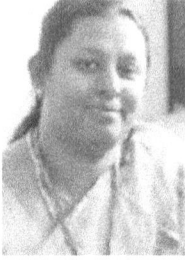

Dr. V. S. Anita Sofia has nearly 23 years of post-graduate teaching experience in computer science. She has indulged in training the postgraduate students. She has published 45 papers in various international journals. Currently, she is working as an associate professor, Department of Computer Applications (MCA), PSG College of Arts & Science, Coimbatore.

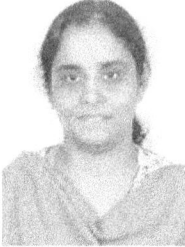

Dr. C. Srimathi is working as a professor at VIT Vellore, Tamil Nadu, India. She received her B.E. in electrical and electronics from Bharathiar University, India, ME (CSE) from Madurai Kamaraj University, India, and Ph.D. from VIT, Vellore. Her research interest includes the Internet of Things, Big Data analytics, and agent-based computing. She works on funded projects sanctioned by government agencies in India.

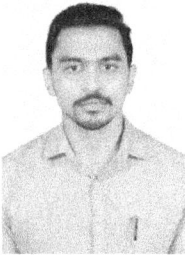

Dr. K. Muthamil Sudar holds a Ph.D. degree in computer science and engineering and has specialized knowledge in the area of network security, software-defined networking, and machine learning techniques. He has over 7 years of teaching and research experience. As an accomplished author, he has successfully published multiple articles in renowned journals and has been a contributor to esteemed IEEE conferences.

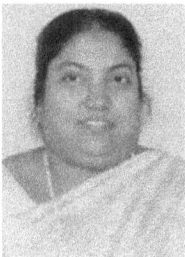

Dr. Hannah Vijaykumar is working as an associate professor and head of the Department of Computer Science, Anna Adarsh College for Women, Chennai. She has 26 years of teaching experience. She obtained her MCA and M.Phil from Bharathidasan University and completed her Ph.D. in 2018 from the University of Madras. Her research domain is software engineering, and her areas of interest include software metrics and their constraints, agile software development and Cloud computing architecture. She has published 3 papers in international journals and 4 papers in international conferences. In addition, she has published 4 book chapters and authored 3 books. She serves as dean of computational studies, Anna Adarsh College for Women, Chennai.

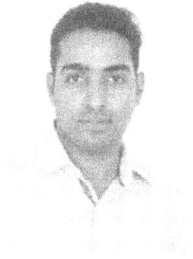

J. Antony Vijay received his master's degree in computer science and engineering from DMI College of Engineering, Anna University, Chennai in 2012. He completed his bachelor's degree in computer science and engineering from DMI College of Engineering, Anna University, Chennai in 2010. He is currently pursuing Ph.D. in computational intelligence from SRM Institute of Science and Technology, Kattankulathur, India. His main research interests are natural language processing, machine learning, deep learning, and computer vision. He has published many journals and book chapters in Scopus-indexed journals.

1 Deep Learning in Healthcare and Clinical Studies

V. Pandimurugan, S. Angayarkanni Annamalai,
G. Saranya, V. Rajaram, and A. Chinnasamy
School of Computing, SRMIST, Kattankulathur, Chennai, India

1.1 INTRODUCTION TO DEEP LEARNING IN CLINICAL TRIALS

In the healthcare sector, artificial intelligence plays a major role in providing better healthcare facilities to people. In particular, deep learning (DL) plays a crucial role in clinical trials. Data collection and selection on medical records and their management is important to extract the right data, and the same can be given to model training and tuning. Whatever data are collected and trained should satisfy validation and process improvement. If not, then data collection must occur again to get the right data. New live data also can be included in the data model for tuning and noise removal processes. DL can streamline the process, which can improve drug production and identification with the help of various medical records and may optimize the treatment level and testing of the various new models [1]. Clinical trial management first identifies the target patients and participant retention. To improve participant retention, reduce the trial burden of the patient, and increase faith in the model to accurately predict, missing data can be approached in the form of data-related assumptions. Intended analytic methods—the DL model—have some constraints for predicting the results of clinical trials. The data may be augmented, or not augmented, so all the data are improved for the denoising method to retain the quality of accuracy. The various roles of the DL process in clinical trials are shown in Figure 1.1.

1.1.1 THE FUNCTION OF DEEP LEARNING

Neural networks are layers of nodes simply because the human brain is made from neurons. Layer nodes that are nearby each other are connected. How deep a community seems relies upon the number of layers it has. An unmarried neuron inside the human mind gets loads of indicators from different neurons. In a synthetic neural community, indicators journey among nodes and follow complementary weights. A biological neuron is shown in Figure 1.2.

A node's effect on the nodes within the layer below it will likely be more potent if it has a bigger weight. The ultimate layer combines the weighted inputs to provide

DOI: 10.1201/9781003469605-1

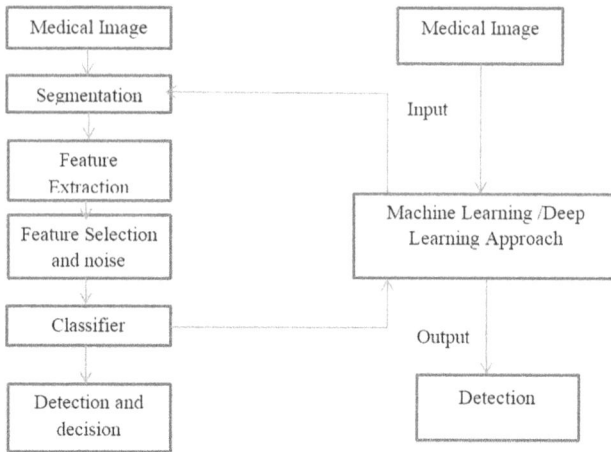

FIGURE 1.1   Role of deep learning process in clinical trials.

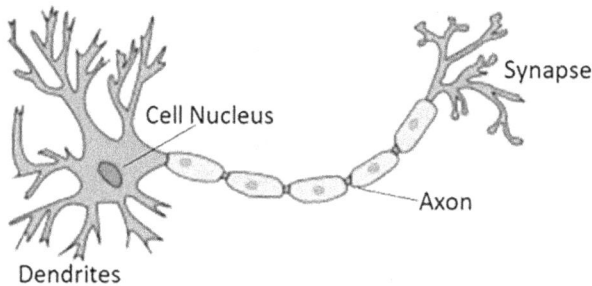

FIGURE 1.2   Structure of a biological neuron.

an output. Deep studying structures require effective hardware due to the fact they system a massive quantity of information and carry out numerous complicated mathematical computations. However, training a neural network might take days or even weeks, even with such sophisticated technology [2]. DL systems receive input in the form of enormous data sets since they require a lot of data to produce accurate results. In order to classify data, artificial neural networks process it using the answers to a sequence of binary yes-or-no questions regarding fantastically hard mathematical calculations. For example, a facial recognition set of rules learns to understand the rims and contours of faces first, observed via means of the faces' greater large features, and ultimately the general representations of faces. As the software program learns, the chance of having the ideal reaction increases. Facial recognition software programs will quickly be gifted at figuring out faces in this scenario.

The recently identified SARS-CoV-2 virus and COVID-19, the disease it produces, have changed the world. The current global health catastrophe, unlike any other in recent memory, is referred to as a pandemic by the World Health

Organization. The virus and the sickness are both mysteries to the scientific community around the world. It is required to concentrate and work internationally at a level that has never been seen before to safeguard the integrity of clinical trials throughout the pandemic, develop and identify treatments, and determine the circumstances in which they are safe and effective. DL models are used for efficient identification of lung-infected areas from chest images, prediction of feasibility analysis of conversion time to a severe stage of illness, natural language processing (NLP)-based disease classification with questionnaire, summarization, and chatbots.

1.1.1.1 Deep Learning at Work: An Example

Consider that one of the goals is to teach a neural network to recognize photographs of dogs. A poodle and a rottweiler are two instances of how dissimilar all dogs are in appearance. Additionally, images show dogs in a variety of lighting and perspective settings. So, it is necessary to put together a training set of pictures that includes a variety of canine faces that anyone would categorize as "canine" and photographs of factors that are not dogs but are labeled (as one would possibly expect) "now no longer canine." The entered photographs are transformed into facts via the means of the neural network. As this fact travels through the network, numerous nodes assign weights to the components. The phrase "canine" is produced via means of the very last output layer, which mixes the facts that, at the start, look unconnected (furry, has a nose, has four legs, etc.).

We will now compare the neural network's answer to the label made by a human. If there is a match, the output is validated. Otherwise, the weightings are adjusted, and the neural network notices the error. To improve its capacity to recognize dogs, the neural network regularly updates the weights in its model. Although it is not clearly mentioned what "makes" a dog, the neural networks utilized in this training process, supervised learning, can nonetheless generate results [3]. They must slowly begin to recognize patterns in the data and learn new information on their own.

1.1.1.2 Deep Learning's Ascent

British mathematician Alan Turing is credited with inventing machine learning when he proposed his artificially intelligent "learning system" in the 1950s. Arthur Samuel advanced the primary totally PC-based instructional program. His set of rules stepped forward through the years as an IBM PC performed checks with it. Over the following decades, different learning systems strategies came and went. Neural networks have been in large part disregarded as machine learning systems by researchers because of the "local minima" problem, in which weightings are erroneously regarded to supply the fewest errors. Computer imagination and prescient and facial recognition are examples of superior machine learning strategies. Real-time face identification in photos is possible thanks to the 2001 invention of Ad boost, a machine learning technique. It was able to filter pictures using decision sets such as "does the image have a bright area between dark regions, maybe indicating the bridge of a nose?" Based on the data movement, whether the data are checked with the images, to make the right decision for identifying the right data [4,5]. Even with the introduction of competitive graphics processing units, the popularity of neural networks did not rise again for several more years. The new equipment allowed researchers to run, edit, and process images using desktop computers instead of supercomputers. The most significant development in neural networks came because of the introduction of massive amounts of labeled data through ImageNet, a collection of millions of annotated photographs from the Internet. The time-consuming task of manually classifying photographs was replaced by crowdsourcing, which gave networks access to an essentially endless supply of training data. Since then, IT firms have made their DL libraries accessible. Microsoft CNTK, Amazon DSSTNE on GitHub, Facebook's open-source Torch plugins, and Google TensorFlow are a few examples.

1.1.2 ACTIVE DEEP LEARNING

As the training model provides, the streaming nodes provide the right picture to gain DL knowledge. As it turns out, gaining DL knowledge is being included in all sorts of programs. Anyone who makes use of Facebook will quickly realize that while you add new photographs, it mechanically recognizes and tags your friends. Digital assistants like Siri, Cortana, Alexa, and Google Now use natural language and recognize voices via DL knowledge. Through Skype, conversations are translated in real time. Numerous email programs have honed their skills to determine unsolicited mail earlier than it even reaches the inbox. PayPal has utilized DL knowledge to thwart fraudulent payments. DL knowledge is being hired with the aid of using Google, especially to provide answers to the usage of cellular search engine technologies. Recently, Google Deep mind's AlphaGo PC program trounced present-day Go champions. DeepMind's WaveNet can produce speech that sounds more natural and just like human speech than different speech structures presently in the marketplace. Google Translate makes use of DL knowledge and photo recognition to translate spoken and written language. Google Planet can be used to pinpoint the region of any photo. Google constructed the TensorFlow deep, gaining knowledge of software program databases to facilitate the introduction of AI applications [6]. DL knowledge remains in its infancy; however, within the near future, it's going to revolutionize society. Around the world, self-driving cars are present in process testing; an incredibly evolved layer of neural networks is being trained to realize items to avoid, note visitors' lights, and realize when to alternate speed. Neural networks are enhanced in all areas, such as marketplace pricing and climate forecasting. Consider the blessings of virtual assistants that could recommend to buyers whether to sell or promote stocks earlier than a hurricane. DL knowledge of structures might even save lives as they predict the potential for evidence-based treatment to help patients and help with the early diagnosis of tumors.

1.1.3 CLINICAL TRIALS FOR MEDICINES, NOT COVID

Travel restrictions, social isolation, or even quarantine were a part of the worldwide community's reaction to the COVID-19 pandemic. All of those factors will notably limit the potential and/or willingness of contributors and personnel to go to medical sites to gather records. Data classification techniques might also change, and a few records can be overlooked (e.g., remotely vs. online only). Additionally, there may be a large possibility that contributors could pass COVID-19 to healthcare workers, especially considering the reality that a few infected people show no signs and symptoms and the virus seems to be contagious earlier than signs and symptoms arise. In reaction to those issues, the U.S. Food and Drug Administration has posted revised suggestions for the behavior of medical studies for the duration of the pandemic [7,8]. All of those issues are likely to result in troubles that taint looking at records and make it tough to interpret medical trial results. These demanding situations, which could range in severity based on the length of the present-day COVID-19 pandemic, the number of affected people, the disease circumstance being studied, and diverse trial layout factors, could also add pressure to the termination of several ongoing medical trials. Once a medical trial is terminated, there may be an absence of records, so it could be tough to acquire and report the findings, especially if the trial terminated in its early stages. For many reasons, some of which are obvious and some of which are not, records collected before the pandemic can be affected more than records collected after the outbreak. For instance, medical sites' daily operations might be significantly damaged, and there may be missed visits, a rise in protocol violations, overdue records entry, and records collected through a whole lot of modalities (together with wide distribution), and sluggish follow-up. Participants might also have stopped providing data once COVID-19 first appeared, have been infected, have been placed on "lock-down," or have been removed from that location to diverse countries, states, counties, cities, and towns. Individuals with SARS-CoV-2 infection might show a huge variety of symptoms; a few patients might show no symptoms in any respect, while others pass away. It might be tough to attribute the drug for outcomes, look at protocol violations, and, as a result, envision the trial's purpose due to this variability. Additionally, it could influence the conduct in each trial; however, the more extreme illnesses are treated and changes to laboratory warnings (e.g., major cancers). These and lots of extra repercussions can be felt for the duration of the epidemic and for a while after as worldwide healthcare structures address the aftermath. When the trial is continued, it will be essential to deal with those demanding situations with the aid of growing powerful and dependable techniques for acquiring insight from records and for fostering confidence in that understanding.

In trials now being carried out, medical trial records evaluation is a less common where the affected person checks in online for the duration of the pandemic, which will result in lacking records. Furthermore, capacity adjustments in frequency earlier than, for the duration of, and after the pandemic would possibly obstruct the previous periods for taking pictures of the affected person's records [9]. Current machine learning strategies might be used to solve these problems. To fill in the gaps left with the aid of using lacking records, machine learning algorithms designed particularly to assign lacking records in temporal record streams might be utilized. When online monitoring changed to have much less widespread use, those techniques allowed for the inference of the affected person's circumstance. Machine learning techniques significantly outperform traditional techniques, together with outcome optimization, pattern completion, and a couple of imputations with the aid of using chained equations, in this problem [10]. These techniques use multi-dimensional recurrent neural networks and generative adversarial imputation nets (Yoon et al. from the UCI Machine Learning Repository). All those techniques are primarily based on the idea that records are incomplete at random, i.e., that the incomplete records have a regarded purpose of becoming independent from the patients' unobserved circumstance. This might also additionally or might not be an affordable assumption inside the context of the pandemic; for instance, a few elements (e.g., local situations and an affected person's chance status) that influence whether visits are canceled are likely to be recorded, while others (e.g., a close relative's infection and problem traveling) might not be. Additionally, this presumption might or might not adhere to present-day trial standards.

The estimation will continue to be complicated if inadequate records will be used for attribution or prediction purposes. To collect those records, it may be required to hyperlink affected persons' statistics from the studies with location-unique operational statistics. Other machine learning models are designed to examine temporal records that have been collected randomly. Since medical trials continue all through the pandemic, the massive variations among the instances earlier than, for the duration of, and after the epidemic should undermine the validity of looking at results. The daily activities of trial contributors, the overall quantity of care they receive, how the underlying treatment is provided, or even the control, are likely to change due to measures taken for the duration of the pandemic. It is critical to differentiate those outcomes from the ones of the drug treatments to prevent having a detrimental effect on medical results or treatment efficacy. This necessitates the software of present-day machine learning strategies to anticipate the treatment outcomes in addition to variables that recall a location's private records for the duration of the pandemic (adjustments in clinical treatment, as well as adjustments in nutrition, exercise, etc., if applicable). Because the true nature of the connection to a situation beyond attention to an outbreak and treatment results is now unknown, machine learning algorithms have an advantage over conventional statistical methods because of their inherent flexibility and data-driven nature. If the trial continues for the duration of the pandemic, it is feasible that participation and enrollment will range (if not stop entirely).

The composition of the affected population will range if specific subgroups are disproportionately impacted with the aid of using those adjustments, and if those confounding outcomes are not taken into consideration within the studies, the anticipated population-level treatment effect can be biased. It will conse-quently be critical to decide the volume of those adjustments, their outcomes at the estimates of treatment results for the diverse subgroups, and the extent of confidence in those estimates. Before drawing inferences from research data that have been discontinued earlier than the supposed goal, we need to first decide what we already recognize and what we no longer recognize based on the records at hand. Machine learning algorithms can address those issues with the aid of estimating more than a few treatment responses. These and other techniques for estimating individualized treatment outcomes (ITE) are used as a place to begin earlier than implementation of subgroups and estimations of various treatment responses. Hill (2011), Athey and Imbens (2016), Alaa and van der Schaar (2017, 2018), and Yoon et al. offer numerous precise techniques for estimating ITE (2018a). For additional statistics, refer to Bica et al. and the earlier stage in "Exploiting Observational Data within the Design of New Trials" (2020). These models can decide whether or not subgroups have connected traits and treatment responses in addition to estimating the treatment responses in every subgroup. Because the trial ended earlier than its supposed goal, records will necessarily be lacking. Additionally, in all likelihood efforts to acquire and report case aspects and results have been impeded by the pandemic's effect on healthcare. There can be issues concerning the accuracy of predictions of curative results as a result.

To deal with those issues and decide between sincere estimates and misguided ones, it's essential to evaluate the confidence in those estimations. For problems like these, the latest machine learning methods were advanced that comprehensively characterize estimation uncertainty. In medical research, which has been abandoned, it could be mainly complicated when the demographic distribution of trial contributors (with the aid of using age, gender, income, geographic region, etc.) differs significantly from the presumed population and/or the population of the real world. Such distortion might have an effect on the reliability and confidence of the extracted data. Therefore, it needs to be taken into consideration the use of the best methodologies; for instance, see Akacha et al. (2020) and the references therein. For comparing underlying uncertainty, covariate shift machine learning methods will also be the best manner to resolve this issue.

1.2 DEEP LEARNING FRAMEWORKS

1.2.1 TENSORFLOW

One of the most well-known machine learning frameworks, it provides a collection of models that have already been trained to help engineers and experts in DL create DL models and algorithms. This open-source framework was the brainchild of the Google Brain team. Machine learning developers can use it in dataflow programs to handle large-scale supervised and unsupervised learning as well as numerical calculation. TensorFlow creates models that combine DL and machine learning and train them to reason and deliver logical results on their own, utilizing enormous amounts of data. It can be run on CPUs and GPUs alike. Keras is a high-level framework built on top of TensorFlow. We will discuss it separately. Figure 1.3 shows the DL framework.

1.2.1.1 Benefits of Utilizing Tensorflow

It works well, offers seamless performance, and enables quick updates because Google supports it. Additionally, it permits the execution of graph subcomponents, which enables computers to extract discrete data.

1.2.1.2 Issues with Tensorflow

TensorFlow is slower and less user-friendly than its competitors, and it is incompatible with Windows platforms.

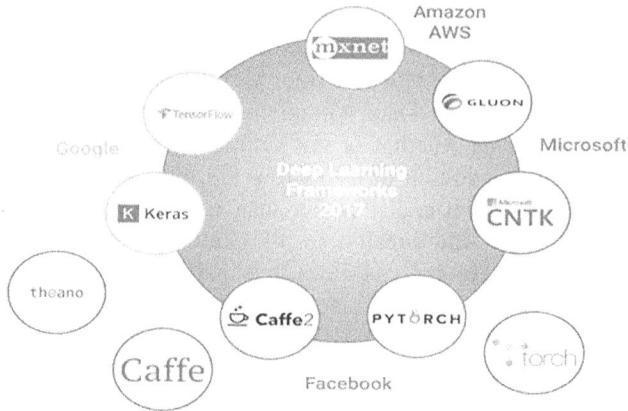

FIGURE 1.3 Deep learning framework.

1.2.2 KERAS

Keras is an open-source framework constructed on top of TensorFlow. Python was used to construct it, and both GPUs and CPUs can effectively use it. After extensive study and revision, Keras became the most popular high-level neural network. François Chollet, a Google developer, designed it to be speedy, user-friendly, and logically modular. Machine learning algorithms can be used in many different industries, such as healthcare, corporate insights, virtual assistants, and sales forecasting. A high-level API called Keras facilitates connections across multiple platforms and backends. It is used by developers for quick prototyping. It provides a range of already trained models.

1.2.2.1 Cons of Keras Use

The Keras framework struggles to handle low-level computing, and finding its flaws is challenging.

1.2.3 MXNET

Developers of DL exclusively use MXNet. Programming languages and a range of GPUs are supported for scalability. Long- and short-term memory networks, convolutional neural networks, and other methods can all be used by MXNet, which is versatile and portable. It is employed in a wide range of sectors, such as manufacturing, healthcare, and transportation.

1.2.3.1 Benefits of Using MXNet

Programming languages supported include R, Scala, Python, JavaScript, C++, and more. It is rapid, effective, and scalable.

1.2.3.2 Cons of Using MXNet

It has less open-source community support than TensorFlow; as a result, bug fixes and feature updates take longer to complete.

1.2.4 Caffe

Convolutional Architecture for Fast Feature Embedding is a machine learning and DL framework built in C++. It is ideal for distributing cutting-edge content, classifying photos, and experimenting with research methods. Academics, small and medium-sized organizations, and startups frequently employ Caffe to perform computer vision and speech recognition tasks. It offers an interface that enables software developers to switch between the CPU and GPU.

1.2.4.1 Benefits of Using Caffe

It is open-source and developer-friendly.

It is well-accepted for systems with limited computing resources.

1.2.4.2 Cons of Using Caffe

It has a steep learning curve.

It is not recommended for use with recurrent neural networks or sequence modeling.

1.2.5 H2O

It is another open-source, business-oriented machine learning framework. It makes it easier to apply predictive analytics with mathematics so that judgments may be made based on precise data. Robot training utilizing data insights is supported by open-source Breed technology, which also supports database independence. The Java-based core of H2O can be accessed or embedded from any other source code or script thanks to the REST API. Experts in machine learning can extend H2O to work with modern programming languages and technologies. Machine learning developers employ it in consumer intelligence in addition to analyzing insurance, advertising technology, risk, healthcare, and fraud.

1.2.5.1 Benefits of Using H2O

H2O is adaptable.

Using H2O for automatic machine learning is efficient.

It is incredibly simple to use for programmers with a variety of programming experiences.

1.2.5.2 Cons of Using H2O

The H2O framework has too little scalability.

1.2.6 Theano

Theano, a machine learning library that was constructed on top of NumPy, is one of the fastest. It was made with CUDA and Python and released under a BSD license. It allows users to optimize mathematical representations in machine learning applications and is used by programmers to handle multidimensional arrays. Both GPU and CPU platforms can be used with Theano; however, when the latter is used, it can provide results faster. This machine learning method can perform tasks 140 times faster when used on GPU architectures. Popular machine learning software called Theano has a wide range of uses in logistical and financial processes.

Tools for unit testing and validation are available in Theano. Both exponential and log functions are supported. Defects can be automatically avoided. Both CPU and GPU architectures are capable of handling data-intensive tasks.

1.2.6.1   Cons of Using Theano

Its compile time is noticeably longer than TensorFlow's.

1.2.7   SHOGUN

It is an extremely venerable and old open-source machine learning library. It integrates a significant variety of data formats and machine learning methods. It was made in C++ and integrated amazingly with C++. Because it treats C++ modestly, it is well-liked in the educational and learning sectors. Shogun also demonstrates compatibility with a variety of other languages, such as Python, C#, Java, Lua, R, and Ruby. Programmers utilize Shogun to process enormous volumes of data for applications using machine learning. On a wide range of systems, developers can do regression, classification, or exploratory analytic activities. Shogun is employed by machine learning developers in their work on NLP, teaching, and research projects.

The appropriateness of Shogun for rapid prototyping, as well as its adaptable and user-driven features, are benefits.

1.2.7.1   Cons of Using Shogun

Compared to TensorFlow or Caffe, Shogun does not have the same level of community support.

1.3   DEEP LEARNING-BASED ELECTRONIC HEALTH RECORDS

Electronic health records (EHRs) and DL have both emerged as major technological advancements in recent years, and they are increasingly being used in the field of preclinical drug discovery. In this context, EHRs play a crucial role in providing access to vast amounts of patient data that can be used to train and validate DL algorithms, while DL algorithms provide a powerful tool for analyzing and processing these data in order to improve drug discovery outcomes. EHR features are shown in Figure 1.4

EHRs provide access to a wealth of patient data, including demographic information, medical history, lab results, and other important clinical information. These data are critical for drug discovery research, as they can be used to identify potential drug targets, evaluate the safety and efficacy of new drugs, and optimize dosing strategies. EHRs can also be used to track the outcomes of drug trials, providing valuable information for further research and development [11,12].

DL algorithms, on the other hand, can process large amounts of data quickly and accurately, providing valuable insights into patient populations and drug interactions. For example, DL algorithms can be used to analyze EHR data to identify

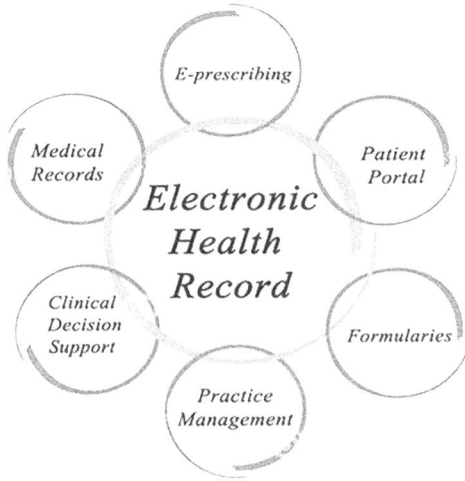

FIGURE 1.4 EHR features.

potential biomarkers that can be used to predict disease progression or response to therapy. This can help to reduce the time and cost associated with traditional drug discovery methods and improve the accuracy of preclinical testing.

In preclinical drug discovery, DL algorithms can be used to analyze EHR data in combination with other data sources, such as genomics, proteomics, and imaging data, to identify novel drug targets and validate existing targets. For example, DL algorithms can be used to analyze gene expression data to identify genetic variations that are associated with disease and to identify potential drug targets based on these variations. This can lead to the development of personalized medicine, where drugs are tailored to the individual needs of each patient based on their unique genetic profile.

Additionally, DL algorithms can be used to analyze EHR data to identify subpopulations of patients who are most likely to respond to a particular drug. This can help to optimize clinical trial design and reduce the risk of adverse events, leading to faster and more cost-effective drug development. Furthermore, DL algorithms can be used to evaluate the safety and efficacy of new drugs by analyzing large amounts of patient data to identify potential side effects and interactions with other drugs.

1.4 ROLE IN PRECLINICAL DRUG DISCOVERY USING DEEP LEARNING

DLs are used to analyze EHR data in preclinical drug discovery. DL algorithms are transforming the field of preclinical drug discovery by providing powerful and efficient solutions for analyzing EHR data. In recent years, DL algorithms have been successfully applied to various applications in the healthcare industry, including NLP, image classification, and prediction of patient outcomes. In this article, we will provide a comprehensive overview of the DL algorithms used for analyzing EHR data in preclinical drug discovery.

1.4.1 CONVOLUTIONAL NEURAL NETWORKS

Convolutional neural networks CNNs are a type of neural network that is specifically designed for image classification tasks. They have been used to extract and analyze medical images from EHR data, such as X-rays, CT scans, and MRI images. CNNs are trained to identify specific patterns in the images, which can be used to predict diseases, diagnose conditions, and assess treatment efficacy.

1.4.2 RECURRENT NEURAL NETWORKS

Recurrent Neural Networks (RNNs) are a type of neural network that is designed for sequence data. They have been used to process EHRs, which typically consist of a large number of sequential data points, such as laboratory test results, patient vital signs, and medication orders. RNNs can analyze the sequential data to predict future events, such as disease progression or patient outcomes.

1.4.3 LONG SHORT-TERM MEMORY NETWORKS

Long short-term memory (LSTM) networks are a type of RNN that are designed to handle long-term dependencies in sequential data. They have been used to analyze EHR data in preclinical drug discovery to identify patterns and relationships in patient data over time [13,14]. LSTMs have also been used to predict patient outcomes, such as hospital readmission or death.

Generative adversarial networks (GANs): GANs are a type of neural network that consists of two components: a generator and a discriminator. They have been used to generate synthetic EHR data, which can be used to train machine learning algorithms and evaluate their performance. GANs can also be used to impute missing data in EHRs, which is a common problem in preclinical drug discovery.

1.4.4 AUTOENCODERS

Autoencoders are a type of neural network that can be used to identify and extract meaningful features from complex data. They have been used to analyze EHR data in preclinical drug discovery to identify the most important features that predict patient outcomes, such as drug efficacy or toxicity.

In conclusion, the integration of EHRs and DL algorithms in preclinical drug discovery is a promising development that has the potential to transform the way drugs are discovered, developed, and approved. DL algorithms are playing a critical role in the field of preclinical drug discovery by providing powerful and efficient solutions for analyzing EHR data. These algorithms have been successfully applied to various applications in the healthcare industry, including NLP, image classification, and prediction of patient outcomes. With continued advancements in both EHRs and DL algorithms, the future of drug discovery is bright and holds great promise for improving human health.

1.5   DATA COLLECTION AND MANAGEMENT

Data collection is the key process, as it is the base on which the analysis is made. To get a holistic view of the healthcare industry, data should be extracted from all aspects like the details of doctors, patients, health records, health equipment, hospitals, location of outbreak, mode of spreading, etc [15,16].

In short, healthcare-related data are collected through questionnaires, lab observations, and clinical documents. In the current era of the digital world, researchers can collect data through mobile apps and web forums.

1.5.1   TYPES OF DATA

Data collected from the healthcare industry are of two types—primary data and secondary data. Primary data are the raw data collected directly from the patients. Vital sources of primary data are x-ray images, which reveal the disease-related parameters, and surveys and questionnaires from patients or doctors, from recorded health data. These data also include key information about the patient like height, weight, blood pressure, blood group, etc.; secondary data refers to when the data are extracted from standard databases, which are composed of standard regulatory bodies like the World Health Organization and state and central government statistics.

1.5.2   DATA COLLECTION METHODS

1. Crowdsourcing of data

    Through the shared platform, a wide range of data can be collected from a variety of contributors globally. This helps to achieve data diversity, which is required to train the model in a better way. But there is no guarantee about the quality of data collected, whereas quantity is satisfiable. Data collection methods are shown in Figure 1.5.

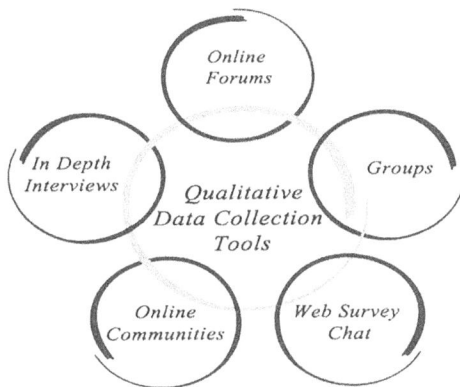

FIGURE 1.5   Data collection.

2. Private way

Although this method is pretty conventional, it is very effective when we need to get sensitive and private data from the targeted contributors. This can be feasible to build smaller datasets only.

3. Pre-existing dataset

When one needs to get refined data of high quality, then the usage of an existing dataset is a better choice. Existing standard datasets have preprocessed and cleaned data samples. This may also give the benefit of easy implementation and the cheapest mode of data collection.

4. Automated tools

Usage of well-developed software tools to collect data from online data sources and social media. This is a better choice of data collection when there is a need to collect secondary data. It is one of the faster modes of data collection.

Random data collection is not building up standard datasets. While collecting data, the quality of the data matters. The collected sample data must be a proper representative of the entire population of the same kind. The integrity of the data should be preserved. Collected data may be of various categories like continuous data, categorical data, and research data. With the help of various information technology, manual surveys and questionnaires are replaced by software-based tools. Mobile-based and Web-based applications are widely popular and reach the masses in a quick time. In this digital era, data collection becomes easier, whereas the selection of qualitative data is the key. It is the best practice to keep the collected raw data as it is.

1.6 OPERATIONAL BARRIERS TO DEEP LEARNING IN CLINICAL RESEARCH

- The accuracy of DL algorithms depends on the quantity of data used for training the model. Again, there is a demand for more medical data.
- Although most hospital records become e-records nowadays, getting medical data breaches data privacy.
- It is crucial to keep healthcare data secure.
- Visualization of the data is the more critical part because most of the health data collected have multidimensional features.
- There is a lack of proper documentation of healthcare data.
- There is a lack of skilled healthcare employees to handle e-data.
- There is no proper integration of systems and policies across the world.
- Patients and caretakers hesitate to use their health data for experimental analysis.
- There is a lack of a strong policy framework to handle health data.
- Human body behavior is unpredictable, although prediction depends on the collected data.
- There is lack of trust within the users and patient community.

- Machine learning-based health diagnosis leads to health disparity.
- There is lack of clarity in data with reference to the gender and nationality of the patient data source.

1.7 DEEP LEARNING ALGORITHMS PROS, CONS, AND APPLICATIONS

Comparison of different deep learning algorithms is depicted in Table 1.1.

TABLE 1.1

Deep Learning Algorithms Pros, Cons, and Applications

Algorithm	Supervised/ Unsupervised	Advantages	Disadvantages	Applications
Backpropagation [17]	Supervised	Easy implementation is possible.	It is performed only on validated data, not training data.	GOCR, used in speech analysis for disease detection
Autoencoders	Unsupervised	It works well for linear functions but is not suitable for nonlinear transformation.	Data-specific loss occurs for the unrivaled information of the data image.	Compression of the data, denoising using Kalman filter
Vartional Autoencoders [18]	Unsupervised	It will be good for image augmentation and image training data models.	Data accuracy for augmented images is not good.	Special tissue and cell detection
RBMS	Unsupervised	It can be used to train the other model. It can be used to extract the data from the query-issued format.	RBMs are tricky to train well. You are unable to track the loss that is required (let alone take derivatives with respect to it).	Applied in the PHR model, better hospital management
CNN [19]	Supervised	The image segment is easy to classify for the fine-tuning of image segregation.	Removal of the redundant pixel value is a big challenge.	NLP classification, image processing
RNN	Unsupervised	It can process input of any length.	It has slow computation, and there is difficulty in training.	Clinical trial cohort selection
LSTM	Unsupervised	It is efficient at modeling complex sequential data.	It is not suitable for data that are not in sequence.	Disease prediction

1.8   CLINICAL TRIALS IN DRUG DELIVERY

Clinical trials are a critical step in the process of developing and bringing new drugs to market. They are used to test the safety and efficacy of a new drug in a controlled environment and provide data that can be used to demonstrate to regulatory agencies that the drug is safe and effective for its intended use. Drug delivery is a rapidly growing field in the pharmaceutical industry, with the goal of improving the effectiveness and safety of drugs by developing new and innovative ways of delivering them to the body [20,21]. This can include using new types of delivery systems, such as nanoparticles, liposomes, or microspheres, as well as developing new routes of administration, such as inhalation or transdermal delivery. Clinical trials for drug delivery are designed to test the safety and efficacy of the new delivery system or route of administration, as well as the drug itself. These trials typically involve many subjects and are divided into several phases [22].

Phase 1 trials are usually the first step in testing a new drug or delivery system in humans. These trials are typically conducted with a small number of healthy volunteers and are designed to test the safety of the drug or delivery system, as well as to determine the optimal dosage.

Phase 2 trials are typically conducted in a larger number of subjects and are designed to test the efficacy of the drug or delivery system in treating a specific condition. These trials also provide additional information on safety, as well as on the optimal dosage and schedule for administration.

Phase 3 trials are usually large, multicenter trials that are conducted in many subjects and are designed to confirm the efficacy and safety of the drug or delivery system. These trials also provide important information on the long-term safety and effectiveness of the drug or delivery system. After Phase 3 clinical trials, the data are sent to the FDA to review and decide whether to approve or not approve the drug for general use.

There are also Phase 4 clinical trials, which are post-approval studies that are conducted after a drug or delivery system has been approved for use by regulatory agencies. These trials are designed to provide additional information on the long-term safety and effectiveness of the drug or delivery system, as well as to gather data on the drug's use in real-world settings. It's important to note that the success rate of drugs in clinical trials is low. It is estimated that only about 12% of drugs that enter clinical trials eventually get approved by regulatory agencies. Drug development phases are shown in Figure 1.6.

Overall, clinical trials in drug delivery are a critical step in the process of developing and bringing new drugs to market. These trials are designed to test the safety and efficacy of new delivery systems and routes of administration, as well as the drugs themselves. The data generated from these trials are used to demonstrate to regulatory agencies that the drug is safe and effective for its intended use.

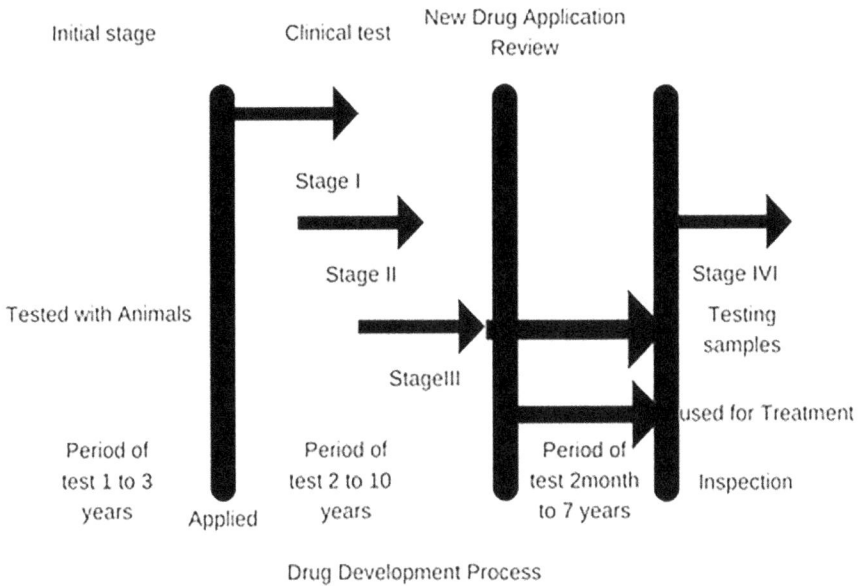

FIGURE 1.6   Drug development phases.

1.9   DEEP LEARNING APPLICATIONS IN HEALTHCARE

DL is a type of machine learning that uses neural networks with multiple layers to learn complex patterns in data. It has been applied in a wide range of fields, including healthcare, and has the potential to revolutionize the way we diagnose and treat diseases. One of the most promising applications of DL in healthcare is medical imaging. DL algorithms can be trained to identify patterns in medical images, such as CT scans or MRIs, that are indicative of specific diseases or conditions. For example, a DL algorithm can be trained to identify tumors in CT scans or detect early signs of Alzheimer's disease in MRI. This can lead to more accurate and faster diagnoses, as well as earlier detection of diseases [23].

Another area where DL is being applied in healthcare is NLP. NLP is a type of artificial intelligence that allows computers to understand and process human language [24]. In healthcare, NLP can be used to extract information from EHRs and other medical documents, such as clinical notes and discharge summaries. This can be used to improve patient care and population health management, as well as to support research [25]. DL is also being used in drug discovery and development. By analyzing large amounts of data from various sources, such as genomic data, drug efficacy data, and clinical trial data, DL algorithms can help identify new drug targets and predict drug efficacy. This can help to speed up the drug development process and lead to the discovery of new and more effective drugs [26].

In addition to the above, DL is also being used in other areas of healthcare, such as:

- Predictive modeling: DL can be used to predict patient outcomes, such as the likelihood of readmission or the risk of developing a specific disease [27].
- Personalized medicine: DL can be used to analyze genomic data and other patient information to develop personalized treatment plans.
- Telemedicine: DL can be used to analyze video and audio data from telemedicine consultations to improve the diagnosis and treatment of patients remotely. Healthcare applications are shown in Figure 1.7.

Despite the many potential benefits of DL in healthcare, there are also some challenges that need to be addressed. One of the main challenges is the need for large amounts of high-quality data to train DL algorithms [28]. Another challenge is the lack of interpretability of DL models, which can make it difficult to understand why a particular decision was made by the model. Overall, DL has the potential to revolutionize healthcare by improving the accuracy and speed of diagnoses, as well as by supporting research and drug development. However, more research is needed to address the challenges of deep DL in healthcare and to fully realize its potential [29,30].

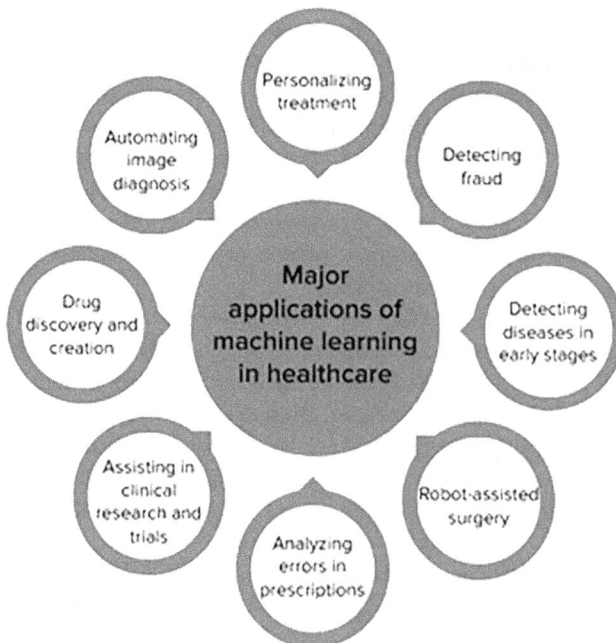

FIGURE 1.7 Applications of ML/DL in healthcare.

1.10 CONCLUSION

In this chapter, we discussed the importance of DL in drug delivery as well as a prediction model to improve drug delivery and healthcare management. EHR plays an important role in health information technology; it will be given more value for predicting diseases and medicine based on earlier records, and how it will be checked with data validation. Data management is important for all applications, and healthcare is the most crucial one, because a lot of mixed data sets must be handled for the different trained models. In the intelligent decision clinical trials model, based on the EHR, personal health record, and electronic medical record, data can be extracted with the different DL and machine learning techniques to be implemented for a better drug delivery system.

REFERENCES

1. Meinl, T., Jagla, B., Berthold, M. R. Integrated data analysis with KNIME. In *Open Source Software in Life Science Research*; Elsevier: Amsterdam, The Netherlands, 2012; pp. 151–171.
2. Alcalá-Fdez, J., Sánchez, L., García, S., Del Jesus, M. J., Ventura, S., Garrell, J. M., Otero, J., Romero, C., Bacardit, J., Rivas, V. M., et al.
3. Alcala-Fdez, J., Garcia, S., Berlanga, F. J., Fernandez, A., Sanchez, L., del Jesus, M., Herrera, F. KEEL: A data mining software tool integrating genetic fuzzy systems. In Proceedings of the 2008 3rd International Workshop on Genetic and Evolving Systems, Witten-Bommerholz, Germany, 4–7 March 2008.
4. Welikala, R. A., Remagnino, P., Lim, J. H., Chan, C. S., Rajendran, S., Kallarakkal, T. G., Zain, R. B., Jayasinghe, R. D., Rimal, J., Kerr, A. R., et al. Automated detection and classification of oral lesions using deep learning for early detection of oral cancer. *IEEE Access*. 2020;8:132677–132693. doi: 10.1109/ACCESS.2020.3010180.
5. Al-Khalifa, K. S., AlSheikh, R. Teledentistry awareness among dental professionals in Saudi Arabia. *PLoS One* 2020;15:e0240825. doi: 10.1371/journal.pone.0240825.
6. Huang, T. K., Yang, C. H., Hsieh, Y. H., Wang, J. C., Hung, C. C. Augmented reality (AR), and virtual reality (VR) applied in dentistry. *Kaohsiung J. Med. Sci.* 2018;34:243–248. doi: 10.1016/j.kjms.2018.01.009.
7. Davis, S. E., Lasko, T. A., Chen, G., Siew, E. D., Matheny, M. E. Calibration drifts in regression and machine learning models for acute kidney injury. *J. Am. Med. Inform. Assoc.* 2017;24(6):1052–1061. doi: 10.1093/jamia/ocx030.
8. Harbour, R., Miller, J. A new system for grading recommendations in evidence-based guidelines. *BMJ*. 2001;323(7308):334–336. doi: 10.1136/bmj.323.7308.334.
9. Pandimurugan, Parvathi, M., Jenila, A. A survey of software testing in refactoring based software models. International Conference on Nanoscience, Engineering and Technology (ICONSET 2011), Chennai, 2011, pp. 571–573. doi: 10.1109/ICONSET.2011.6168034.
10. Parvathi, M., Pandimurugan. A study on soil testing using SOA and its future considerations. 2012 International Conference on Computing, Electronics and Electrical Technologies (ICCEET), Kumaracoil, 2012, pp. 894–899. doi: 10.1109/ICCEET.2012.6203895.
11. Hussain, A., Raja, M., Vellaisamy, P., Krishnan, S., Rajendran, L. Enhanced framework for ensemble effort estimation by using recursive-based classification. *IET Soft*. 2021;15:230–238. doi: 10.1049/sfw2.12020.

12. Pandimurugan, V., Jain, A., Sinha, Y. IoT based face recognition for smart applications using machine learning. 2020 3rd International Conference on Intelligent Sustainable Systems (ICISS), Thoothukudi, India, 2020, pp. 1263–1266. doi: 10.1109/ICISS49785.2020.9316089.

13. Lakshmanan, S. K., Shakkeera, L., Pandimurugan, V. Efficient auto key based encryption and decryption using GICK and GDCK methods. 2020 3rd International Conference on Intelligent Sustainable Systems (ICISS), Thoothukudi, India, 2020, pp. 1102–1106. doi: 10.1109/ICISS49785.2020.9316114.

14. Meenakshi, N., Pandimurugan, V., Sathishkumar, L., Chinnasamy. Optimal routing methodology to enhance the life time of sensor network. *Materials Today: Proceedings*. 2021, ISSN 2214-7853. doi: 10.1016/j.matpr.2021.02.752.

15. Kumar, L. S., Hariharasitaraman, S., Narayanasamy, K., Thinakaran, K., Mahalakshmi, J., Pandimurugan, V. AlexNet approach for early stage Alzheimer's disease detection from MRI brain images. *Materials Today: Proceedings*. 2021, ISSN 2214-7853. doi: 10.1016/j.matpr.2021.04.415.

16. Kumar, L. S., Pandimurugan, V., Usha, D., Nageswara Guptha, M., Hema, M. S. Random forest tree classification algorithm for predicating loan. *Materials Today: Proceedings*. 2021, ISSN 2214-7853. doi: 10.1016/j.matpr.2021.12.322.

17. Scott, I., Carter, S., Coiera, E. Clinician checklist for assessing suitability of machine learning applications in healthcare. *BMJ Health & Care Informatics*. 2021;28(1):e100251.

18. Kraft, S. A. Respect and trustworthiness in the patient-provider-machine relationship: applying a relational lens to machine learning healthcare applications. *Am. J. Bioeth.* 2020;20(11):51–53.

19. Sarkar, S. K., Roy, S., Alsentzer, E., McDermott, M. B., Falck, F., Bica, I., Hyland, S. L. Machine learning for health (ML4H) 2020: advancing healthcare for all, in: Machine Learning for Health. *PMLR*. 2020, November, pp. 1–11.

20. Haleem, A., Javaid, M., Singh, R. P., Suman, R. Applications of artificial intelligence (AI) for cardiology during COVID-19 pandemic. Sustainable Operations Comput. 2021;2:71–78.

21. Revuelta-Zamorano, P., Sánchez, A., Rojo-Álvarez, J. L., Álvarez-Rodríguez, J., Ramos-López, J., Soguero-Ruiz, C. Prediction of healthcare-associated infections in an intensive care unit using machine learning and big data tools XIV Mediterranean Conference on Medical and Biological Engineering and Computing 2016, Springer: Cham. 2016, pp. 840–845.

22. Ramachandran, A., Adarsh, R., Pahwa, P., Anupama, K. R. Machine learning-based techniques for fall detection in geriatric healthcare systems 2018 9th International Conference on Information Technology in Medicine and Education (ITME), IEEE. 2018, October, pp. 232–237.

23. Hassan, M. M., Peya, Z. J., Mollick, S., Billah, M. A. M., Shakil, M. M. H., Dulla, A. U. Diabetes prediction in healthcare at early stage using machine learning approach 2021 12th International Conference on Computing Communication and Networking Technologies (ICCCNT), IEEE. 2021, July, pp. 1–5.

24. Singh, R. P., Javaid, M., Haleem, A., Vaishya, R., Bahl, S. Significance of health information technology (HIT) in context to COVID-19 pandemic: potential roles and challenges. *J. Ind. Integration Manage.* 2020;5(4):427–440.

25. Cho, S. Health record tracking enhancement based on multimedia and machine learning for mobile healthcare: trends and challenges. Proceedings of the 3rd International Workshop on Multimedia for Personal Health and Health Care, 2018, October, p. 1.

26. Khaleghi, T., Abdollahi, M., Murat, A. *Machine learning and simulation/optimization approaches to improve surgical services in healthcare Analytics, Operations, and Strategic Decision Making in the Public Sector*, IGI Global. 2019, pp. 138–165.

27. Mohan, S., Thirumalai, C., Srivastava, G. Effective heart disease prediction using hybrid machine learning techniques. *IEEE Access*. 2019;7:81542–81554.

28. Pandimurugan, V., Rajasoundaran, S., Routray, S., Prabu, A. V., Alyami, H., Alharbi, A., Ahmad, S. Detecting and extracting brain hemorrhages from CT images using generative convolutional imaging scheme. *Comput. Intell. Neurosci.* 2022;2022, Article ID 6671234, 10 pages. doi: 10.1155/2022/6671234.

29. Lucas, C. A., Hadley, E., Chew, R., Nance, J., Baumgartner, P., Thissen, R., Tatum, A. Machine learning for medical coding in healthcare surveys. *Vital Health Stat.* 2021;189:1–29.

30. Sathiyamoorthi, V., Ilavarasi, A. K., Murugeswari, K., Ahmed, S. T., Devi, B. A., Kalipindi, M. A deep convolutional neural network based computer aided diagnosis system for the prediction of Alzheimer's disease in MRI images. *Measurement*. 2021;171:108838, ISSN 0263-2241. doi: 10.1016/j.measurement.2020.108838.

2 Deep Learning Framework for Classification of Healthcare Data

Hannah Vijaykumar and K. Maheswari
Anna Adarsh College for Women, Chennai, India

S. Vahini Ezhilraman
Shri Krishnaswamy College for Women, Chennai, India

2.1 INTRODUCTION

For women, among the commonly diagnosed diseases in the present-day world is breast cancer. Cancer in the breast happens when the cell tissues of the breast become abnormal. These abnormal cells form a tumor inside the surface of the breast. The tumor is detected by the clinical breast test; yet, the detection tends to be very low, and finding the abnormal areas is quite challenging using traditional techniques. Therefore, the machine learning techniques help the doctors to discover the existence of the tumors, thus quickening the treatment process. The machine learning techniques perform disease prediction with the extracted features from the suspicious regions using mammography images.

Convolutional neural network, popularly known as CNN [1], is one of the well-known techniques developed by the experts to categorize the entire mammography images for identifying the cancer. Deep CNN failed in developing an assembled classifier that combines the mammogram images to achieve optimal performance. The upgraded version of CNN technique for classification of breast cancer was developed [2]. This upgraded version is somewhat enhanced in increasing its accuracy level. However, in this technique, the time complexity was not at all reduced.

Another improved technique for identifying or mining the features of the breast cancer images was introduced as the Convolutional Sparse Auto-Encoder (CSAE) [3] technique. Yet, the efficiency in accurate prediction risk in the disease is unaddressed. Besides, a new hybrid feature extraction of three outputs and CNN segmentation were introduced [4] for finding breast cancer. But this newly designed method takes more time to identify breast cancer.

A multiclass support vector machine (MSVM) with deep learning approach is introduced [5] in automated mammogram detection. This approach failed to

DOI: 10.1201/9781003469605-2

accurately validate huge datasets in less time complexity. One of the classification algorithms of random forest was introduced in [6] for predicting the factors for cancer, but the rate in error was not reduced in disease prediction. To categorize the images related to breast cancer, an integrated CNN and LSTM [7] was developed and introduced. However, this integrated designed model did not attain much success in improving its classification performances. Coding Network with Multilayer Perceptron (CNMP) technique is combined with a deep learning approach [8] for medical image classification with extracted features, but this multilayer technique also failed in achieving its expected classification accuracy rate.

An end-to-end multilevel algorithm [9] was developed for enhancing the accuracy level of the classification process. However, this algorithm has not succeeded in reducing the FPR in the process of such classification. Therefore, a combination of new convolutional neural network and small SE-ResNet component [10] was designed for further classifying the breast cancer images. But similar to the above techniques, this new enhanced technique also failed in minimizing the training error.

2.2   LITERATURE REVIEW FOR RELATED WORKS

One of the classifiers of support vector machine with elastic net (EnSVM) was designed in [11] for breast predicting risk of patients, but the feature extraction was not done for accurate prediction. A convolutional method was developed in [12], detecting breast cancer through image classification. Breast cancer detection time was not minimized while considering large training samples. A novel method was introduced [13] for finding the breast lesions from the ultrasound images using local configuration pattern features. The method failed in finding the accurate classification of images in larger databases.

The innovative technique of discrete orthonormal S-transform (DOST) was introduced in a two-dimensional method, which mined the [14] features from digitally driven mammograms for breast cancer identification. It failed to reduce the time in detecting breast cancer. Deep learning approach was developed in [15] breast cancer deduction. Even though the learning approach increased in accuracy, complexity in time did not decrease.

The new deep learning approach introduced [16] for identifying use in transfer learning. Still, the accuracy in classification had no improvement. A stacked sparse autoencoder (SSAE) was introduced [17] in efficiently detecting cancer using high-level features, though accuracy was not achieved with minimum error rate. Though a convolutional method [18] is used to identify the mammogram images along the breast cancer images, it has not achieved expected success in minimizing the time of feature extraction in detecting breast cancer.

Deep convolutional with advanced technique is used [19] to identify breast cancer with the deep feature extraction. The impact in time complexity problems remained the same. A dual contourlet transform and improved*K*nearest neighbor (KNN) were developed [20] for analyzing the mammogram and achieving higher breast cancer diagnosis accuracy. However, its FPR was not minimized as expected.

The technique of extracting image features using the machine learning process was introduced by Barisoni et al. allows for tissue interrogation by both biologically and clinically homogeneous disease categories to identify patient risk. Again the false positive rate remained unaddressed.

The issues of the existing reviews were overcome by developing a novel ensemble classification technique called Coiflet wavelet feature extraction-based deep learning (CWFE-DL) technique. The brief description of CWFE-DL technique with necessary diagrams is presented in the following section.

2.3 COIFLET WAVELET FEATURE EXTRACTION BASED DEEP LEARNING

Breast cancer is always a mortal disease, and the accurate finding can save humans' lives. To prevent the cancer in advance, predicting both the ordinary as well as unusual or cancer tissues is more important. Therefore, to predict such diseases like tumors, imaging such regions of the body facilitates the medical doctor for similar prognosis. The innovative machine learning approach selects particular parts and collects them more reliably and predicts the damage of the tissue. The proposed approach is represented in diagrammatic form in Figure 2.1.

The overview of CWFE-DL approach predicts the tumor from the input images with higher accuracy. The technique includes the three processes, namely image collection, feature extraction, and classification. Breast images are taken as $i_1, i_2, \ldots i_n$ gathered in a digital mammography database. After that, the unwanted part is removed from the input image, and the quality images are the result for accurate classification. The features from the input breast images of size, shape, texture, color, and edge are extracted for predicting the disease using a Coiflet wavelet transform. The feature extraction is used for identification of malignant parts at an early period. Finally, classification is performed using DN with the extracted features and prediction with lesser complexity.

2.3.1 COIFLET WAVELET TRANSFORM BASED FEATURE EXTRACTION

The proposed CWFE-DL technique performs the feature extraction to predict the normal and abnormal images with minimum time. Feature extraction is a

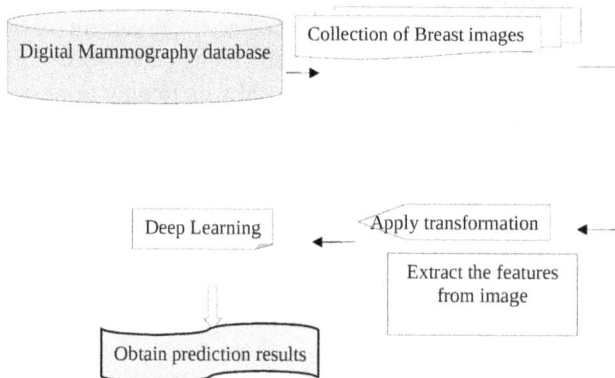

FIGURE 2.1 Overview of CWFE-DL.

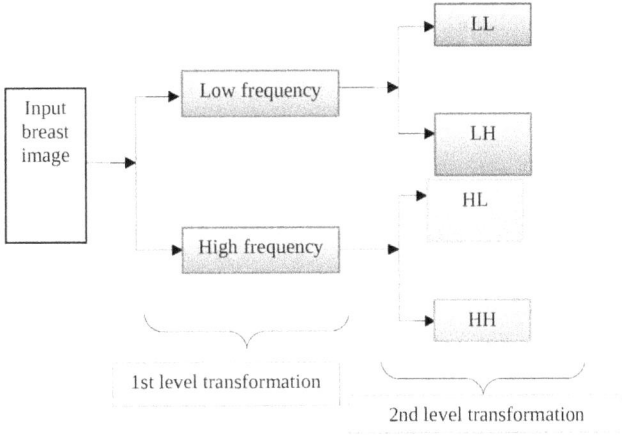

FIGURE 2.2   Transformation levels of Coiflet wavelet transform.

dimensionality reduction technique, and it is useful when the image sizes are large. The proposed CWFE-DL technique uses the Coiflet wavelet transform for image feature extraction. The original image is submerged as a Coiflet wavelet, which subbands into low (L) and high (H) frequencies. The levels of Coiflet wavelet transformation are given in Figure 2.2.

In the first-level transformation, the input image is decomposed into two frequency levels.

$$y = x(t) * g(t - k) \tag{2.1}$$

In Equation (2.1), y denotes an output of the finest level transformation, $x(t)$ denotes an input image, and $g(t)$ denotes a low pass filter. In the second-level transformation, the image is decomposed by 2 and obtains four subbands $\{LL, LH, HL, HH\}$. Filtering of lower level pass and higher level of pass is evaluated using in the following equation,

$$y_L = x(k) * g(2t - k) \tag{2.2}$$

$$y_H = x(k) * h(2t - k) \tag{2.3}$$

In (2.2) and (2.3), y_L denotes an output of lower-level filter, y_H indicates higher level filter g denotes a low pass filter (i.e., scaling function), and high pass filter as h(wavelet function), $2t$ denotes a decomposition by 2. After performing the decomposition, wavelet coefficient behavior of each subband is significant for extracting the features in multi-resolution levels. In addition, the statistical behavior of wavelet coefficients in each subband at various decomposition levels is necessary for feature extraction. The Coiflet wavelet coefficients is mathematically expressed as follows,

$$\beta_r = (-1)^r * D_{m-1-r} \tag{2.4}$$

In (2.4), β denotes Coiflet wavelet coefficients, r represents the coefficient index, D denotes a scaling function (i.e., low pass filter), and m represents the wavelet index. The coefficient extracts the features from the input image for breast cancer prediction with minimum time complexity.

Algorithm 1:
Input: Number of input images $D_1, D_2, D_3, ...D_n$, extracted features

Output: Improve classification accuracy

Begin

\\ feature extraction and Deep Learning Techniques

- **For each breast image**
- Perform first level transformation 'y' obtain L and H subbands
- Perform second-level transformation y_L, y_L obtain four subbands LL, LH, HL, HH with different resolutions
- Extract features using Coiflet wavelet coefficients
- Apply deep learning to classify the features
- Detect the breast cancer images
- **End for**

Algorithm 1 describes the process of Coiflet wavelet feature extraction-based deep learning technique. The input images are collected from the database. After that, the Coiflet wavelet transformation is applied to decompose the images into different subbands and extract the features from an input. The output of the mined features, the classification technique is performed to predict cancer disease at an earlier stage using an ensemble technique with minimum time.

2.3.2   DEEP LEARNING

For detecting the malicious blood-related diseases and particularly detecting the cancer, an innovative performance was proved by the technology of neural network and machine learning for healthcare. Thus, this new technology attracts the researchers to work on medical image analysis using the deep learning techniques. Among cancer-related diseases, breast cancer still remains the cause for the women's mortality. Though in countries like the USA such deaths are reduced with the help of mammography screening test methods, such deaths are inevitable. In this screening method they found both high false positive as well as false negative cases. Generally the specificity and sensitivity of such screening found in the US is 88.9% and 86.9%, respectively, which results in difficulty of predicting the cancer. Therefore, it is now needed for increasing the accuracy level of the screening process with the help of CAD and some of the software were introduced related to diagnosis in the early 1990s.

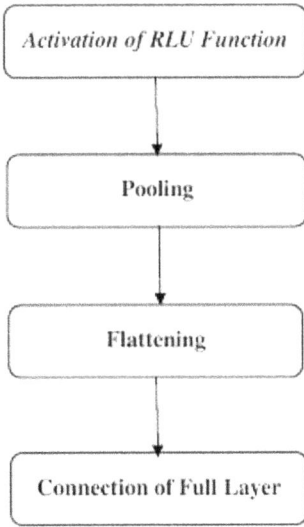

| Activation of RLU Function |
| Pooling |
| Flattening |
| Connection of Full Layer |

FIGURE 2.3   Processing of CNN.

2.3.2.1   Enhanced Technique of Machine Learning

CNN is an enhanced version of machine learning technique. The most preferable method for recognition of medical images is through computer vision. This CNN technique consists of different layers that extract and process the significant features of such medical images. Experts formulated four major steps for the working of CNN technique. The processing of CNN is shown in Figure 2.3.

Step 1. **Activation of Rely Function with the Operation of Convolution Technique**

The convolution operation technique aims to find the existing features of the suspected medical images by applying the feature detectors for preserving the distinct association with the pixels. In this method, the activation of the Rely function is used for breaking the linearity of the image and needs to enhance its non-linearity, due to its highly non-linear feature.

Step 2. **Pooling**

One of the down-sampling operations is the Pooling technique. As there are very few parameters in this method, this technique decreases the dimensions and calculation of the sampling as well as overfitting. This method is more tolerant in its distortion and variation.

Step 3. **Flattening**

The Flattening technique is utilized for pooling the output of the single-dimension matrix, before its further processing.

Step 4. **Connection of Full Layer**

In the fourth step, the further process of Flattening output is fed into a neural network, which is a fully connected form of the above layers. These layers are further utilized to classify and recognize such medical images deeply.

2.3.3 DATASET

Experimental evaluation of the proposed technique is implemented in MATLAB®, and some samples of suspected images of breasts are collected from a digital database site [21]. These images are used for predicting cancer diseases at an earlier stage. The collected images are preprocessed to remove the noise in an image. Then the extracted features from the images have to apply in classification. The early detection can choose the different input images and various simulation purposes. Ranges from 10 to 500 images selected to perform classification.

2.4 ANALYSIS AND EVALUATION OF PERFORMANCE RESULTS

Analysis and the evaluation of CWFE-DL approach is compared with other similar techniques like deep convolutional neural network, CNNI-BCC. The simulation work is applied in MATLAB, and the input images are collected from the DDSM (Digital Database for Screening Mammography) website [22]. The collected breast images are applied and predict the diseases as normal or cancerous at an earlier stage. At first, the input images are preprocessed to remove the noise in an image. After that, the extracted images are further processed for the classification (CWFE-DL) of such images to detect breast cancer at an early stage. The ten different simulation runs are performed in input images. For simulation purposes, the input samples vary for each run (i.e., the count of input images is chosen differently in each run). The sample applied for from 20 to 200 input images to perform classification.

Performance analysis and results are agreed for certain metrics like false positive rate, accuracy, and time consumption. Based on the metrics, comparison is applied for the techniques: CWFE-DL, Deep CNN, and CNNI-BCC.

2.4.1 COMPARISON ANALYSIS AND RESULTS

The comparison of the techniques CWFE-DL, Deep CNN, and CNNI-BCC are discussed in this section based on the metrics like time complexity, false positive rate, and accuracy. The analyzed output displayed in both tables and graphical representation along with the sample calculations are given in each subsection.

2.4.2 PERFORMANCE ANALYSIS OF CLASSIFICATION ACCURACY

The ratio of correctly classified breast images is divided from the total number of sample images taken for calculating its accuracy. Formula for calculating the accuracy rate of the breast cancer images are given below:

$$classification\ accuracy = \left[\frac{Number\ of\ breast\ images\ correclty\ classified}{n}\right] * 100 \quad (2.5)$$

In (2.5), n denotes total sample images. Classification accuracy is represented by percentage (%). The example of classification accuracy calculation is given below.

Example for classification accuracy calculation:

- **CWFE-DL:** The sample images taken as 20. The properly classified image is 18, and the remaining is not correct. Then the accuracy of classification is calculated using the formula,

$$classification\ accuracy = \frac{18}{20} * 100 = 90\%$$

- **Deep CNN:** There are 20 images taken for a sample out of 20 images. Fifteen images are classified correctly; the remaining are not correct. Then classification accuracy is calculated.

$$classification\ accuracy = \frac{15}{20} * 100 = 75\%$$

- **Existing CNNI-BCC:** Here 20 images are giving input for the 17 images that are classified in the right manner. Then apply the mathematical formula to calculate the classification accuracy,

$$classification\ accuracy = \frac{17}{20} * 100 = 85\%$$

Let us take the breast images of 20. Accuracy of classification is calculated in all the comparison techniques such as CWFE-DL, Deep CNN, and CNNI-BCC. The proposed CWFE-DL technique correctly classified 18 breast images, and their accuracy is 90%. Whereas the correctly classified breast images of Deep CNN, CNNI-BCC technique are 15 and 17 along with their accuracy are 75% and 85%, respectively. The prediction of breast cancer is compared with two more methods along with CWFE-DL, whose result is calculated with higher accuracy level. In Figure 2.4, all the techniques' accuracy rates are reported with a different number of breast images.

Algorithm of CWFE-DL
Input: Number of input images $D_1, D_2, D_3, ... D_n$

Output: Improved Accuracy and less time complexity

Step 1. for each breast image apply Coiflet wavelet feature extraction
Step 2. Images are decomposed into subbands

Number of breast images	Classification accuracy (%)		
	CWFE-DL	**Deep CNN**	**CNNI-BCC**
20	90	75	85
40	88	73	83
60	90	77	85
80	94	78	86
100	92	80	88
120	93	82	89
140	91	79	84
160	94	83	87
180	92	81	84
200	93	85	88

FIGURE 2.4   Classification Accuracy.

Step 3. the subbands images are applied into feature extraction
Step 4. the feature extracted images are applied into Deep-CNN
Step 5. the input image applies activities of RLU function
Step 6. then the pooling function performed
Step 7. the output of the pooling function applied into flattening function
Step 8. connected the full layer1
Step 9. again the output of full layer1 is connected into the full layer2
Step 10. the images are detected into the breast images

Algorithm of Deep CNN
Input: Number of input images D_1, D_2, D_3, ... D_n

Step 1. For each breast image applied into Deep-CNN
Step 2. The input image applies Convolutional Layer 1
Step 3. The output of CL1 is the input for pooling function
Step 4. Then the flattening function is performed based on RLU1
Step 5. The output is applied into the fully connected layer
Step 6. Finally, the breast images are detected

Algorithm of CNNI-BCC
Input: Number of input images D_1, D_2, D_3, ... D_n, extracted features

Step 1. For each breast image applied into CNN
Step 2. The input image applies Convolutional Layer 1

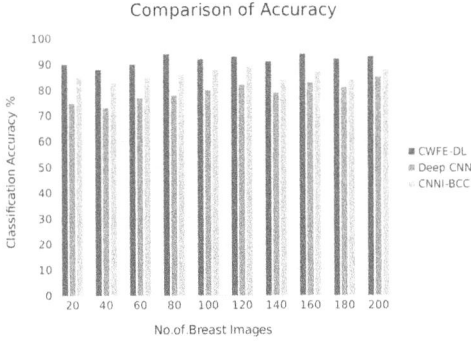

FIGURE 2.5   Comparison of accuracy of classification.

Step 3. The output of Convolutional Layer 1 is next applied into pooling function
Step 4. Then the flattening function is performed based on RLU1
Step 5. The feature extracted images are applied into Classification techniques
Step 6. The breast images are detected

Figure 2.5 shows the classification accuracy of CWFE-DL, Deep CNN, and CNNI-BCC. The analysis is applied for all the methods and the sample images taken in a series from 20 to 200. When comparing Figure 2.5 the accuracy is better than the other two methods, and the outcome clearly shows CWFE-DL technique achieves higher classification accuracy. The graphical representation of the comparison of accuracy is given in Figure 2.5.

From Figure 2.5 the comparison of classification accuracy is drawn. In the x-axis the series of sample images is represented, and in the y-axis, classification accuracy are represented. The output shows that the higher accuracy is achieved in the method CWFE-DL [23,24]. The average of accuracy is calculated, and CWFE-DL approach significantly improved accuracy of classification in 16%, 7% while comparing Deep CNN and CNNI-BCC correspondingly.

2.4.3   PERFORMANCE ANALYSIS FOR FALL-OUT

The fall-out of defined as is classifying the incorrect images (i.e., breast images) and the ratio of sample images (i.e., images). The calculation for false rate of classification,

$$false \; positive \; rate = \left[\frac{Number \; of \; breast \; images \; incorreclty \; classified}{n} \right] * 100 \quad (2.6)$$

In (2.6), n represents the sample images. The measurement of fall-out is incorrectly classified images and it is represented in percentage.

Example of Fall-out Calculations:

- **CWFE-DL:** The Sample of classified images is 20. Out of 20, 2 images are not correctly classified. Out of 20 images, the total number of incorrectly classified breast images are 2. The measurement of false positive rate is calculated as follows:

$$False\ positive\ rate = \frac{2}{20} * 100 = 10\%$$

- **Deep CNN:** The input of breast sample images incorrectly specified is 5 and the total images taken as 20. Then false positive rate is measured as follows,

$$False\ positive\ rate = \frac{5}{20} * 100 = 25\%$$

- **CNNI-BCC:** Number of breast input images not correctly classified is 3 and the sample of image are 20. The calculation for fall-out of CNNI-BCC is given below

$$False\ positive\ rate = \frac{3}{20} * 100 = 15\%$$

Comparison table of fall-out rate is shown in Figure 2.6, which describes the different techniques of incorrected images and the sample images. Let us consider the 20 breast images in the first iteration. The fall-out rate of the proposed CWFE-DL method is 10% minimizes the incorrect classification, 25% for Deep CNN and 15% for CNNI-BCC.

Sample breast images	Fall-Outrate Comparison		
	CWFE-DL	**Deep CNN**	**CNNI-BCC**
20	10	25	15
40	13	28	18
60	10	23	15
80	6	21	14
100	8	20	12
120	7	18	11
140	9	21	16
160	6	18	13
180	8	19	16
200	7	16	13

FIGURE 2.6 Comparison of Fall-Out Rate.

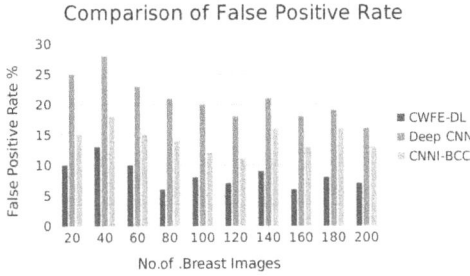

FIGURE 2.7   Graphical representation of fall-out.

The graphical representation shown in Figure 2.7 describes the comparison of various fall-out rates. Various inputs of sample images are represented in the axis "X" and false positive rate is given in the axis "Y." The fall-out rate is defined in percentage (%). The above graph clearly displays that the CWFE_DL methods have lesser incorrected images when compared with the other techniques like 60% for Deep CNN and 42% for CNNI-BCC.

2.4.4   PERFORMANCE RESULTS CLASSIFICATION TIME

The classification of the images taken for a time refers to the total time of classification and the product of time taken to classify the single image. The calculation for computing classification time is given in Equation 2.7.

$$TC = n * t \,[classifying\ single\ image] \tag{2.7}$$

In (2.7), TC denotes the classification total time, n represents the sample images and t taken as a single breast image classification time. The complexity of the total process of time is signified into milliseconds (ms) [25].

Sample mathematical calculation for time complexity:

- **CWFE-DL:** The number of sample input images are 20 and the product of time to process of an individual image is 1.1 millisecond. The complete involvedness of Time taken for the process is calculated as follows:

$$TC = 20 * 1.1ms = 22ms$$

- **Deep CNN:** Let us consider the number of sample input 20. The classifying time for Deep CNN technique for a single image is 1.7 ms. The value is applied for the below calculation,

$$TC = 20 * 1.7ms = 34ms$$

Sample Images	Comparison Table of Time complexity (ms)		
	CWFE-DL	**Deep CNN**	**CNNI-BCC**
20	22	34	28
40	28	40	32
60	39	50	45
80	44	54	48
100	52	65	59
120	58	70	62
140	63	74	70
160	70	88	77
180	77	90	85
200	85	96	92

FIGURE 2.8   Time Complexity.

- **CNNI-BCC:** Let us consider the number of input images 20. The single image to classify the method of CNNI-BCC is 1.4ms. The calculation for the overall classification time is given in Figure 2.8.

$$TC = 20 * 1.4ms = 28ms$$

To evaluate the time complexity of image classification, proposed CWFE-DL technique and existing methods are implemented in MATLAB simulator with sample breast images series like 20–200. Experimental results of time complexity using proposed CWFE-BAC technique are compared against the existing Deep CNN and CNNI-BCC. While considering 20 breast images for calculating the time complexity, the proposed CWFE-DL technique takes 22 ms for classifying the 20 input images as normal or abnormal. Whereas 34 ms and 28 ms taken by the Deep CNN and CNNI-BCC for classifying the input images. From these results, CWFE-DL method is lesser time complexity than the other methods. Graphical representation of time complexity is shown in Figure 2.9.

Figure 2.9 portrays time complexity resulting in three different methods with numbers of the breast images in the range of 20–200 taken from the mammographic medical images. The time complexity in the disease prediction is minimized using CWFE-DL technique than the existing techniques. The CWFE-DL technique aims to help experts of healthcare industries to identify malignant tumors by classifying cancer through the implementation of feature extraction. The CWFE-DL technique uses the Coiflet wavelet transform for feature extraction. The Coiflet wavelet

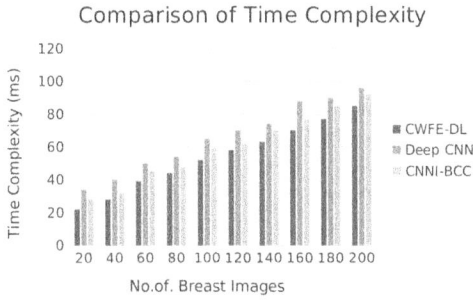

FIGURE 2.9 Comparison results of time consumption.

transform initially decomposes the input images into different submethods using two-level transformations. After that, Coiflet wavelet coefficient is used for extracting the features shape, size, color, and texture from an input image using scaling function and wavelet function. The extracted features are applied for classification, and the images are predicted for lesser time like 20% and 11% like Deep CNN and CNNI-BCC, respectively. The output clearly shows CWFE-DL technique efficiently predicts breast cancer disease with lesser time consumption.

2.5 CONCLUSION

The effective technique named CWFE-DL is presented for breast cancer disease prediction of better accuracy and lesser complexity to process. This chapter helps the medical doctors in determining breast cancer lesion from an input image. The unwanted noisy images are canceled and to improve the quality of image for accurate disease prediction. The Coiflet wavelet transformation is applied and extracted the quality enhanced output images for minimizing the disease prediction time. Finally, the ensemble classifiers accurately predict the cancer disease or normal by constructing the weak learners and voting scheme. Based on the classification results, the breast cancer is accurately predicted with minimum error rate. The various analysis and results of the CWFE-DL approach compared with the other classification methods for various metric. The Database collected for Screening Mammography digital images. The outcome of CWFE-DL experiment shows the effective advancement of accurate classification with minimum time complexity.

REFERENCES

1. Xiaofei Zhang, Yi Zhang, Erik Y. Han, Nathan Jacobs, Qiong Han, Xiaoqin Wang, Jinze Liu, "Classification of Whole Mammogram and Tomosynthesis Images Using Deep Convolutional Neural Networks", IEEE Transactions on Nano Bioscience, Volume 17, Issue 3, July 2018, Pages 237–242
2. Fung Fung, Ting Yen, Jun Tan, Kok Swee Sim, "Convolutional Neural Network Improvement for Breast Cancer Classification", Expert Systems with Applications, Elsevier, Volume 120, 2019, Pages 103–115

3. Michiel Kallenberg, Kersten Petersen, Mads Nielsen, Andrew Y. Ng, Pengfei Diao, Christian Igel, Celine M. Vachon, Katharina Holland, Rikke Rass Winkel, Nico Karssemeijer, Martin Lillholm, "Unsupervised Deep Learning Applied to Breast Density Segmentation and Mammographic Risk Scoring", IEEE Transactions on Medical Imaging, Volume 35, Issue 5, 2016, Pages 1322–1331

4. Cuiru Yu, Houjin Chen, Yanfeng Li, Yahui Peng, Jupeng Li, Fan Yang, "Breast Cancer Classification in Pathological Images Based on Hybrid Features", Multimedia Tools and Applications, Springer, 2019, Pages 1–21

5. Prabhpreet Kaur, Gurvinder Singh, Parminder Kaur, "Intellectual detection and validation of automated mammogram breast cancer images by multi-class SVM using deep learning classification", Informatics in Medicine Unlocked, Elsevier, 2019, Pages 1–19

6. Mogana Darshini Ganggayah, Nur Aishah Taib, Yip Cheng Har, Pietro Lio, Sarinder Kaur Dhillon, "Predicting Factors for Survival of Breast Cancer Patients Using Machine Learning Techniques", BMC Medical Informatics and Decision Making, Springer, Volume 19, Issue 48, 2019, Pages 1–17

7. Abdullah-Al Nahid, Mohamad Ali Mehrabi, Yinan Kong, "Histopathological Breast Cancer Image Classification by Deep Neural Network Techniques Guided by Local Clustering", BioMed Research International, Hindawi, Volume 2018, March 2018, Pages 1–20

8. Zhi Fei Lai, HuiFang Deng, "Medical Image Classification Based on Deep Features Extracted by Deep Model and Statistic Feature Fusion with Multilayer Perceptron", Computational Intelligence and Neuroscience, Hindawi, Volume 2018, September 2018, Pages 1–13

9. Jinjin Hai, Hongna Tan, Jian Chen, Minghui Wu, Kai Qiao, Jingbo Xu, Lei Zeng Fei Gao, Dapeng Shi, Bin Yan, "Multi-Level Features Combined End-to-End Learning for Automated Pathological Grading of Breast Cancer on Digital Mammograms", Computerized Medical Imaging and Graphics, Elsevier, Volume 71, January 2019, Pages 58–66

10. Yun Jiang, Li Chen, Hai Zhang, Xiao Xiao, "Breast Cancer Histopathological Image Classification Using Convolutional Neural Networks with Small SE-ResNet Module", PLoS One, Volume 14, Issue 3, 2019, Pages 1–21

11. Wenqing Sun, Tzu-Liang (Bill) Tseng, Wei Qian, Edward C. Saltzstein, Bin Zheng, Hui Yu, Shi Zhou, "A New Near-Term Breast Cancer Risk Prediction Scheme Based on the Quantitative Analysis of Ipsilateral View Mammograms", Computer Methods and Programs in Biomedicine, Elsevier, Volume 155, 2018, Pages 29–38

12. Teresa Araújo, Guilherme Aresta, Eduardo Castro, José Rouco, Paulo Aguiar, Catarina Eloy, António Polónia, Aurélio Campilho, "Classification of Breast Cancer Histology Images Using Convolutional Neural Networks", PLoS One, Volume 12, Issue 6, 2017, Pages 1–14

13. U. Rajendra Acharya, Kristen M. Meiburger, Joel En Wei Koh, Edward J. Ciaccio, N. Arun Kumar, Mee Hoong See, Nur Aishah Mohd Taib, Anushya Vijayananthan, Kartini Rahmat, Farhana Fadzli, Sook Sam Leong, Caroline Judy Westerhout, Angela Chantre-Astaiza, Gustavo Ramirez-Gonzalez, "A Novel Algorithm for Breast Lesion Detection Using Textons and Local Configuration Pattern Features With Ultrasound Imagery", IEEE Access, Volume 7, 2019, Pages 22829–22842

14. Shradhananda Beura, Banshidhar Majhi, Ratnakar Dash, Susnata Roy, "Classification of Mammogram Using Two-dimensional Discrete Orthonormal S-Transform for Breast Cancer Detection", Healthcare Technology Letters, Volume 2, Issue 3, 2015, Pages 46–51

15. Nadia Brancati, Giuseppe De Pietro, Maria Frucci, Daniel Riccio, "A Deep Learning Approach for Breast Invasive Ductal Carcinoma Detection and Lymphoma Multi-Classification in Histological Images", IEEE Access, Volume 7, 2019, Pages 44709–44720

16. Sana Ullah Khan, Naveed Islam, Zahoor Jan, Ikram Ud Din, Joel J. P. C Rodrigues, "A Novel Deep Learning Based Framework for the Detection and Classification of Breast Cancer Using Transfer Learning", Pattern Recognition Letters, Elsevier, Volume 125, 2019, Pages 1–6

17. Jun Xu, Lei Xiang, Qingshan Liu, Hannah Gilmore, Jianzhong Wu, Jinghai Tang, Anant Madabhushi, "Stacked Sparse Autoencoder (SSAE) for Nuclei Detection on Breast Cancer Histopathology Images", IEEE Transactions on Medical Imaging, Volume 35, Issue 1, 2016, Pages 119–130

18. Gabriele Valvano, Gianmarco Santini, Nicola Martini, Andrea Ripoli, Chiara Iacconi, Dante Chiappino, Daniele Della Latta, "Convolutional Neural Networks for the Segmentation of Microcalcification in Mammography Imaging", Journal of Healthcare Engineering, Hindawi, Volume 2019, April 2019, Pages 1–9

19. Hongmin Cai, Qinjian Huang, Wentao Rong, Yan Song, Jiao Li, Jinhua Wang, Jiazhou Chen, Li Li, "Breast Microcalcification Diagnosis Using Deep Convolutional Neural Network from Digital Mammograms", Computational and Mathematical Methods in Medicine Hindawi, Volume 2019, March 2019, Pages 1–10

20. Min Dong, Zhe Wang, Chenghui Dong, Xiaomin Mu, Yide Ma, "Classification of Region of Interest in Mammograms Using Dual Contourlet Transform and Improved KNN", Journal of Sensors, Hindawi, Volume 2017, November 2017, Pages 1–15

21. A. Singhai, S. Aanjankumar, S. Poonkuntran, "A Novel Methodology for Credit Card Fraud Detection using KNN Dependent Machine Learning Methodology", *2023 2nd International Conference on Applied Artificial Intelligence and Computing (ICAAIC)*, Salem, India, 2023, pp. 878–884, 10.1109/ICAAIC56838.2023.10141427.

22. L. Barisoni, K. J. Lafata, S. M. Hewitt, A. Madabhushi, U. G. Balis, "Digital Pathology and Computational Image Analysis in Nephropathology", Nature Reviews Nephrology, Volume 16, Issue 11, 2020, Pages 669–685

23. T. Anitha, S. Aanjankumar, S. Poonkuntran *et al.*, "A Novel Methodology for Malicious Traffic Detection in Smart Devices Using BI-LSTM–CNN-Dependent Deep Learning Methodology." Neural Comput & Applic, Volume 35, 2023, Pages 20319–20338, 10.1007/s00521-023-08818-0.

24. V. Sathiyamoorthi, A.K. Ilavarasi, K. Murugeswari, Syed Thouheed Ahmed, B. Aruna Devi, Murali Kalipindi, "A Deep Convolutional Neural Network Based Computer Aided Diagnosis System for the Prediction of Alzheimer's Disease in MRI Images", Measurement, Volume 171, 2021, 108838, ISSN 0263-2241, 10.1016/j.measurement.2020.108838.

25. http://marathon.csee.usf.edu/Mammography/Database.html.

3 Leveraging Deep Learning in Hate Speech Analysis on Social Platform

R. Manikandan

School of Business and Management, Christ University, Bangalore

S. Hariharasitaraman

Department of Computing Science and Engineering, VIT Bhopal University, India

S. Ramkumar and R. Gobinath

School of Sciences, Department of Computer Science, Christ University, Bangalore

3.1 INTRODUCTION

Social networking sites (SNS) act as a strong platform and a medium of communication broadcast. The growth of the Internet and usage of SNS have facilitated people to a large extent. The platforms have also opened up avenues for many people around the globe for expressing themselves without resistance. This also has the risk of circulating offensive and threatening posts, termed "cyber-bullying," well used on the Internet. Hate texts are the words or groups of words that are used by people to express their opinions with vulgarity. The opinions in general target either other people, products, or any organization with different views [1,2]. SNS have become a comfortable and easier medium for posting such harmful content that can lead to other cybercrimes. Also, the ability to hide the identity in posts has made it easy for aggressive commenters. Figure 3.1 shows the hate text reviews in SNSs.

Presently, hate texts are being posted more frequently, which mandates modern techniques to automatically detect and delete such posts before it reaches many users. Much research is being carried out in SNS [3] as these generate large volumes of data that can be analyzed for patterns and insights. These sites are also being experimented with for detecting undesired actions such as posting hate comments [4]. These abusers find it easier to get away without being caught as most

DOI: 10.1201/9781003469605-3

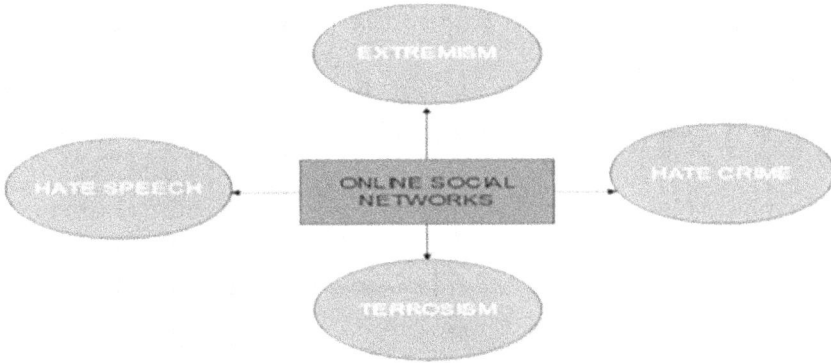

FIGURE 3.1 Hate text review in SNSs.

of the service providers maintain anonymity, and the origin of such contents are hidden and left untraceable. Many SNSs also do not spend much energy in deleting such posts due to ignorance or for any popularity. One of the ways to handle the issue is to come up with automation techniques that can perform analysis, recognize, and finally eliminate such vulgar messages. Usage of natural language processing and machine learning techniques has been largely used by researchers [5,6] for bringing out such detection techniques. Although there is an increase of similar works in the similar field, issues come up as the data are scattered and of different forms and languages [7]. Research that proposes feature extraction through machine learning helps to some extent in coming out with derivatives for the detection of distinct and important properties of information.

The tasks performed through this research resulted in the generation of a variety of features that are relevant to the original list of features. Although it is complex for arriving at such a subset of features, models that can predict such features have seen remarkable achievement in the context of accuracy and classification. Traditional methods included in social media analysis are the bag of words, N-grams, uni-grams, and TFIDF, and semantic and syntactic analysis [8]. This chapter concentrates on Twitter data.

Classification of tweets shall be on the classes that already exist with pre-determined steps such as pre-processing, feature detection, and extraction and decomposition [9]. These processes are then carried out with different schemes for the improvisation in levels of accuracy. Machine learning methods help to classify the available data that are based on a learning scenario. Supervised methods such as SVM are largely deployed in classification. These produce classified outputs based on pre-determined labels. These are simple and binary classifiers that form a hyperplane through the process of separating the members of its class from its input universe.

SVMs are also used in non-linear mapping, which helps to map the input space to a high-dimensional feature space. These planes are then separated through the maxima margin of a hyperplane, a linear way of combining the data points [10]. The SVMs are also used for detecting the points of information for representing the separated hyperplane. Figure 3.2 depicts the proposed model for detecting hate texts.

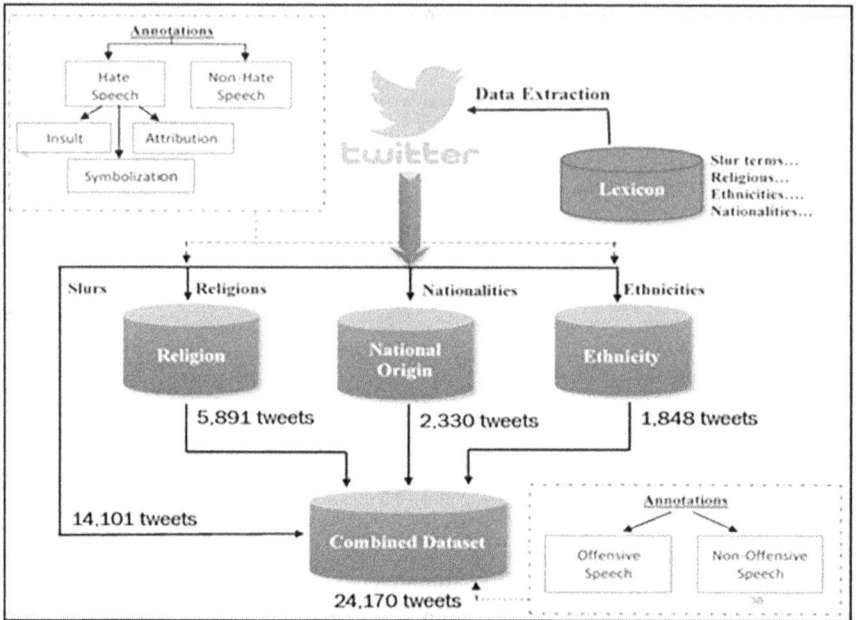

FIGURE 3.2 Hate text detection model.

The important issue taken in this chapter is to work on the problem of automatic detection of hate texts in the Twitter data set. The proposed work uses improved principle component analysis (IPCA) and modified convolution neural network (MCNN) for improving the hate text detection performance. The chapter is organized such that Section 3.2 projects the prominent literature in the field of study, followed by the detailed explanations and hypothesis of the proposed methods from Section 3.3, followed by result discussion and conclusion.

3.2 RELATED WORK

In [11], the authors have proposed a novel method using PCA to detect hate text against minorities. Here, the research focused on data from Facebook and identified the regular expression through primitive pre-processing methods. The proposed method used word-to-vector embedding technique and the uni-grams model. The features were identified using DNN and GRN and using a few variants of RNN. The detected hate content was then subjected to clustering for predicting the target. The data set used was customized and generated using web crawlers on Facebook pages. The use of the word-to-vector model produced better results than other models while the RNN paved the way for more accuracy in classification.

The concept of crowdsourcing was presented in [12] wherein the authors made use of them to collect and classify the hate texts such as offensive and non-offensive. The authors have used a multi-level classifier for classification accuracy. The model paved the way for classifying words under class labels such as racism, homophobic, etc

Principal component analysis was used in [13] for effective feature extraction from tweets. The proposed method used different graphical plots of parallel coordinates. These techniques achieved dual objectives of both automation and filtering. Here, the variables that had larger variances did not support multi-variable classifications, but PCA helped to overcome the issues in feature extraction. The parallel coordinate methods significantly helped in achieving better performance. The methods also proved to be effective in the classification of multi-variable data.

In [14], the authors have made use of the LDA for extracting useful data from features that are not considered in PCA and which has small variance in the class constructors. The authors were sure that these discarded features shall have some useful information, and they were extracted through LDA. The technique was named PDCA, which increased the accuracy of classification when compared to that of PCA and LDA separately. They took a particular community post on Facebook for their experiment. Another supervised technique proposed using N-grams was introduced in [15]. This study helped to remove the redundant features and introduced a new lexicon for semantic analysis. The proposed lexicon was developed in such a way that it only considers the items related to a brand, which helps in complexity reduction but then provides a wide range of topics. The proposed lexicon performance was then compared with other standard methods that use SVM. The results were impressive and the introduction of the DNA2 ML algorithm was also found to be effective when used along with the proposed lexicon in terms of sentiment analysis and outperforms SVM.

In [16], CNN was used for the investigation of pre-trained data from Twitter, the proposed model showed that DLT can perform more efficiently in recognizing hate texts when there are many domains under consideration. The work provided ways for further exploration of using neural networks for promoting accurate content classification in large datasets.

3.3 PROPOSED METHODOLOGY

From the knowledge through existing literature, it is known that there is a large scope for increasing the accuracy in the detection of hate texts. Also, it is seen from the existing works that the computational complexity was not fairly discussed and attended to. Taking these scopes, this chapter proposes a combination of improved principle component analysis (IPCA) and modified convolutional neural network (MCNN) for overall performance improvement in detecting hate texts. The IPCA algorithm is used for efficient feature extraction and MCNN for better classification accuracy.

3.3.1 PRE-PROCESSING

Normalization is used as a prominent pre-processing method in this work. It is important to remove the noise and to clean the data as it largely affects the classification accuracy. The vector space between the features shall also be considered to be kept short as it affects the computational time. The steps involved in pre-processing include segmentation, stop-word removal, and stemming. The complex tweets are broken down into simple sentences using segmentation. The NLTK tokenizers are used for splitting the tweets at the word level. Words having a different kind of behavior such as verbs, nouns, etc. are considered as one. All the pre-fix and suffixes of words are removed through the process of pruning. Grammar errors are ignored in this case, which brings together two concepts: term frequency (TF) and document frequency (DF). The term frequency is the number of times a certain term appears in a document. The frequency of occurrence of a term in a document reflects its importance. Term frequency depicts each text in the data as a matrix, with rows representing the number of documents and columns representing the number of distinct terms across all documents. The amount of words that include a specific phrase is referred to as document frequency. The term's document frequency reflects how common it is. The weight of a term is inverse document frequency (IDF), which seeks to minimize the weight of a term if the phrase's occurrences are low.

The POTTER [17] method is adopted for the Pruning process. There is another study called TF-IDF, a text vectorizer that converts text into a useful vector is the term frequency-inverse document frequency.

The tweet taken for the experiment may also have words of less importance as the classification is considered and thus need not be considered. The proposed work used the efficiency of the NLTK library [18] to remove such stop words and for reducing the impact on classification. The N-gram model is then used for tokenization. The final step in pre-processing includes normalization. The minimum-maximum normalization is used in this work for the linear transformation of data [19] into a pre-defined boundary. Normalization is represented in Equation (3.1).

This normalization can be depicted as Equation (3.1)

$$N' = \left(\frac{N - MIn(N)}{Max(A) - Min(A)} * (B - D) + D \right) \qquad (3.1)$$

Here, N'–denotes the output, which is normalized. $[B, D]$ – denotes the pre-defined boundary and A denotes the actual data that requires transformation. The transformation is executed through this method by taking the Standard Deviation (SD) for getting the normalized output values. Normalization is done to eliminate the features that are non-effective and noisy.

The experimented results of TFIDF are given below,

Step 1: Four sample tweets/Texts were taken, and we need to vectorize these texts using NLTK as given in Table 3.1.

Step 2: Create a TF matrix where rows are documents and columns are distinct terms throughout all Texts. Count word occurrences in every text as mentioned in Table 3.2.

TABLE 3.1

Sample Tweets

Text1	Air quality in the sunny island improved gradually throughout Wednesday.
Text2	Air quality in Singapore on Wednesday continued to get worse as haze hit the island.
Text3	The air quality in Singapore is monitored through a network of air monitoring stations located in different parts of the island
Text4	The air quality in Singapore got worse on Wednesday.

TABLE 3.2
Term Count of Tokens

S.No	Token	Term Count			
		Text1	Text2	Text3	Text4
1	air	0.10	0.07	0.10	0.11
2	quality	0.10	0.07	0.05	0.11
3	sunny	0.10	0.00	0.00	0.00
4	island	0.10	0.07	0.05	0.00
5	improved	0.10	0.00	0.00	0.00
6	gradually	0.10	0.00	0.00	0.00
7	throughout	0.10	0.00	0.00	0.00
8	wednesday	0.10	0.07	0.00	0.11
9	singapore	0.00	0.07	0.05	0.11
10	continued	0.00	0.07	0.00	0.00
11	worse	0.00	0.07	0.00	0.11
12	haze	0.00	0.07	0.00	0.00
13	hit	0.00	0.07	0.00	0.00
14	monitored	0.00	0.00	0.05	0.00
15	network	0.00	0.00	0.05	0.00
16	monitoring	0.00	0.00	0.05	0.00
17	stations	0.00	0.00	0.05	0.00
18	located	0.00	0.00	0.05	0.00
19	different	0.00	0.00	0.05	0.00
20	parts	0.00	0.00	0.05	0.00

Step 3: Compute inverse document frequency (IDF) as given in Equation 3.1, the results are given in Table 3.3.

Step 4: Multiply TF with IDF the Tweets are vectorized as given in Table 3.4.

3.3.2 IMPROVED PRINCIPLE COMPONENT ANALYSIS (IPCA) FOR FEATURE EXTRACTION

Extracting features is important to retrieve the impact of data attributes from a large data set. PCA performs multi-variable data analysis for extracting the linear features. It detects the correlation among the features in given data, which are called observed variables. PCA generally ignores the features that have fewer variations when a subset of features is generated. Hence, it minimizes the dimensionality of feature space and extracts only the variables that are co-related to construct a feature with minimal space [20,21]. In the proposed methodology, the improved PCA is introduced to produce feature vectors from a large data set. The issue with primitive PCA is that these do not consider features that have minor variations among them. The hypothesis here is that these features may also have important information which helps in better classification. The proposed IPCA reduces the value of the

TABLE 3.3

IDF Computation

S.No	Token	Text1	Text2	Text3	Text4	Document Count	IDF
		Term Count					
1	air	0.10	0.07	0.10	0.11	4.00	0.00
2	quality	0.10	0.07	0.05	0.11	4.00	0.00
3	sunny	0.10	0.00	0.00	0.00	1.00	0.60
4	island	0.10	0.07	0.05	0.00	3.00	0.13
5	improved	0.10	0.00	0.00	0.00	1.00	0.60
6	gradually	0.10	0.00	0.00	0.00	1.00	0.60
7	throughout	0.10	0.00	0.00	0.00	1.00	0.60
8	Wednesday	0.10	0.07	0.00	0.11	3.00	0.13
9	Singapore	0.00	0.07	0.05	0.11	3.00	0.13
10	continued	0.00	0.07	0.00	0.00	1.00	0.60
11	worse	0.00	0.07	0.00	0.11	2.00	0.30
12	haze	0.00	0.07	0.00	0.00	1.00	0.60
13	hit	0.00	0.07	0.00	0.00	1.00	0.60
14	monitored	0.00	0.00	0.05	0.00	1.00	0.60
15	network	0.00	0.00	0.05	0.00	1.00	0.60
16	monitoring	0.00	0.00	0.05	0.00	1.00	0.60
17	stations	0.00	0.00	0.05	0.00	1.00	0.60
18	located	0.00	0.00	0.05	0.00	1.00	0.60
19	different	0.00	0.00	0.05	0.00	1.00	0.60
20	parts	0.00	0.00	0.05	0.00	1.00	0.60

Eigenvector by influencing the normalization of vectors. Considering that x_{ij} as the xth element in the jth feature, then SD $\sqrt{\lambda_x}$ to be applied to the feature vector. Then, Equation (3.2) represents the resultant feature vector.

$$M_j' = \left[\frac{M_{iio}}{\lambda_n}, \frac{m_j}{\lambda_1}, \dots \frac{m_{i(n-1)}}{\lambda_{m-n}} \right] \qquad (3.2)$$

The resultant normalization of the feature vectors then creates new other subspaces for the features. This work concentrates on the normalization of these subspace features through their corresponding Eigenvalues square, which are then followed through calculations of distances between features that are used for training and testing. The linear IPCA modification is represented in Equation (3.3).

$$M = T * N \qquad (3.3)$$

Here, M represents the transformation matrix, T denotes the vectors, and N represents the feature vectors that are transformed. The matrix M then takes the form as in Equation (3.4).

TABLE 3.4
Cross Product of TF x IDF

S.No	Token	Term Count				Document Count	IDF	TF x IDF			
		Text1	Text2	Text3	Text4			Text1	Text2	Text3	Text4
1	air	0.10	0.07	0.10	0.11	4.00	0.00	0.00	0.00	0.00	0.00
2	quality	0.10	0.07	0.05	0.11	4.00	0.00	0.00	0.00	0.00	0.00
3	sunny	0.10	0.00	0.00	0.00	1.00	0.60	0.06	0.00	0.00	0.00
4	island	0.10	0.07	0.05	0.00	3.00	0.13	0.01	0.01	0.01	0.00
5	improved	0.10	0.00	0.00	0.00	1.00	0.60	0.06	0.00	0.00	0.00
6	gradually	0.10	0.00	0.00	0.00	1.00	0.60	0.06	0.00	0.00	0.00
7	throughout	0.10	0.00	0.00	0.00	1.00	0.60	0.06	0.00	0.00	0.00
8	Wednesday	0.10	0.07	0.00	0.11	3.00	0.13	0.01	0.01	0.00	0.01
9	Singapore	0.00	0.07	0.05	0.11	3.00	0.13	0.00	0.01	0.01	0.01
10	continued	0.00	0.07	0.00	0.00	1.00	0.60	0.00	0.04	0.00	0.00
11	worse	0.00	0.07	0.00	0.11	2.00	0.30	0.00	0.02	0.00	0.03
12	haze	0.00	0.07	0.00	0.00	1.00	0.60	0.00	0.04	0.00	0.00
13	hit	0.00	0.07	0.00	0.00	1.00	0.60	0.00	0.04	0.00	0.00
14	monitored	0.00	0.00	0.05	0.00	1.00	0.60	0.00	0.00	0.03	0.00
15	network	0.00	0.00	0.05	0.00	1.00	0.60	0.00	0.00	0.03	0.00
16	monitoring	0.00	0.00	0.05	0.00	1.00	0.60	0.00	0.00	0.03	0.00
17	stations	0.00	0.00	0.05	0.00	1.00	0.60	0.00	0.00	0.03	0.00
18	located	0.00	0.00	0.05	0.00	1.00	0.60	0.00	0.00	0.03	0.00
19	different	0.00	0.00	0.05	0.00	1.00	0.60	0.00	0.00	0.03	0.00
20	parts	0.00	0.00	0.05	0.00	1.00	0.60	0.00	0.00	0.03	0.00

$$(\lambda L - s)T = 0 \tag{3.4}$$

In the above equation, where the squares of matrices are denoted by L have the diagonal identity, s denote the covariance matrix of the actual data, and T denotes the eigenvalues. The eigenvalues are computed using the Equation (3.2) and can be represented as $T = [T_1, \quad T_2, \dots \dots, T_n]$.

The proposed IPCA transforms the dataset, and the matrix of transformation is the training set expressed in Equations (3.5) and Equation (3.6)

$$M = T'N \tag{3.5}$$

$$Q_{Nm} = a_1 v_1 + a_2 v_2 + \dots + a_N v_N \tag{3.6}$$

Equations (3.3) and (3.5) are compared to detect the matrices that are transformed and that arise from the covariant matrix and form the complete hate text data. The important advantage of using IPCA is that it helps in reducing the dimension and minimizes the loss of information. Although it is based on PCA, the IPCA is a mathematical approach that helps to map the high dimensional features to the linear problem where fewer dimensions are achieved through eigenvalues of the covariant matrix. Hence, IPCA achieves feature extraction with less probability of errors as it considers the ignored features of PCA also. The algorithm for IPCA is given below.

Algorithm 1: Modified Principle Component Analysis

1. Begin
2. Calculate the mean of T' of the given data set T and subtract it from T
3. Get the new matrix M
4. Obtain the covariance of the matrix C
5. Obtain the Eigenvectors from the new matrices which are
6. Obtain the EigenValues from C
7. Finally, Eigenvectors are calculated for covariance matrix
8. Transform M into Linear vectors using (5)
9. Keep larger EigenValues for forming Low dimension data set
10. Any vector V can be written as a linear combination of Eigenvectors using (6)
11. Extract the top matches
12. Extract the most important features
13. End

3.3.3 MODIFIED CNN FOR CLASSIFICATION

The proposed MCNN helps to classify the data set taken for testing under two class labels namely YES and NO. The CNN used consists of an input, output, and multiple hidden layers that do the job of pooling and convolution. The neurons are

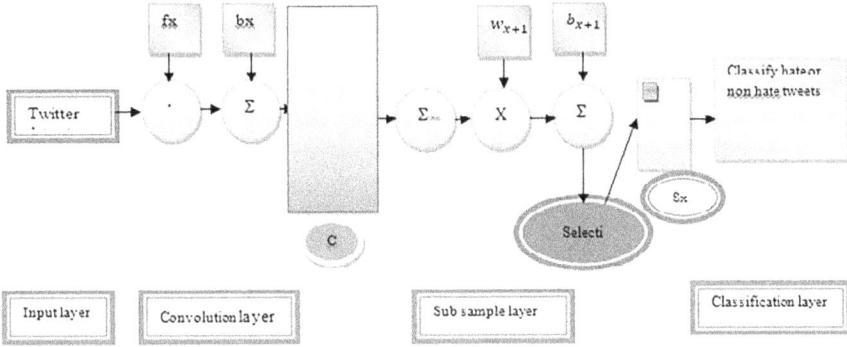

FIGURE 3.3 Architecture diagram of MCNN.

simulated in this layer, which is then passed to the other layers. The proposed architecture is presented in Figure 3.3.

The proposed CNN shall inherit either local or global layers for pooling that joins with the clusters of output neurons. The cluster average is responsible for mean pooling while the fully connected layers take the responsibility of mapping the other neurons in the preceding layer. Unlike the conventional CNN [22–25], the proposed MCNN has different layers each meant for a specific purpose, which can analyze even data of high dimensions efficiently. The shared parameters help to reduce the total parameters to be considered. The MCNN gets its inputs, which are the tweets from the input data set that are in turn transformed to the subsequent layers. This layer also defines the initial parameters such as the scales and filters for producing the feature maps, which helps to extract only the key features, thus reducing the total complexity in computation.

The activation is done in the convolutional layer. This activation function maps the output to a given set of inputs, thus creating a nonlinear framework. Back-propagation is used to assign and update the values of the feature. The proposed method uses the gradient method to activate the function for a given neural network. Weights are then added to values to form the output, which is defined in Equations (3.7) and (3.8).

$$F(m) = f\left(\sum_{i=1}^{j=m} k_i(m)y(m)\right) \tag{3.7}$$

where

$$F(m) = \{+1 \quad if\, m \geq 0 - 1 \quad if\, m < 0 \tag{3.8}$$

where m denotes the index of iteration.

Equation (3.9) denotes the updation of connected weights

$$j_i(m+1) = j_i(m) + \eta(e(m) - x(m)x_i(n)), \quad i = 1, 2, .. N \qquad (3.9)$$

These weighted features are then fed to the proposed MCNN for obtaining better accuracy in classification. A function is introduced to ensure that the data being analyzed are the same. All the feature maps that are generated through the convolution are then again sampled. A fitness value is proposed for MCNN to classify the tweets as HATE or NONHATE through a genetic fitness measure for selecting the accurate features.

A couple of samples are then taken for the genetic operator, which then evolves as future chromosomes. This process is iterated until the best fitness is identified. The selection operator is defined as in Equation (3.10)

$$Q(m_i) = \frac{f(m_i)}{\Sigma_{i=1}^{j} f(m)} \qquad (3.10)$$

Here $Q(c_i)$ represents the chances that a given chromosome is within the population m. This ensures that those chromosomes with large fitness are only selected so that the children have more fitness even after crossover.

Algorithm 2: Steps in MCNN
    Input: Data, Population, Training, and Testing data
    Objective function: Accuracy of the fitness
    Output: HATE or NONHATE

1. Begin
2. Activate the procedure for Twitter data
3. Do – Population initialization
4. While M<= MAX, Perform
5. Conversion of input as sub-layers
6. Classify as HATE and NONHATE using (10)
7. Calculate fitness using (11)
8. If Best, Goto 11 else
9. Identify more relevant features
10. M=M+1
11. Do Training and Testing
12. Return the features with high accuracy
13. Copy the classification label for all of the feature
14. END

During the evaluation of fitness in all of the MCNNs, a new child is generated because of the genetic operations while it increases the count by one, and once the maximum number of generations is reached, the process is stopped. The complete workflow is shown in Figure 3.4.

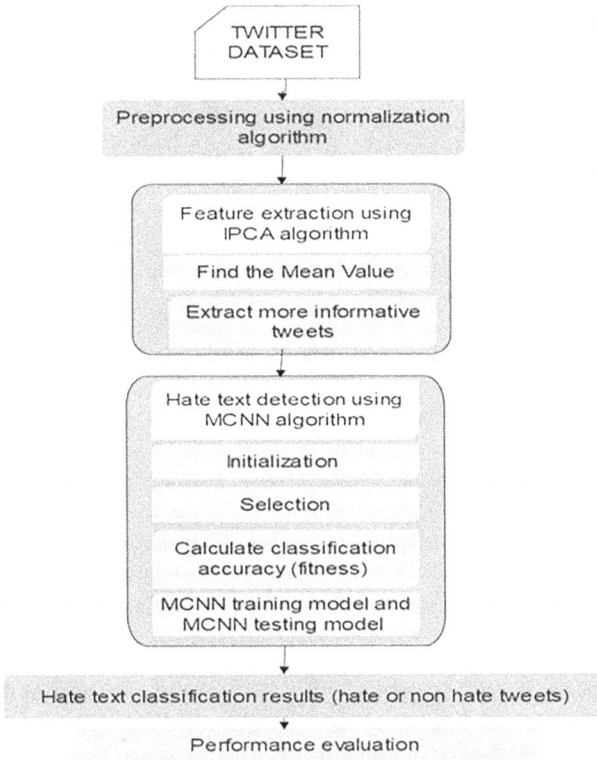

FIGURE 3.4 Workflow of the proposed methodology.

3.4 PERFORMANCE EVALUATION

The data for the study are taken from publicly available tweets [26]. The sample size had about 14500 tweets, which are classified into three classes (HATE, NONHATE, and NORMAL). The study revealed that 16% of the tweets have HATE text, 33% of NONHATE, and the remaining are NORMAL tweets. The performance of the proposed work is then compared with traditional methods such as SVM and RNN. Precision, recall, and F-measure were taken as performance measures.

3.4.1 PRECISION

It is the ratio of the total positive prediction of a model to total positive instances. It is normally used when the cost of FP is more. Precision is calculated as

$$Precision = TP/TP + FP \qquad (3.11)$$

3.4.2 RECALL

It is the ratio of true positive to that of the sum of true positive and true negative. It is largely used when the cost associated with FN is high

$$Recall = TP/TP + FN \tag{3.12}$$

3.4.3 F1 SCORE

It is a measure of accuracy and is represented as

$$F = \cfrac{1}{2\left(\frac{1}{RECALL}\right) + 1/Precision} \tag{3.13}$$

3.4.4 ACCURACY

It is the percentage of test tuples that are classified properly by any algorithm.

$$Accuracy = No \ of \ TP + no \ of \ TN/No \ of \ TP + FN + FP + TN$$

3.5 RESULTS AND DISCUSSION

The following table provides the comparative analysis of the performance of the proposed method IPCA+MCNN with that of the standard methods like SVM and RNN and Figure 3.5(a-d) shows the graphical representation of the same [27].

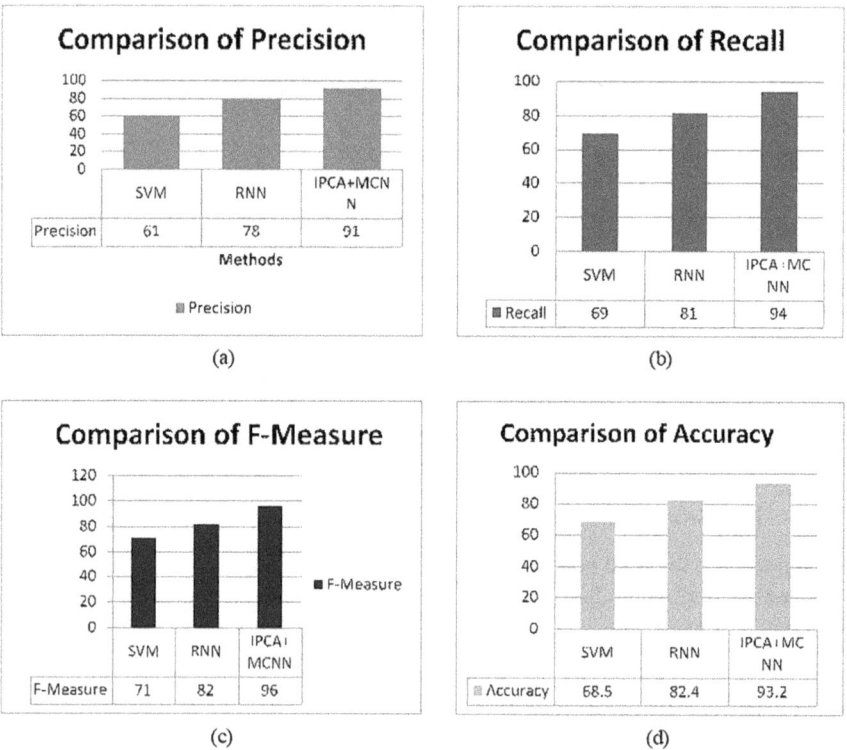

(a)

(b)

(c)

(d)

FIGURE 3.5 Comparison of (a) precision, (b) accuracy, (c) F-measure, and (d) recall.

TABLE 3.5
Comparison of IPCA-MCNN, SVM, and RNN

Methods	Precision	Recall	F-Measure	Accuracy
SVM	61	69	71	68.5
RNN	78	81	82	82.4
IPCA+MCNN	91	94	96	93.2

The experimental demonstration and benchmarking of the proposed work are given below for RNN [27], the merit of Tensorflow-Python 3, parameters and functions utilized, as well as the LSTM built-in layer. The final RNN model was made up of eight LSTM layers, each followed by a dropout in the range of 0.1–0.5. The batch size was 128, and each sequence had 120 data values. There are two dense layers: the first has an input size of 32 and an activation function, followed by a dropout of 0. The last dense layer features a softmax activation function and an input size of 2. The model is built with an Adam optimizer, which has a learning rate of 10–4 and a decay rate of 1e-6, and the loss function is sparse categorical cross-entropy. Each model was trained for a total of ten epochs [28].

The SVM was constructed in Python3 using Scikit-learn, and the data were pre-processed similarly to the RNN. Scikit-learn SVM is used to import the SVM.SVC technique, with parameter C set to 1, kernel set to "RBF," and gamma set to 0.1. The C parameter is an error term penalty parameter, and gamma defines how far the impact of a single training example is. The kernel argument specifies which kernel function should be used.

The RNN technique was evaluated using TensorFlow's evaluate function on each of the models with the highest validation accuracy. For the SVM, a similar technique was employed, in which the Scikit-learn predict method was applied with the test data for each fold, and the best prediction model was picked for evaluation with the test data. We next calculated the average prediction accuracy, recall and F-measure, maximum prediction accuracy, and minimum prediction accuracy using the prediction accuracies acquired from these two methods. A confusion matrix was used to evaluate both models further, displaying how the models forecast by providing data from each prediction compared to the true values (Table 3.5).

It is evident from the results that the proposed method IPCA+MCNN is better than the other standard methods such as SVM and RNN.

3.6   CONCLUSION

The proposed work is intended to classify the HATE TEXTs from the Twitter dataset. IPCA and MCNN are used for accurately classifying the text data. Pre-processing is done through normalization and traditional approaches such as pruning and stop word removal. Tokenization is done through the uni-gram model. The features are extracted using IPCA and then passed on to MCNN for classification. The significance of the proposed work is the introduction of IPCA, which is a mathematical function that maps the features with high dimension to a lower dimension using linear transformation. The MCNN helps to achieve maximum accuracy in classification. The experimental results have proven that the proposed method performs better than SVM and RNN. The future scope of the work includes the possibility of using fuzzy clustering or better optimization when large data are involved.

REFERENCES

1. S. Alami and O. Elbeqqali, "Cybercrime profiling: Text mining techniques to detect and predict criminal activities in microblog posts", In Proc. 10th Int. Conf. Intell. Syst., Theories Appl. (SITA), Oct. 2015, pp. 1–5.
2. Q. Huang, R. Chen, X. Zheng, and Z. Dong, "Deep sentiment representation based on CNN and LSTM", In Proc. Int. Conf. Green Informat., Aug. 2017, pp. 30–33.
3. J. Wang, L.-C. Yu, K. R. Lai, and X. Zhang, "Dimensional sentiment analysis using a regional CNN-LSTM model", In Proc. 54th Annu. Meeting Assoc. Comput. Linguistics, 2016, pp. 225–230.
4. R. Gobinath and M. Hemalatha, "An optimized k-harmonic mean based clustering user navigation patterns", In 2013 IEEE Int. Conf. Comput. Intell. Comput. Res., Enathi, India, 2013, pp. 1–4. 10.1109/ICCIC.2013.6724155.
5. S. Somasundaram and R. Gobinath, "A hybrid convolutional neural network and deep belief network for brain tumor detection in MR images", Int. J. Recent Technol. Eng. (IJRTE), 8 (2S4), 979–985, 2019.
6. W. Mengqiao, Y. Jie, C. Yilei, and W. Hao, "The multimodal brain tumor image segmentation based on convolutional neural networks", In 2017 2nd IEEE Int. Conf. Comput. Intell. Appl. (ICCIA), 2017, September, pp. 336–339. IEEE.
7. D. Sarkar, "Text analytics with python: A practical real-world approach to gaining actionable insights from your data," Apress Book copyright, 2016.
8. D. Kondor *et al.*, "Using robust PCA to estimate regional characteristics of language use from geo-tagged Twitter messages", In 2013 IEEE 4th Int. Conf. Cogn. Infocommun. (CogInfoCom), Budapest, Hungary, 2013, pp. 393–398. 10.1109/CogInfoCom.2013. 6719277.
9. E. J. Candès, X. Li, Y. Ma, and J. Wright, "Robust principal component analysis", JACM, 58 (3), 11, 2011.
10. E. Alothali, K. Hayawi, and H. Alashwal, "Hybrid feature selection approach to identify optimal features of profile metadata to detect social bots in Twitter", Soc. Netw. Anal. Min., 11, 84, 2021. 10.1007/s13278-021-00786-4.
11. E. Alothali, Z. Nazar, E. A. Mohamed, and A. Hany, "Detecting social bots on Twitter: A literature review", In 2018 Int. Conf. Innov. Inform. Technol. (IIT), IEEE, 2018, pp. 175–180. 10.1109/INNOVATIONS.2018.8605995.
12. C. Cai, L. Linjing, and Z. Daniel, "Behavior enhanced deep bot detection in social media", In 2017 IEEE Int. Conf. Intell. Secur. Inf. (ISI), IEEE, 2017, 128–130. 10. 1109/ISI.2017.8004887.
13. Z. Gilani, W. Liang, C. Jon, A. Mario, and F. Reza, "Stweeler: A framework for Twitter bot analysis", In Proc. 25th Int. Conf. Companion World Wide Web—WWW '16 Companion, New York, New York, USA, ACM Press, 2016, pp. 37–38. 10.1145/ 2872518.2889360.
14. N. Dugué, A. Perez, M. Danisch, F. Bridoux, A. Daviau, T. Kolubako, S. Munier, and H. Durbano, "A reliable and evolutive web application to detect social capitalists", In Proc. IEEE/ACM ASONAM, ACM, 2015, pp. 741–744.

15. C. Edwards, A. Edwards, P. R. Spence, and A. K. Shelton, "Is that a bot running the social media feed? Testing the differences in perceptions of communication quality for a human agent and a bot agent on Twitter", Comput. Human Behavior, 33, 372–376, 2014.
16. A. Hasan, S. Moin, A. Karim, and S. Shamshirband, "Machine learning-based sentiment analysis for Twitter accounts", Math. Comput. Appl., 23, 11, 2018. 10. 3390/mca23010011.
17. M. A. Razzaq, A. M. Qamar, and H. S. M. Bilal, "Prediction and analysis of Pakistan election 2013 based on sentiment analysis", In Proc. 2014 IEEE/ACM Int. Conf. Adv. Social Networks Anal. Mining (ASONAM 2014), Beijing, China, 17–20 August 2014, pp. 700–703.
18. R. Miranda Filho, J. M. Almeida, and G. L. Pappa, "Twitter population sample bias and its impact on predictive outcomes: A case study on elections", In Proc. 2015 IEEE/ACM Int. Conf. Adv. Social Netw. Anal. Mining (ASONAM), Paris, France, 25–28 August 2015, pp. 1254–1261.
19. A. Esuli and F. Sebastiani, Sentiwordnet: A High-Coverage Lexical Resource for Opinion Mining. Institute of Information Science and Technologies (ISTI) of the Italian National Research Council (CNR): Pisa, Italy, 2006.
20. M. Ibrahim, O. Abdillah, A. F. Wicaksono, and M. Adriani, "Buzzer detection and sentiment analysis for predicting presidential election results in a Twitter nation", In Proc. 2015 IEEE Int. Conf. Data Mining Workshop (ICDMW), Atlantic City, NJ, USA, 14–17 November 2015, pp. 1348–1353.
21. R. Rezapour, L. Wang, O. Abdar, and J. Diesner, "Identifying the overlap between election result and candidates' ranking based on hashtag-enhanced, lexicon-based sentiment analysis", In Proc. 2017 IEEE 11th Int. Conf. Semantic Comput. (ICSC), San Diego, CA, USA, 30 January–1 February 2017, pp. 93–96.
22. F. H. Khan, S. Bashir, and U. Qamar, "Tom: Twitter opinion mining framework using a hybrid classification scheme", Decis. Support Syst., 57, 245–257, 2014.
23. S. Neelakandan, M. Sridevi, S. Chandrasekaran, K. Murugeswari, A. Kumar Singh Pundir, R. Sridevi, and T. Bheema Lingaiah, "Deep learning approaches for cyberbullying detection and classification on social media", Comput. Intell. Neurosci., 2022, Article ID 2163458, 13 pages, 2022. 10.1155/2022/2163458.
24. K. Maheswari and S. Ramkumar, "Analysis of error rate for various attributes to obtain the optimal decision tree", Int. J. Intell. Enterprise, 9(4), 458–472, Oct. 2022. 10.1504/IJIE.2022.10048744.
25. K. Maheswari, P. Packia Amutha Priya, S. Ramkumar, and M. Arun, "Missing data handling by mean imputation method and statistical analysis of classification algorithm", In EAI Int. Conf. Big Data Innov. Sustainable Cogn. Comput., 2020, pp. 137–149, Springer Innovations in Communications and Computing Book Series, 1st Edition, ISBN: 978-3-030-19562-5_14. 10.1007/978-3-030-19562-5.
26. E. Agirre and P. Edmonds. Word Sense Disambiguation: Algorithms and Applications. Springer Science & Business Media: Berlin, Germany, 2007; Volume 33.
27. M. Khan, S. Hariharasitaraman, S. Joshi, V. Jain, M. Ramanan, A. Sampathkumar, and E. Ahmed, "A deep learning approach for facial emotion recognition using principal component analysis and neural network techniques", Photogrammetric Record, 37, 435–452, 2022. 10.1111/phor.12426.
28. S. Franzén, A. K. Kozlov, and Ö. Ekeberg. A Comparative Analysis of RNN and SVM, 2019.

4 Medical Image Analysis Based on Deep Learning Approach for Early Diagnosis of Diseases

S. Balasubramaniam

School of Computer Science and Engineering, Kerala University of Digital Sciences, Innovation and Technology (Digital University of Kerala), Thiruvananthapuram, Kerala, India

A. Prasanth

Department of ECE, Sri Venkateswara College of Engineering, Sriperumbudur, Tamil Nadu, India

K. Satheesh Kumar

School of Computer Science and Engineering, Kerala University of Digital Sciences, Innovation and Technology (Digital University of Kerala), Thiruvananthapuram, Kerala, India

Kavitha V.

Department of CSE, University College of Engineering, Kanchipuram, Tamil Nadu, India

4.1 INTRODUCTION

Medical imaging has become a major field of study since Roentgen's 1895 discovery of X-ray radiation. Medical image analysis uses clinical images to solve clinical problems. The goal is to efficiently extract information for better clinical diagnosis. Diagnostic imaging techniques such as computed tomography, magnetic resonance imaging, positron emission tomography, ultrasound, mammography, and X-ray techniques that have been developed and implemented during recent years for the purpose of illness detection, diagnosis, and treatment [1]. In order to make use of this ever-increasing data, to study it, and to show it in a way that is suitable for the medical mission, medical image processing is required. Medical image processing's main goal is to improve content interpretation, unlike general image processing, which can enhance a picture's aesthetics or create art. The image may be enhanced to highlight certain elements, and information may be extracted

DOI: 10.1201/9781003469605-4

manually or automatically. Medical imaging has traditionally been interpreted by radiologists and doctors at hospitals and clinics. Due to pathologic variations and human expert fatigue, however, researchers and doctors are starting to reap the rewards of using computer-assisted therapy. With the emergence of artificial intelligence (AI) approaches, computational medical image processing is catching up to medical imaging technology [2].

Medical image analysis is a key research and development topic due to biomedical engineering breakthroughs. Medical image analysis using machine learning (ML) is one cause for this improvement. Medical image analysis utilizing ML relies heavily on the identification and acquisition of features that faithfully represent recurring structures or patterns within the data being analyzed. Due to the fact that historically, relevant or task-related features were generated mostly by human specialists based on their understanding of the target domains, it has been difficult for non-experts to utilize ML techniques for their own study [3]. A neural network can automatically learn features using deep learning for ML, unlike approaches that use hand-crafted characteristics. These qualities are difficult to choose and calculate. Deep convolutional networks are utilized for medical picture analysis. Applications include segmentation, anomaly detection, disease classification, computer-aided diagnosis, and retrieval. Large amounts of data, high-performance CPUs and GPUs, and learning algorithms have contributed to deep learning's remarkable success. It is possible to generate higher-level features from lower-level features by using the hierarchical feature representations discovered by deep neural networks. Deep learning is made possible by learning hierarchical feature representations from data to achieve its unprecedented success in AI applications and major problems. Segmentation, registration, fusion, annotation, examination of microscope images for purposes of diagnosis (by computer-aided diagnosis), prediction (via prognosis); detection of lesions and landmarks (via lesion detection and landmark detection); are all examples of how deep learning is put to work in the medical imaging industry [4].

Medical image analysis helps radiologists and physicians improve diagnosis and therapy. Medical image analysis is essential for computer-aided detection (CADx) and diagnosis (CAD), which directly affect clinical diagnosis and therapy. Medical imaging provides body images. Medical imaging helps radiologists and doctors improve diagnosis and therapy. Medical imaging is essential to disease diagnosis and treatment. These include X-ray, CT, MRI, PET, ultrasound, and hybrid modalities. These methods help diagnose and research organ anatomy and function.

Figure 4.1 shows a typology of radiology and laboratory-generated medical imaging modalities for various body sections.

Modern healthcare requires medical imaging. CADx relies on ML for tumor segmentation, cancer diagnosis, classification, image guided therapy, medical picture annotation, and retrieval.

Image analysis methods include the following:

Image enhancement: Removing noise, background inhomogeneities, and other distortions and enhancing contours and other features.
Image segmentation: Identifying the shape of a body part, such as an organ.

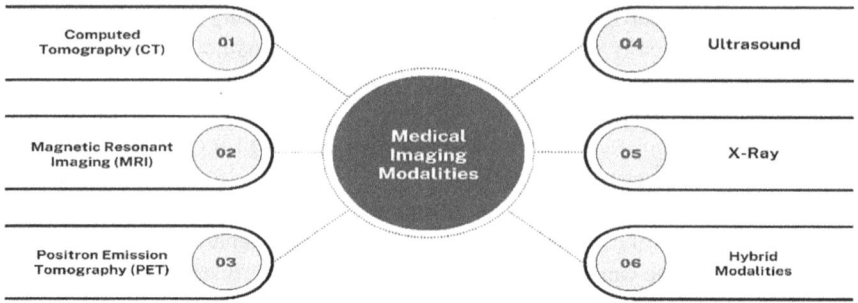

FIGURE 4.1   Medical imaging modalities.

Acquiring a registration of images: Modifying an image to match a reference image spatially. For PET/CT imaging, this is necessary.

Quantification: The measurement of geometrical features like dimensions including length, width, and angularity, as well as physiological characteristics like blood flow and tissue make-up of anatomical structures.

Ideation: Rendering of picture data in several dimensions (including volume rendering) and virtual models of internal organs and other anatomical aspects (e.g., surface models).

Detection: Finding characterization of diseased features like tumors and vascular blockages.

Figure 4.2 shows the different medical imaging applications.

Recent advances in deep learning algorithms for image recognition coincide with a surge in electronic medical records and diagnostic imaging. Medical image analysis

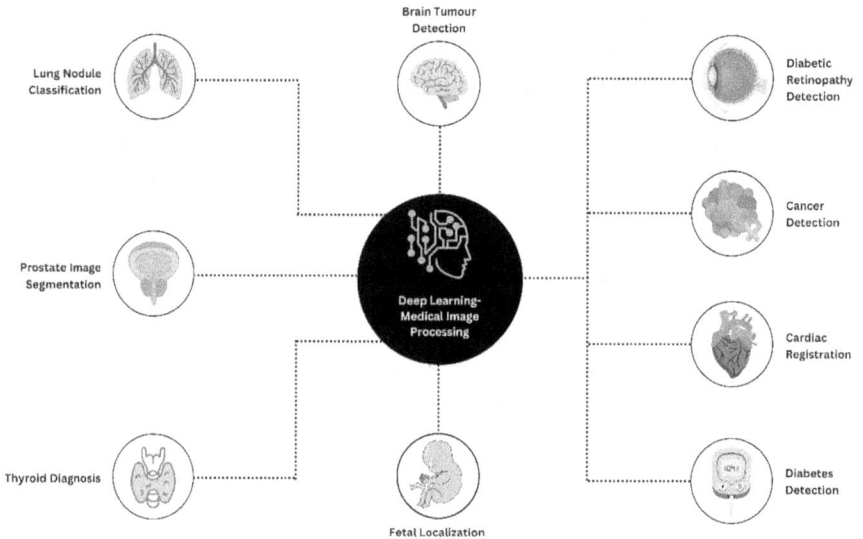

FIGURE 4.2   Medical imaging applications.

has relied on ML and AI-powered systems for decision making from its inception. These methods include low-level processing of pixels, engineering of features, and supervised learning of classifiers, and convolutional neural networks (CNN)-based feature learning. Deep learning-based image-based diagnosis, disease prognosis, and risk assessment are improving. With the rapid rise of AI, especially deep learning, sophisticated deep learning-based algorithms for medical image analysis have become a hot topic in academia and industry. Thus, intelligent healthcare helps clinicians use medical big data [5].

4.2   MEDICAL IMAGE ANALYSIS

Medical image analysis is the process of using a database of 3D images of a patient's body (often from a CT or MRI scanner) to make diagnoses, plan treatments (like surgery), or conduct research. Radiologists, engineers, and physicians process medical images to comprehend patient anatomy. Medical image processing offers non-invasive interior anatomy study. Multi-dimensional models of needed organs can be constructed then researched for improving patient care, medical device and drug delivery systems, and diagnosis. It has become a major medical progress instrument [6].

4.2.1   CORE AREAS OF MEDICAL IMAGE ANALYSIS

Figure 4.3 shows some principles and ways for organizing medical image processing. These areas influence image formation, computing, and management.

Medical image analysis steps are structurally classified in Figure 4.4.

Image generation solves a mathematical inverse problem through data capture and reconstruction. Picture computing enhances image interpretation and extracts

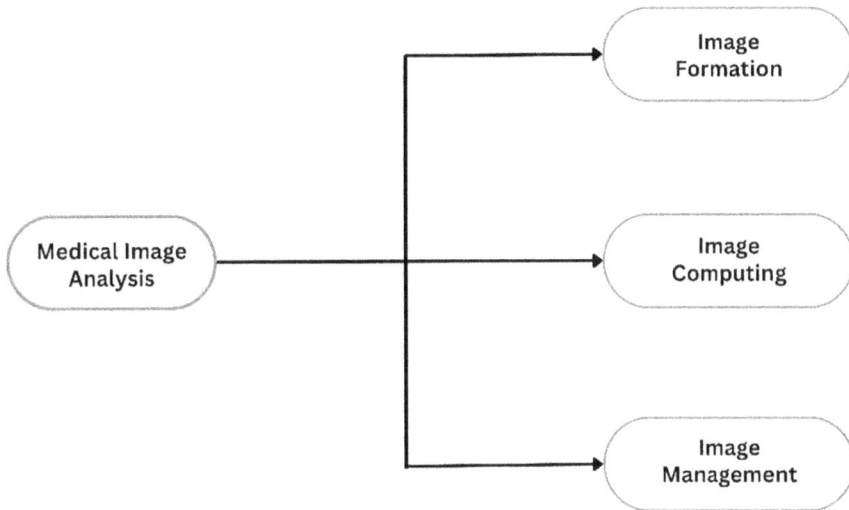

FIGURE 4.3   Major process in medical image analysis.

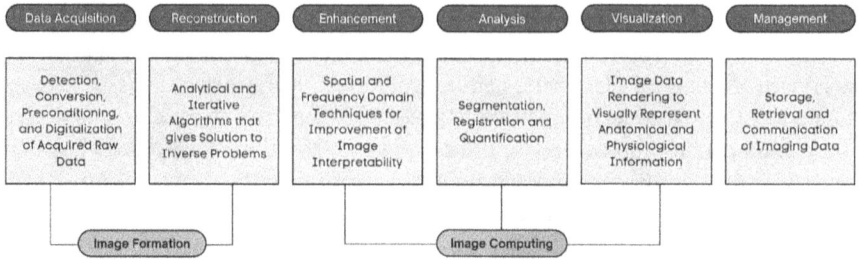

FIGURE 4.4 Structural classification of steps in medical image analysis.

therapeutically useful data. Image management compresses, archives, retrieves, and shares captured images and generated data.

4.2.1.1   Image Formation

Data acquisition and picture reconstruction solve a mathematical inverse issue in image generation.

4.2.1.1.1   Data Acquisition

Image data capture contains the original data on body interior physical quantities. Using this data, further image processing steps can be tailored to their specific needs. Different imaging modalities may be able to detect distinct physical quantities according to distinct physical principles. Ultrasonography uses the acoustic echoes, while magnetic resonance imaging uses the characteristics of a radio-frequency signal created by excited atoms. The incident photon energy that is utilized in digital radiography (DR) and computed tomography (CT). Regardless of imaging method, data acquisition involves detection, conversion into an electrical signal, preconditioning, and digitization of a physical quantity.

4.2.1.1.2   Image Reconstruction

Mathematical image reconstruction is the process of making a picture from scratch. This technique also combines several data sets from different viewpoints or time steps for multidimensional imaging. Medical image processing's core topic is inverse issues. Analytical and iterative strategies are utilized to solve these difficulties. Analytical approaches utilized in tomography, MRI, and ultrasonography include filtered back projection (FBP), Fourier transform (FT), and delay and sum (DAS) beamforming. Elegant and computationally efficient, these methods are based on idealized models and cannot handle complex elements like measurement noise, statistical characteristics, and imaging system physics. Iterative methods overcome those limits to increase noise insensitivity and recreate an ideal image from incomplete raw data. Based on the original object model with expected coefficients, iterative approaches construct projections using a system and statistical noise model. When there is a disparity between the predicted future and the actual data, new coefficients are required to be added to the object model. Iterations of this process are taken until the minimum cost function is found between the estimated and actual values, causing the reconstruction process to converge to the final image.

4.2.1.2   Image Computing

Picture computing enhances image interpretation and extracts therapeutically useful data. Image computing extracts therapeutically relevant information from reconstructed imaging data using computer and mathematical methodologies. These methods improve imaging, analysis, and visualization [7].

4.2.1.2.1   Enhancement

Image augmentation improves information interpretation by refining transform representations. It uses frequency- and spatial-domain approaches. Spatial domain approaches optimize contrast by directly manipulating image pixels. The logarithmic, histogram, and power law transformations are utilized by these techniques. Using filters, images can be refined and smoothed using a frequency domain method. These techniques reduce noise and inhomogeneity, optimize contrast, enhance edges, eliminate artefacts, and improve other important features for image analysis and interpretation.

4.2.1.2.2   Analysis

Image segmentation, registration, and quantification are the major approaches used in image analysis, which is the core of image computing. Image segmentation divides the image into anatomical structures. Image registration is crucial for analyzing temporal changes or images from distinct modalities. Quantification establishes structure attributes like volume, diameter, content, and anatomical or physiological information. All of these processes affect image inspection quality and medical results.

4.2.1.2.3   Visualization

Anatomical and physiological imaging data can be displayed visually in predetermined dimensions via visualization. Visualization can help with segmentation, registration, and result display at both the beginning and end of imaging analysis.

4.2.1.3   Image Management

In the end, data storage, retrieval, and transmission are the remaining steps in medical image processing. There are a number of methods and protocols for managing images. Storage and transmission of medical pictures are supported by both the picture archiving and communication system (PACS) and the digital imaging and communication in medicine (DICOM) standard, both of which are products of medical imaging technology, while PACS also provides inexpensive access to images from several modalities. These processes are sped up by image compression and streaming technologies.

4.2.2   Major Challenges in Health Picture Analysis

Accuracy of visual information and the amount of information included within it has been vastly enhanced by recent improvements in hardware. Reduced scanning times, improved image quality, and hybrid ultrasound–mammography–computed tomography–magnetic resonance imaging (CT–MRI) systems are all benefits of

Data Fusion	CADe/CADX	Data-Driven Image Analysis	AI	Cloud Computing
Multimodal, Multiplane, and other Multifunctional and Multidimensional Data Fusion Techniques that Provide More Complete Information.	Computer-Aided Detection (CADe) and Computer-Aided Diagnosis (CADx) to Support the Interpretation of Medical Images to Achieve More Reliable and Accurate Diagnostic Results.	Model-Based Image Analysis and Machine Learning Methods Leveraging Training Data to Identify Patterns for Interpreting New Imaging Results.	Artificial Intelligence (AI) Technique for Workflow and Capacity Management.	Migration from PACS to Cloud-Based Radiological Information System (RIS) for Intelligent Management of Big Data.

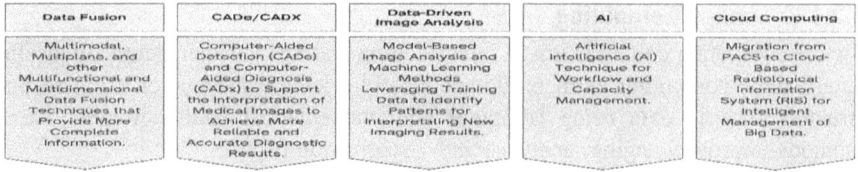

FIGURE 4.5 Major trends in medical image analysis.

integrated front-end solutions. Nowadays, it's more common to use fast iterative algorithms to rebuild images rather than analytic methods. They boost PET image quality, reduce CT X-ray dose, and compress MRI sensing. Data-driven signal models solve inverse problems better than human-defined models. Computational technologies must improve as imaging technology gathers more data and algorithms get more complicated. A wider range of research-to-application choices is now possible because of more powerful graphics processors and multiprocessing approaches. Figure 4.5 shows some of the significant trends and problems of this image computing and image management revolution. Data fusion, computer-aided detection, diagnosis, data drive image analysis, AI, and cloud computing are examples [8].

4.3 ARTIFICIAL INTELLIGENCE

The subject of AI in health is rapidly expanding, inspiring optimism, and posing puzzling questions. The ability of a machine to simulate human cognitive capacities is known as AI. AI is a broad category of approaches. One of these that is particularly pertinent to the medical industry is ML. The emergence of "big data," or the creation and analysis of very large databases, along with the phenomenal expansion in processor computing power and new deep learning techniques, have helped medical ML applications succeed. These technical developments made it possible for algorithms to process images and sounds, and to be included into both automated professional workflows and the digital tools we use every day. The volume, complexity, and variability of raw data in the medical profession are all currently growing dramatically. Big data analysis that is efficient and medically relevant is a significant problem for public health. In this area, AI offers three bright perspectives: automating medical image analysis; risk prediction using correlation analyses; and genomic analysis and phenotype-genotype association research. There is a branch of AI known as ML that allows computers to acquire new skills without being hand-coded with instructions. In order to analyze data patterns and enable machines to respond to various scenarios, ML employs sophisticated algorithms that repeatedly iterate through enormous data sets. In ML, you'll find that there are three primary subfields: supervised learning, unsupervised learning, and reinforcement learning [9].

4.3.1 SUPERVISED LEARNING

The group of systems and procedures called supervised learning develop predictive models utilizing data points with predetermined outputs. The model is developed through training using a suitable learning method (e.g., neural networks, linear

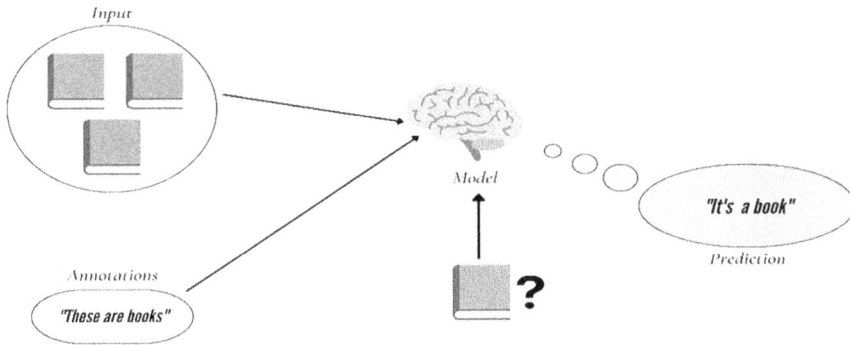

FIGURE 4.6 System for supervised machine learning.

regression, or random forests), which often employs some sort of optimization procedure to reduce a loss or error function. The usual supervised ML configuration is shown in Figure 4.6. Classification and regression are two major types of supervised learning.

4.3.1.1 Classification

Algorithms classify test data into categories. They identify entities in the collection to determine their labels and descriptions. Linear classifiers, SVM, decision trees, k-nearest neighbor, random forest, and others are classification methods.

4.3.1.2 Regression

Regression analysis dependent-independent relationships. It's often used for sales revenue forecasts. Regression methods predict continuous values. Regression can forecast housing values depending on size, cost, etc.

4.3.2 UNSUPERVISED LEARNING

Unsupervised ML uses no training dataset. Instead, models uncover data patterns and insights. Learning new things in the brain is similar [10]. Figure 4.7 illustrates typical unsupervised ML setup. Clustering and association include unsupervised learning.

4.3.2.1 Clustering

To analyze and manipulate unlabeled data, it involves finding similar structures. Without input-output mapping, the computer learns properties and trends in clustering. Clustering uses unsupervised ML because the samples are unlabeled. Clustering becomes classification when instances are labeled. Density-based, distribution-based, centroid-based, hierarchical-based, K-means, DBSCAN, and Gaussian mixture model methods are clustering techniques.

4.3.2.2 Association

Finding rules that explain significant portions of your data, such as customers of X also purchasing Y, are examples of the kind of problems that can be solved by

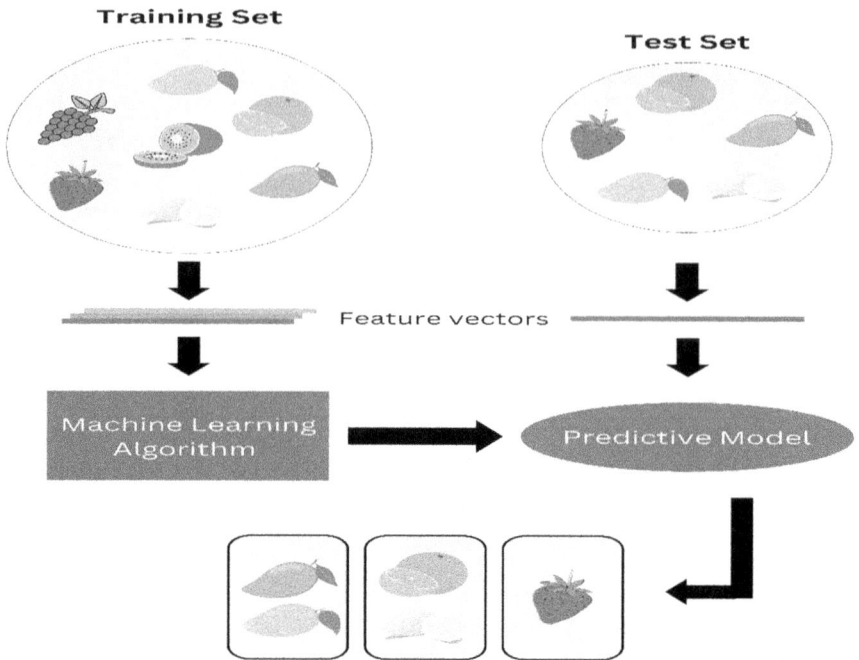

FIGURE 4.7   Unsupervised machine learning setup.

applying association rule learning techniques. Large companies utilize market-based analysis to demonstrate product relationships.

4.3.3   REINFORCEMENT LEARNING

Reinforcement learning trains a model to find the best solution by making a series of decisions. Model a problem environment here. Without human input, the model solves problems in this environment. We simply reward it for actions that move it toward its goal or punish it for actions that move it away. Figure 4.8 illustrates reinforcement learning.

Table 4.1 shows the distinguishing factors of supervised, unsupervised, and reinforcement learning.

4.3.4   NEURAL NETWORKS

Neural networks refers to a network of artificial neurons or nodes modeled after animal brains. Much of modern AI is based on it. We present important basics to help comprehend neural networks, repeat successful medical imaging neural networks, and motivate further neural network development. Beginning with a theoretical model of a single neuron, we proceed to explain several types of neural networks and describe their architectures, learning algorithms, operational principles, and practical applications [11].

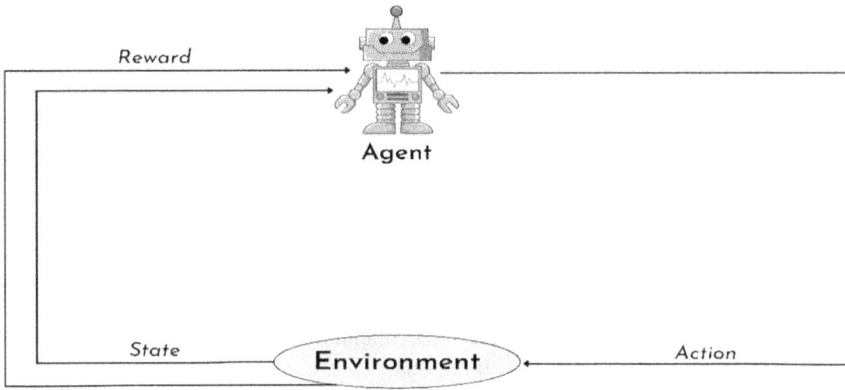

FIGURE 4.8 Reinforcement learning setup.

TABLE 4.1
Difference between Supervised, Unsupervised and Reinforcement Learning

Supervised Learning	Unsupervised Learning	Reinforcement Learning
Data provided with specified target values.	The data provided is unlabeled data, the output values are not specified, machine makes its own prediction	The machine learns from its environment using rewards and errors
Used to solve continuous values and category-based issues	Used to solve concordance and grouping issues	Used to solve reward-based issues
The information is categorized	The information is not categorized	There is no use of fixed parameters.
Outside authority monitoring	No outside authority for monitoring	No outside authority for monitoring
Converts labeled input to a known output in order to solve problems.	Solves problem by understanding patterns and discovering outputs	Follows trial and error problem solving approach

4.3.4.1 Basic Structure

Figure 4.9 is a theoretical representation of a neuron's fundamental structure, in which X (x_i, $i = 1, 2, \ldots, n$) are inputs and Y are outputs. The activation function f has given to the sum of each input's weight w_i and the bias b associated with each neuron. Therefore, the following Equation (4.1) can be used to express the connection between input and output:

$$y = f\left(\sum_{i=1}^{n} w_i x_i + b \right) \qquad (4.1)$$

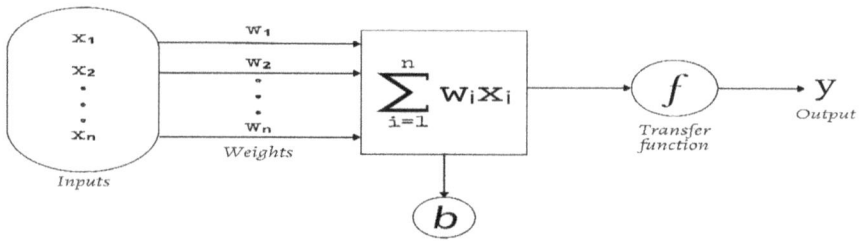

FIGURE 4.9 The model of a neuron.

Up until this point, researchers have experimented with the step, sigmoid, tanh, ReLU, and leaky ReLU activation functions.

Three types of neural networks—feedforward, feedback, and self-organizing—have been developed to tackle this problem. When it comes to training neural networks, medical image processing often employs one of two methods: supervised learning or unsupervised learning. Networks are trained with inputs and outputs in supervised learning (targets). There will be a set of input values and one or more output values for each training case; by iteratively adjusting weights and biases between the neurons, we may reduce the average output error across all training examples. One subfield of ML is unsupervised learning, in which the identifying labels or labels themselves are absent from the training data. Instead, we focus on defining a function that assesses the network's fitness or precision. This function, also known as a cost function, often employs input values and the value(s) produced by the network to calculate a price for the current setup; its form and implementation are application-specific. By definition, in unsupervised learning, input vectors for the training set will be optimized so that their total cost is either minimized or maximized.

4.3.4.2 Feed-Forward Network

The feed-forward network is the most popular neural network topology used in medical imaging applications. The layers of these models typically include an input layer, a concealing layer or layers, and an output layer. A feed-forward network is one in which neurons in each layer can only communicate with their immediate superiors. Due to the one-way nature of these connections, the signals or data being processed can only travel from the input layer to the hidden layer(s) and then to the output layer. Figure 4.10 depicts the conventional layout of a feed-forward system.

When training feed-forward networks, the weight and bias values of individual neurons are often updated in real time using a supervised learning process called backpropagation. In order to close the gap between the network's actual and desired output values, the method iteratively modifies the connection weight values of neurons.

When it comes to feed-forward networks, multilayer perceptrons (MLPs) are a subtype that employs many layers and has nonlinear neurotransmission of its buried levels. MLPs can correlate training patterns with outputs even when the data are not linearly separable. Medical imaging lends itself nicely to feed-forward networks due to the fact that both inputs and outputs are numbers, and because pairs of input/output vectors provide a concrete foundation for supervised learning.

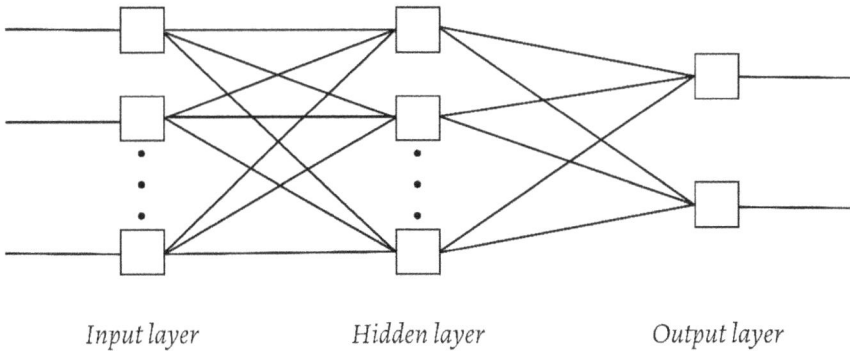

Input layer   *Hidden layer*   *Output layer*

FIGURE 4.10   Neural network with feedback loop.

4.3.4.3   Feed-Back Network

By looping back through the network, values from the hidden and output layers are supplied back into the network at earlier stages in a feed-back (or recurrent) neural network, permitting two-way exchange of information. They are in a constant process of transition toward a new, stable state. Before the input is altered and a new equilibrium is established, they tend to stay put at the equilibrium point. They have great processing potential, but they can also become very intricate.

4.4   DL-BASED ARCHITECTURES FOR ANALYZING HEALTH IMAGES

To those in the know, "deep learning" is the branch of ML in which a complex, multi-layered neural network is used to solve problems and acquire knowledge from massive datasets. By repeatedly analyzing data with a predetermined framework, deep learning algorithms aim to arrive at the same conclusions as people would. Deep learning accomplishes this by employing complex algorithmic structures known as neural networks. Classification, regressing, clustering, re-creating images with less artefacts, detecting and removing lesions, and segmenting are just some of the many tasks that deep learning is designed to accomplish. In deep learning, many linear and non-linear processing units are combined in a deep architecture to model high-level abstraction contained in the data. Many deep learning methods are already in use, and they can be put to use in large settings. Deep learning models can be broken down into two categories: those that rely on human input for training data, and those that do not.

4.4.1   Deep Learning Models with Supervision

4.4.1.1   Convolutional Neural Networks (CNN)

When it comes to ML techniques for analyzing medical images, CNNs have received the most attention. This is due to the fact that, unlike other image filtering methods, CNNs are able to maintain important spatial relationships between pixels. The spatial relationships between anatomical structures are vital in radiography, whether it be the transition from bone to muscle at a bone's border or the transition

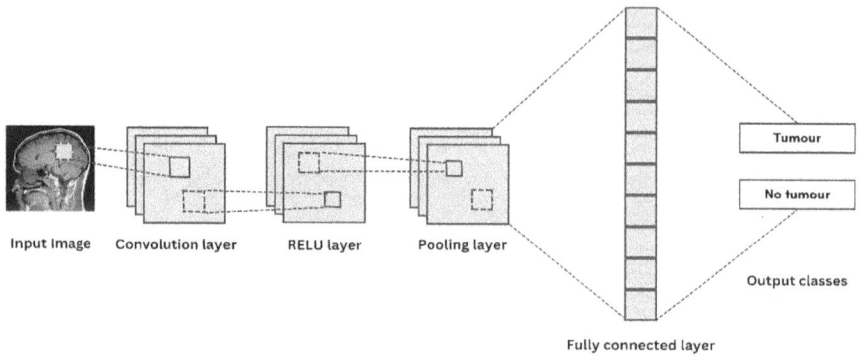

FIGURE 4.11   A schematic depiction of CNN.

from normal to malignant lung tissue at the lung's periphery. Layers of rectified linear units (RELUs), pooling, and convolutions are all employed in deep neural networks by CNN to convert a raw pixel image into a more useful representation, as shown in Figure 4.11. To determine which class an input most closely fits into, as soon as the information is collected, it is transferred to a fully connected layer where class scores or probabilities are assigned.

4.4.1.2   Recurrent Neural Networks (RNN)

Traditional uses of RNNs have involved the analysis of sequential data. RNNs are useful for text analysis because of their ability to generate text, which has led to their application in areas as varied as automated linguistic processing, linguistic modeling, text prediction, and image caption synthesis. Simple RNN contextual "memory" is achieved by adding each layer's output to the next input and then feeding that information back into the layer. LSTM networks and gated recurrent units (GRUs) have evolved from standard RNNs to circumvent issues of temporal backpropagation with vanishing gradients. These are improvements on RNNs, which allow them to retain knowledge about long-term dependencies while selectively forgetting other information. Historically, RNNs have been employed mostly for segmentation in analysis of medical pictures as a topic of study.

4.4.1.3   Transfer Learning with CNNs

To get around the problem of not having enough training data, researchers came up with a technique called transfer learning, in which an algorithm learned using a dataset that is very loosely connected to the original dataset and a labeled training dataset. The basic idea is to use the training's emphasis on a set of weights of a CNN to another (perhaps unrelated) dataset to train a second CNN on labeled medical data. Only the final fully connected layer of the CNN is off-limits for weight adjustments. While CNNs are often employed in analysis of medical pictures, transfer learning techniques can be implemented with any standard ML methodology. In general, unlike when beginning with a blank slate to train a CNN, the results were better when more layers were transferred over from another CNN. Contrasted with other computer vision tasks, medical picture processing requires careful calibration of numerous layers.

4.4.2 Unsupervised Deep Learning Models

4.4.2.1 Autoencoders

Autoencoders are able to learn unsupervised interpretations of the data inputs as features without requiring labeled data. So, in essence, it's a model that takes in unstructured input, processes it to derive meaningful codes, and then applies those codes to the reconstruction of new data. The premise behind autoencoders is that the encoded output should closely resemble the input data; hence, autoencoder models typically incorporate a cost function that penalizes the model when the two do not match. Autoencoders are helpful due to their many built-in advantages. First, they are used as feature detectors that can pick up encodings on their own, without being given any labels to follow. Furthermore, because codings typically exist in a lower dimension, they simplify and reduce the dimensionality of the model. Third, the output of an autoencoder is information highly like original information because they must reconstruct outputs. These characteristics are especially helpful in the challenging area of analyzing health images, where labeled data is in short supply. Figure 4.12 illustrates several examples of network architectures.

Autoencoders are distinguished from other neural network architectures by the need for a similar number of neurons to be used in the input and output layers.

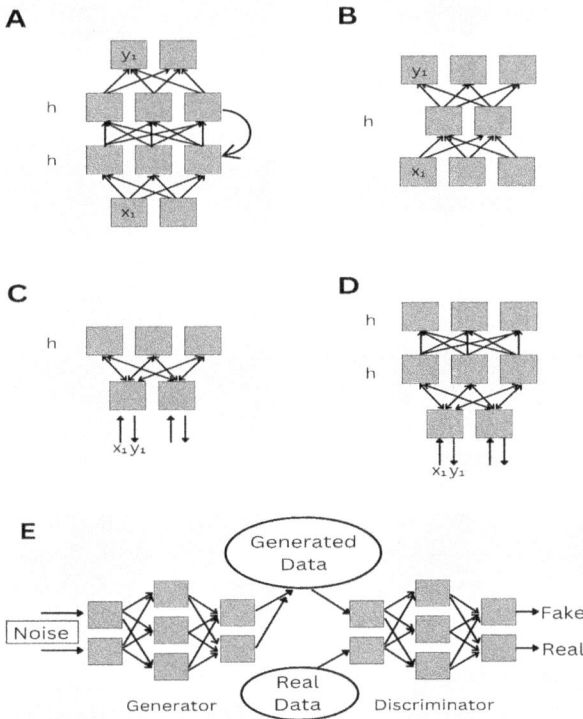

FIGURE 4.12 A) RNN, B) autoencoder, C) restricted Boltzmann machine, D) deep belief network, E) generative adversarial network.

Autoencoders, like CNNs, use underlying depths that can be layered to improve performance. There is often a path of contemplation across a concealed layer in a stacked autoencoder's (SAE) middle layer, making the architecture symmetrical. Techniques such as transfer learning, training multiple autoencoder subsets independently, and layer-by-layer weight tying can be used to improve an autoencoder's performance.

Constraints are necessary to coax models into learning relevant representations. The denoising autoencoder is an example of a method that employs hidden layers of Gaussian noise to improve accuracy. The similar result can be achieved by using a technique called dropout, which involves arbitrarily by silencing some of the brain's earliest buried layers of neurons. It compels the model to pick up efficient codings to reproduce the clean inputs at the output layer. Second, sparse autoencoders are another type of encoding method in which a certain number of neurons in the deeper levels are intentionally disabled. To prevent the model from becoming overly dependent on a small number of activated neurons, you can implement a cost function that penalizes the model when the number of activated neurons reaches a certain value. An increasingly popular and cutting-edge unsupervised learning architecture is the variational autoencoder (VAE). Stochastic gradient descent can be used to train VAEs, which consist of a Bayesian inference encoder network and a decoder network to form a generative model. The encoder network uses a Gaussian distribution to approximate the distribution of latent space variables onto which input data is projected.

4.4.2.2 Restricted Boltzmann Machines

Open and hidden layers make up restricted Boltzmann machines (RBMs), Those are bidirectional graphical models that generate stochastically and probabilistically; they are based on the original Boltzmann machine, which was invented in 1985. These layers have external connections but no internal communication. RBMs employ the backward pass of input data to reconstruct and estimate the probability distribution of the original input.

4.4.2.3 Deep Belief Networks (DBNs)

In deep belief networks (DBNs), one RBM's hidden layer output feeds into the next RBM's output layer input, allowing for fast training with contrast-divergence algorithms. This newfound interest in deep learning can be attributed in large part to DBNs. It was possible to train DBNs greedily, incrementally, with lower layers responsible for learning fundamental characteristics and higher layers for more complex ones, simulating the natural hierarchy of data in the actual world. As an alternative, a semi-supervised deep learning architecture can be created by coupling DBNs with layers of supervised RBMs.

4.4.2.4 Generative Adversarial Networks (GANs)

Unsupervised learning techniques like generative adversarial networks (GANs) show potential for applications like medical image analysis. GAN is a type of generative model, not unlike a VAE. GANs are made up of two competing models that are trained at the same time. These models can be multilayer perceptrons like

CNNs, or they can be completely different types of models. The models can be viewed as adversaries in a contest with no winners. In the context of convolutional neural networks, a generator is something that creates fake training images. The second CNN is a discriminator, and it determines whether or not a picture is part of the training set or was generated by the generator. The ideal outcome of this adversarial setup would be for the discriminator to be unable to distinguish between a real and a produced image.

4.5   DEEP LEARNING-BASED MEDICAL IMAGE ANALYSIS TECHNIQUES

Deep learning outperforms traditional ML. Since then, computational medical imaging researchers have investigated how deep learning can be applied to CT, MRI, PET, and X-ray pictures. Deep learning is applied to image registration and localization, object recognition, organ segmentation, and computer-assisted disease prognosis and diagnosis.

4.5.1   DEEP LEARNING FOR IMAGE REGISTRATION

Common in the area of image analysis, health pictures registration involves calculating coordinate transform between two medical pictures in order to bring them into better spatial alignment with one another. This type of optimization is usually done iteratively using a specific (non-)parametric transformation and a fixed measure like the L2-norm. Despite the fact that deep learning is typically applied to more prominent issues like segmentation and lesion identification. The best registration performance has been attained using deep networks, according to the research. Most of the recent research has focused on one of two approaches: Deep learning networks can directly forecast transformation parameters or determine a similarity measure between two images to drive an iterative optimization technique [12].

4.5.2   DEEP LEARNING FOR IMAGE LOCALIZATION

Pre-processing segmentation activities or clinical workflows for therapy planning and intervention include positioning anatomical items like organs or landmarks in space or time. Medical imaging localization frequently involves the segmentation of 3D volumes. Several approaches have been proposed that use deep learning algorithms to parse 3D data, but they always boil the space down to a series of 2D orthogonal planes. Using convolutional neural networks to classify 2D images looks to be the most popular approach for localizing organs, regions, and landmarks. Newer publications, however, build on this idea by adapting the learning process to place a greater emphasis on precise localization, and they show promise. They prove that deep learning strategies can be modified for use in numerous localization applications. We anticipate that such approaches will be researched further (e.g., multiple landmarks) [13].

4.5.3 Deep Learning for Detection of Objects

Among the many labor-intensive aspects of diagnosis, object/lesion recognition in images is crucial. In most cases, the tasks include finding and labeling tiny lesions throughout a full image. There is a long history of research into automated lesion detecting systems, typically with the dual goals of improving output and reading faster. The radiology workflow relies heavily on the localization and interpolation of anatomical components in medical pictures. To fulfill these goals, radiologists typically look for "anatomical signatures," or features in images that uniquely identify a given anatomical structure. Can these anatomical signatures be automatically learned by a computer? How many anatomical signatures can be recovered by computational procedures is crucial to the success of such approaches. Instead of using custom image filters to isolate anatomical signatures, as was common in earlier research, deep learning-based approaches have emerged as the norm for 2 factors: (a) DL-based methods have advanced to the point where they can be applied to worldly concerns, and (b) a growing number of medical image data sets are now accessible, paving the way for researchers to delve into massive medical picture databases [14].

4.5.4 Deep Learning for Organ Segmentation

In heart or brain analysis, medical pictures can be segmented to quantify clinical factors like volume and form. Segmentation is described as the process of selecting the group of voxels that compose the object's boundary or its interior. Since applying DL to health imaging typically focuses on segmentation, there has been the greatest experimentation with different approaches, such as the creation of novel architectures for segmentation based on CNNs and the widespread use of RNNs. When it comes to medical image analysis, the alternative CNN architecture known as UNet is the most well-known of the bunch. The equal number of up sampling and downsampling layers is one of U-most net's innovative architectural features. UNet mixes adversarial convolution and deconvolution layers with learned up sampling layers using so-called skip connections. This joins together characteristics of both the narrowing and widening routes. From a training standpoint, this means that UNet can analyze full images/scans in a single forward pass, yielding a segmentation map immediately. As a result, unlike patch-based CNNs, UNet can benefit from considering the entire image. Due to the proliferation of RNNs, mechanism of timekeeping in space H&E-histopathology pictures can now be segmented of the perimysium using RNNs. This network remembers its predecessors in both the current patch's rows and columns. Bidirectional input from both left and right neighbors is incorporated by applying the RNN four times in opposite directions and then feeding the combined result into a fully connected layer. The applications of DL and similar techniques for health picture segmentation has increased dramatically. There are now specialized architectural approaches that aim squarely at the segmentation problem. In several cases, these have even outperformed the results of fCNNs; thus, they are clearly on the right track [15].

4.5.5 APPLYING DEEP LEARNING TO HELP PREDICT AND DIAGNOSE ILLNESSES WITH COMPUTERS

The purpose of CADe is to detect questionable areas in structural pictures and raise clinician awareness of them. CADe was developed to improve illness detection by decreasing false-negative rates attributable to human error or exhaustion. Recent developments in deep learning have made CADe a viable option in medical imaging, albeit it has been around for some time have made it more useful in a variety of clinical settings. Standard CADe consists of the following steps: Features, which might be morphological or statistical data, are utilized to represent candidate regions, which are then input into classification models such as SVM, which then outputs or makes conclusions about the presence of disease. Deep learning can use feature representations that were created by humans. There are many examples of groups successfully applying their own deep models, among them are the classification of interstitial lung disease in CT pictures, the diagnosis of cerebral microbleeds, and the diagnosis of lesions associated with multiple sclerosis in MR images for the purpose of diagnosis [16].

4.5.6 ARTIFICIAL INTELLIGENCE-ASSISTED DISEASE DIAGNOSIS AND CLASSIFICATION USING DEEP LEARNING

It's not uncommon for people to refer to classification as "computer-assisted diagnosis" (CADx). CADx offers a second, unbiased opinion on the diagnosis of an illness based on imaging data. Malignant lesion classification and disease diagnosis from a single image are two of CADx's most important uses. Historically, CADx systems have been built around the incorporation of human-designed, domain-expert-engineered features. Recently, CADx systems have benefited greatly from the implementation of deep learning techniques [17]. Content-based image retrieval, picture production, augmentation, and merging image data with reports are some of the additional deep learning-based medical imaging applications.

4.6 DEEP LEARNING-BASED CLINICAL APPLICATIONS FOR EARLY DISEASE DIAGNOSIS

This section provides a synopsis of the ways in which deep learning has aided medical imaging's numerous clinical application domains. In particular, this section discusses the AI techniques applied to the analysis of medical photographs for diagnostic purposes for some of the most common disorders, such as those affecting the brain, heart, eyes, abdomen, breasts, and chest [18].

4.6.1 BRAIN

Deep neural networks (DNNs) have been widely employed for brain imaging processing across many different fields of use. Segmentation of brain tissue and architectural components, as well as the categorization of Alzheimer's disease, are frequent subjects of study. In addition, the processes of lesion identification and classification are critical. Many problems associated with analyzing brain images are now totally solved by DNNs. To date, CNNs have been deployed by the best performing teams during 2014/2015 brain tumor identification competitions (BRATS), 2015 longitudinal MS lesion segmentation challenge (ISLES), and the 2013 MR brain image segmentation challenge (MR brains). The majority of these approaches center on analyzing MR scans of the brain, deep learning is not just useful for statistical analysis, but also MRI; CT and US scans of the brain should see similar improvements [19].

4.6.2 EYE

Recently, advanced-level ML algorithms applied understanding of eye images, despite the fact that significant progress has been made in ophthalmic imaging in recent years. The majority of studies use basic convolutional neural networks to analyze color fundus images (CFI). Segmentation of anatomical features, retinal abnormality detection, eye illness diagnosis, and overall picture quality evaluation are just few of the many applications covered [20]. Kaggle's 2015 diabetic retinopathy detection competition used over 35,000 color fundus photos to train algorithms to assess disease severity in 53,000 test photographs. Sixty-one percent of competing teams used deep learning, and four of them outperformed humans with the help of end-to-end convolutional neural networks. Recently, Gulshan et al. (2016) conducted an in-depth examination of effectiveness of the Google Inception v3 network [21], and resulted in the same conclusion as a group of seven highly trained ophthalmologists.

4.6.3 CHEST

The most common topic of discussion in radiography and CT thoracic image analysis is the detection, characterization, and classification of nodules. Many studies either supplement pre-existing feature sets with features obtained from deep networks or compare CNNs to traditional ML techniques utilizing hand-crafted features. Several research groups have found that chest X-rays can identify numerous diseases using a single system. The use of CT for the diagnosis of interstitial lung disorders is an active area of study. Multiple works have taken advantage of the fact that chest x-rays are the most often performed radiologic examination in order to hone their own CNN image analysis and RNN text analysis systems. Additional study in this area is anticipated in the near future.

4.6.4 BREAST

Breast imaging was one of the early areas where DNNs were used. With the recent resurgence of interest, significant improvements have been made over the state of the art, allowing ROIs to match the performance of human readers. Since most methods for examining the breast only use two dimensions, procedures proven effective with natural photographs can be used with relative ease. Aside from that one exception, only breast cancer detection is addressed, which itself is broken down into three subtasks: imaging breast tissue, identifying mass-like lesions, identifying micro-calcifications, and ranking the images according to their potential. As the most frequently used screening method, mammography has received the most attention. Tomosynthesis, ultrasound, and shear wave elastography, as well as breast MRI utilizing deep learning, are anticipated to receive further investigation in the future.

4.6.5 CARDIAC

AI techniques have been applied to various facets during heart picture interpretation, imaging techniques, such as echocardiography, CAT scanning, and MRI. Doctors can learn more about heart muscle shape and function, determine what's causing a patient's heart failure, look for signs of tissue damage, and so on by using automated analysis of pictures from the aforementioned modalities. Despite the fact that MRI is the most studied modality and left ventricle segmentation is the most common task, there are a wide variety of applications that can be carried out. These include segmentation, tracking, slice classification, image quality assessment, automated calcium scoring, coronary centerline tracking, and super-resolution.

Most of the research relied on simple 2D CNNs and slice-by-slice evaluations of 3D and, in some cases, 4D data; DBNs were used in a select few studies. In compound segmentation frameworks, DBNs are exclusively applied for extracting the features. Two works stand out for their creative application of CNNs and RNNs: one established repeated linkage inside the UNet framework for sectioning off the left ventricle, while the other used a CNN to detect and label blood vessels. while the other used RNNs to learn what information to retain from one segmentation to the next. Another architecture uses a regular 2D CNN with a long short-term memory unit to perform temporal regression, allowing for the detection of individual frames within a cardiac sequence.

4.6.6 ABDOMEN

The liver, kidneys, bladder, and pancreas were the most commonly discussed abdominal organs in articles that attempted to localize and divide them. The standard of care for analyzing the prostate is magnetic resonance imaging (MRI), while for all other organs, CT is the gold standard. Diverse applications have been made to the colon alone, but they have all taken a rather simple approach, making use of CNN for feature extraction and then using those features to classify data. It has recently been discovered that a 3D fCNNs very similar to UNet has risen to the top. This study takes an intriguing tack by creating a hybrid of ResNet and UNet architecture [22] by substituting a sum operation for U-concatenation net's function.

4.7 CONCLUSION AND FUTURE DIRECTIONS

Using computational modeling for medical image processing has improved both clinical applications and fundamental research tremendously. New possibilities for analyzing medical photos based on their morphological and/or textural patterns have been made available by recent advances in deep learning. In many medical applications, deep learning techniques have already reached technically advanced efficiency. In technically-assisted visual perception, where massive amounts of training data (such as the over a million annotated photos in ImageNet) led to revolutionary advances in performance; a huge collection of medical pictures that can be viewed by the public would also lead to enhanced performance. Features that are represented in a data-driven manner, in particular when applied with unmonitored fashion, improved precision; however, building a new methodological framework with domain expertise is recommended. In order to avoid the need to train deep models that are exclusive to a given scanning modality, we need to create algorithmic strategies that can efficiently manage images gathered using many scanning protocols. Finally, fMRI image analysis utilizing deep learning to uncover previously unseen patterns, it remains difficult to intuitively grasp and interpret the generated models [23,24].

Deep learning models have been quite successful in medical image processing; however, the primary limitation of this discipline is the lack of large-scale medical datasets. Domain transfer, which takes a model learned on natural images and applies it to medical image applications or moves it to a different image modality, is one approach inspired by the concept of transfer learning. Federated learning is another approach, which allows training to be carried out between different data centers in concert. There has been a recent push when referring to the analysis of medical images to compile benchmark datasets. Class imbalance is another significant difficulty encountered by analysts of medical images. Different studies on novel loss function design have been offered to address this issue. These include focal loss, grading loss, contrastive loss, and triplet loss.

Thanks to the proliferation of cutting-edge deep learning techniques, medical image analysis has achieved remarkable success on many fronts, including precision, efficiency, stability, and scalability. This chapter covered the recent developments of deep learning-based approaches in clinical applications such as picture classification, object finding, segmentation, and registration. Particularly, uses of imaging analysis in diagnosis in human cardiovascular, neurological, and gastrointestinal systems were investigated in depth. Diseases of the eye, heart, and brain, among others, are presented with cutting-edge research in their respective field.

REFERENCES

1. Ritter, F., et al. (2011). "Medical Image Analysis." IEEE Pulse, 2(6), 60–70.
2. Shen, D., et al. (2017). "Deep Learning in Medical Image Analysis." In Annual Review of Biomedical Engineering, 19, 221–248.
3. Anwar, S. M., et al. (2018). "Medical Image Analysis using Convolutional Neural Networks: A Review." Journal of Medical Systems, 42, 226.
4. Ker, J., et al. (2018). "Deep Learning Applications in Medical Image Analysis." IEEE Access, 6, 9375–9389.
5. Fourcade, A., & Khonsari, R. H. (2019). "Deep Learning in Medical Image Analysis: A Third Eye for Doctors." Journal of Stomatology, Oral and Maxillofacial Surgery, 120(4), 279–288.
6. Litjens, G., et al. (2017). "A Survey on Deep Learning in Medical Image Analysis." Medical Image Analysis, 42, 60–88.

7. de Bruijne, M. (2016). "Machine Learning Approaches in Medical Image Analysis: From Detection to Diagnosis." Medical Image Analysis, 33, 94–97.

8. Wells, W. M. (2016). "Medical Image Analysis – Past, Present, and Future." Medical Image Analysis, 33, 4–6.

9. [Online] Analog Devices. (Accessed on November 30, 2022). "Medical Image Processing: From Formation to Interpretation." Available at: https://www.analog.com/en/technical-articles/medical-image-processing-from-formation-to-interpretation.html

10. Duncan, J., & Ayache, N. (2000). "Medical Image Analysis: Progress Over Two Decades and the Challenges Ahead." IEEE Transactions on Pattern Analysis and Machine Intelligence, 22(1), 85–106.

11. Jiang, J., et al. (2010). "Medical Image Analysis with Artificial Neural Networks." Computerized Medical Imaging and Graphics, 34(8), 617–631.

12. Kazeminia, S., et al. (2020). GANs for medical image analysis, Artificial Intelligence in Medicine, Volume 109, 2020, 101938, ISSN 0933-3657, https://doi.org/10.1016/j.artmed.2020.101938.

13. Chen, M., et al. (2021). "Deep Feature Learning for Medical Image Analysis with Convolutional Autoencoder Neural Network." IEEE Transactions on Big Data, 7(4), 750–758.

14. Liu, X., et al. (2021). "Advances in Deep Learning-Based Medical Image Analysis." Health Data Science, 2021, 8786793.

15. Son, J., et al. (2011). "The Recent Progress in Quantitative Medical Image Analysis for Computer Aided Diagnosis Systems." Health Informatics Research, 17(3), 143–149.

16. Balasubramaniam, S., & Satheesh Kumar, K. (2023). "Optimal Ensemble Learning Model for COVID-19 Detection using Chest X-ray Images." Biomedical Signal Processing and Control, 81, 104392.

17. Poudel, R. P. K., et al. (2017). "Recurrent Fully Convolutional Neural Networks for Multi-slice MRI Cardiac Segmentation." Reconstruction, Segmentation, and Analysis of Medical Images, RAMBO HVSMR 2016, Lecture Notes in Computer Science, 10129.

18. Kong, B., et al. (2016). "Recognizing End-diastole and End-systole Frames via Deep Temporal Regression Network." In Medical Image Computing and Computer-Assisted Intervention, 264–272.

19. Sahiner, B., et al. (1996). "Classification of Mass and Normal Breast Tissue: A Convolution Neural Network Classifier with Spatial Domain and Texture Images." IEEE Transactions on Medical Imaging, 15, 598–610.

20. Kooi, T., et al. (2016). "Large Scale Deep Learning for Computer Aided Detection of Mammographic Lesions." Medical Image Analysis, 35, 303–312.

21. Gulshan, V., et al. (2016). "Development and Validation of a Deep Learning Algorithm for Detection of Diabetic Retinopathy in Retinal Fundus Photographs." JAMA, 316, 2402–2410.

22. Yu, L., et al. (2017). "Volumetric Convnets with Mixed Residual Connections for Automated Prostate Segmentation from 3D MR Images." Thirty-First AAAI Conference on Artificial Intelligence.

23. Balasubramaniam, S., et al. (2022). "Feature Selection and Dwarf Mongoose Optimization Enabled Deep Learning for Heart Disease detection." Computational Intelligence and Neuro Science, 1–11.

24. Sathiyamoorthi, V., Ilavarasi, A. K., Murugeswari, K., Ahmed, S. T., Devi, B. A., Kalipindi, M. (2021). "A Deep Convolutional Neural Network Based Computer Aided Diagnosis System for the Prediction of Alzheimer's Disease in MRI Images." Measurement, 171, 108838, ISSN 0263-2241, 10.1016/j.measurement.2020.108838.

5 A Study of Medical Image Analysis using Deep Learning Approaches

Syed Saba Raoof, M. A. Saleem Durai, and C. Srimathi
SCOPE, Vellore Institute of Technology, Katpadi, Vellore, Tamil Nadu, India

Robin Doss
Center of Cyber Security Research and Innovation, CSRI, Deakin University, Geelong, Australia

M. A. Mohammed Sahul Hameed
SSL, Vellore Institute of Technology, Katpadi, Vellore, Tamil Nadu, India

5.1 INTRODUCTION

Deep learning (DL) and machine learning (ML) approaches, image processing techniques, and medical data provide the highest potential for establishing a positive and beneficial impact on human beings in a relatively short period. Computer vision (CV) and image processing techniques include image pre- and post-processing, image data retrieval, image generation, and image visualization and analysis. Particularly, medical image processing is enhanced and widened by integrating various diverse domains of artificial intelligence (AI), image mining, natural language processing, CV, and pattern recognition. DL is the frequently utilized technique to assist the medical field through precise decisions. In healthcare, DL has a wide range of applications from disease diagnosis, and drug discovery, to remote patient monitoring. At present physicians have access to a vast amount of data from diverse sources, including radiography scans, genetic sequences, and various diagnostic imaging.

Since the last few decades, medical diagnostic imaging methods have been employed for early disease identification, diagnosis, and medication. These methods include angiography, positron emission tomography, CT (computed tomography), echocardiography, X-ray, MRI (magnetic resonance imaging), PET (positron

DOI: 10.1201/9781003469605-5

emission tomography), and ultrasound. The traditional method for analyzing and visualizing medical images before CAD has been done manually by doctors and radiologists. Researchers and medical professionals commenced exploiting the CAD due to considerable pathological variances, time-consuming, and expert intensive. Medical image processing has not advanced quickly as diagnostic imaging technology, but due to DL and ML in medical image analysis gained popularity. In the early 1970s medical image analysis evolved [1–3] and in the 1990s CAD was evolved by researchers [4] through the association of DL and ML with CAD and mathematical models. The pipeline of CAD systems for disease diagnosis models follows certain steps: data acquisition, data pre-processing, object detection and segmentation, feature engineering, and classification.

DL techniques can be applied for the classification, detection, segmentation, and diagnosis of medical images [5,6]. A handful of DL algorithms have been developed such as ResidualNet, AlexNet, GoogleNet, DenseNet, VGG, CapsuleNet, and so on. A DL convolutional neural network (CNN) improves and eases the task of detection, segmentation, and classification by employing various activation and dropout functions that clinch the problems raised during training the model and regularizing the network models. CAD aims to achieve an agile and precise diagnosis model for higher-quality treatment of people at once. The research work presents the different DL techniques utilized for lung cancer diagnosis and prediction. DL uses many layers among which permit abundant steps for processing non-linear information along with the hierarchical models to be present that are used for pattern classification and feature learning. Learning models relying on data representation can be determined by representation learning. A recent literature survey asserts that DL-based representation learning models include a feature hierarchy, which helps to define high-level concepts from low-level and vice versa. Some researchers had stated that DL is an extensive learning approach that can have the ability to solve all types of problems in various fields. Currently, DL is being practiced in almost all fields. Thus, DL is often known as a universal learning approach.

DL is mostly preferred when compared to other recognized ML algorithms since its performance is high at large datasets. Various ML algorithms' performance decreases as data increases such as naive Bayes, random forest (RF), support vector machine (SVM), decision tree, etc [7]. Whereas the DL algorithm works well and demonstrates the best performance metrics even on large datasets. Figure 5.1 shows comparison of DL vs. ML algorithms performance by Andre Ng.

5.2   DEEP LEARNING

Similar to ML, DL techniques are classified as supervised, semi-supervised, and reinforcement/unsupervised as shown in Figure 5.2. Also, to this classification, there is one more category of DL, namely reinforcement learning (RL), which is most probably considered as a part of semi-supervised learning and even as unsupervised learning sometimes.

   a. **Supervised Learning:** It is a learning technique that uses labelled data to train the model. This type of learning has input sets and equivalent outputs.

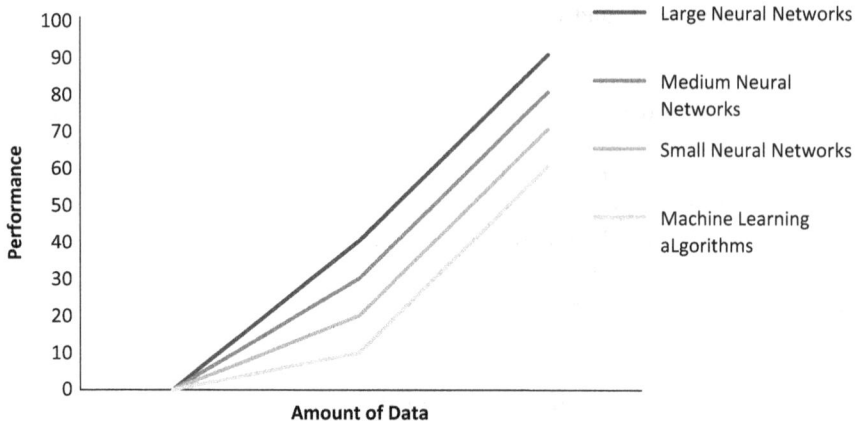

FIGURE 5.1 Performance comparison of deep learning algorithms vs. machine learning algorithms by Andre Ng.

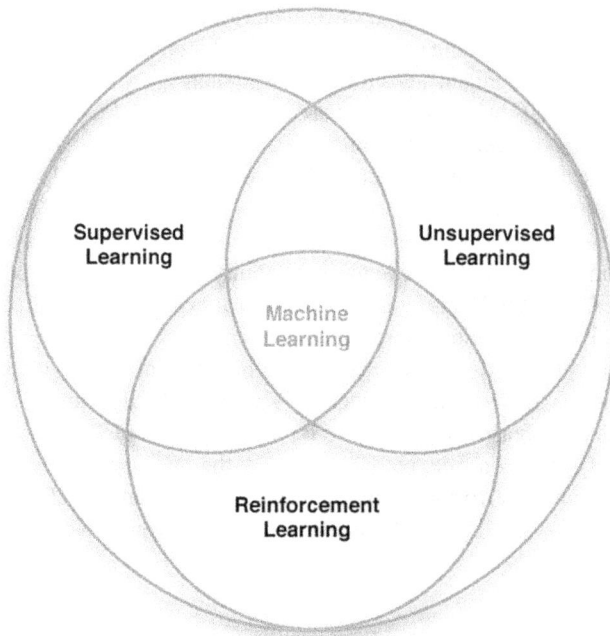

FIGURE 5.2 Deep learning classification.

Supervised learning permits a collection of data and production output from previous experiences and optimizes performance with this technique. There are distinct supervised learning approaches like CNN, deep neural networks (DNNs), recurrent neural networks (RNNs), long short-term memory (LSTM), ResNet (residual networks), and GRU (gated recurrent units) [8].

b. **Unsupervised Learning:** These learning methods are capable of learning and training the model without using labels. Important features of these algorithms are learned to identify the unknown relationships from the input data. Generative learning and dimensionality reduction approaches are known as unsupervised learning techniques. AE, RNN, LSTM, and restricted Boltzmann machines (RBM) are some of the unsupervised learning algorithms.

c. **Semi-supervised Learning:** This is a type of learning that works on both labeled and unlabeled data, that is integration of supervised and unsupervised algorithms (partially labeled datasets). Sometimes, in certain cases, RNN and LSTM are used as semi-supervised learning, whereas deep reinforcement learning (DRL) and GAN are also used.

d. **Deep Reinforcement Learning (DRL):** It is a learning approach that is utilized in anonymous environments [9]. This technique is considered semi-supervised learning in some cases. There are several semi-supervised and unsupervised algorithms that are developed on the basis of DRL. This type of learning doesn't have a direct loss function; hence, learning in this environment is harder when compared to traditional supervised approaches.

5.3 DEEP LEARNING IN MEDICAL FIELD

According to the literature review, scholars and analysts developed various applications in medical imaging for automatic CAD systems. The primary task of medical images in radiology is classifying and identifying disease categories [10]. Medical images originated from various imaging techniques like CT, MRI, X-ray, microscopic, and ultrasound.

CAD aims to procure an agile and accurate diagnosis to assure enhanced treatment of a group of people at a time. Furthermore, effective automatic processing without humans reduces the manual errors caused by humans, and even processing time and cost is reduced. Data scarcity and class imbalance are the limitations in medical image processing. Most often in the case of large datasets, there are not enough labels for training the model. In this scenario, it requires an immersive effort and time of domain experts, and even it is an expensive process. To eradicate this problem data augmentation and transformation techniques like scaling, rotation, translation, and data cleaning are employed. The class imbalance problem is addressed by patch-based approaches.

Before DL innovation, various traditional ML and image processing methods had been provided for medical image segmentation, classification, and detection, for example, random forest (RF), decision trees, SVM, nearest neighbor (NN), Bayesian classifier, and so on. However, DL is not only restricted to medical imaging, the different DL-based techniques are implemented in distinct fields including data acquisition, segmentation, classification, automatic labeling and captioning, computer-aided detection and diagnosis, reading assistants, and automatic dictation, advanced electronic health recording (EHR), and precision imaging for personalized medicine [11–15].

The following sections discuss the DL topics in detail, where DL techniques had been implemented successfully and demonstrated excellent results for medical imaging for segmentation, classification, and detection tasks.

5.4 DEEP LEARNING APPROACHES FOR ANALYZING MEDICAL IMAGES

5.4.1 CONVOLUTIONAL NEURAL NETWORKS (CNN)

CNN is a neural network architecture designed for data processing, which is in the form of arrays, and images (i.e., structured data). CNN algorithms are most broadly applied for CV and image processing; these algorithms have become advanced algorithms for various applications like image segmentation and classification [16]. This type of algorithm works very well for defining the patterns from input images, for example, points, lines, circles, gradients, and even on the face, skin, and eyes. Unlike former CV algorithms, CNN can be applied directly to unprocessed images without performing any pre-processing techniques [17].

This network contains various convolutional layers arranged on each other, where every layer can recognize complex shapes. The ability of CNN originates from a specific layer known as the convolutional layer. The application of convolutional layers in CNN reflects the working of a human being's visual cortex, where a sequence of layers manipulates an input image and recognizes complicated features.

5.4.1.1 Architecture

Like a neural network, CNN comprises several hidden layers known as convolutional layers; the linear function here determines the stride convolutions to extract the features from an image, as shown in Figure 5.3. It even includes a pooling layer that computes other functions like min pool, average pool, and max pool to compress the image size so that computational speed can be increased; this is done by the feature extraction method. Seventeen more layers are known as a fully connected layer similar to the hidden layer; here, the sum of each output layer is flattened and passed as input to the succeeding layer, followed by an activation function.

5.4.1.2 Convolutional Layer

In CNN layers where the linear function is used is known as the convolutional layer. Every node in hidden layers extracts various features by implementing image processing techniques like feature extraction. For instance, the first node from the first layer can extract the vertical edges, whereas the second node can extract the horizontal edges, and so on. The kernel is used to extract these features. Figure 5.3 explains how strided convolutions work. The input image is at the bottom, and the output image after applying convolution is at the top.

5.4.1.3 Pooling Layer

This layer is estimated subsequently to be the convolutional layer. The main aim of the pooling layer is dimensionality reduction. Pooling is done in three ways (i.e., average pooling, min pooling, and max pooling). The function of max pooling is to

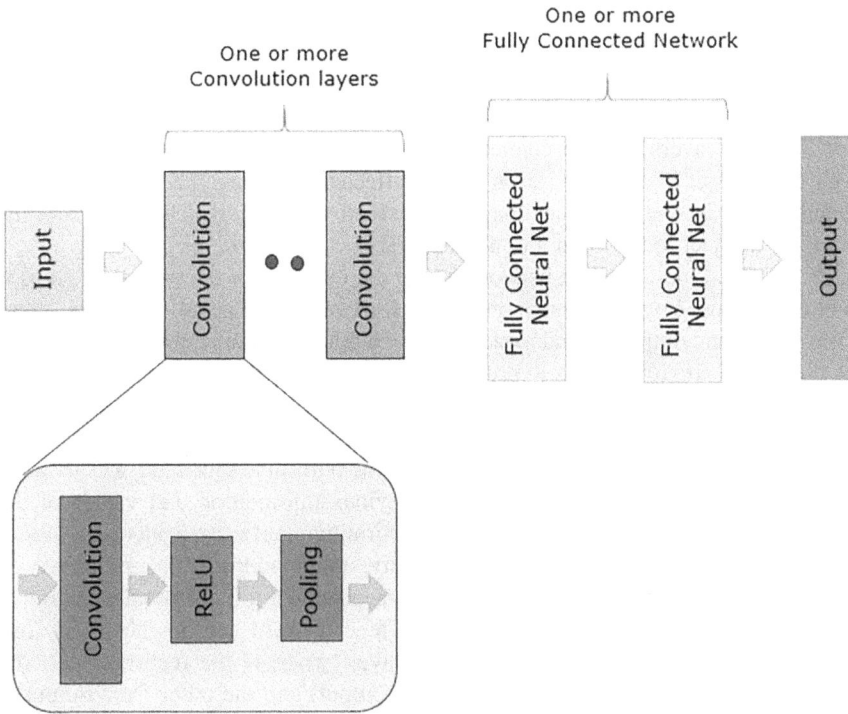

FIGURE 5.3 Architecture of CNN with various layers (i.e., input layer, convolutional layers) where different operations are performed like activation, pooling, and convolution; hidden layers (fully connected layers, and output layers).

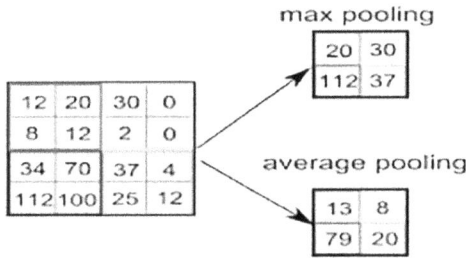

FIGURE 5.4 Pooling layer working.

extract the highest range of pixels from a feature scale, whereas the function of average pooling is to compute the average value of pixels that have been extracted. Figure 5.4 demonstrates the working of max and average pooling.

5.4.2 RECURRENT CONVOLUTIONAL NEURAL NETWORK (RCNN)

Recurrent convolutional neural networks (RCNN) can be mixed with different models; for example, some researchers proposed recurrent convolutional neural networks, and others abbreviated as region-based CNN, recursive CNN, and recurrent CNN. In a mixed CNN and RNN model, the positive features of RNN are utilized to improve the efficiency of CNN. The key features of RCNN are recurrent convolutional layers (RCL; i.e., recurrent connections are introduced into convolutional layers). These connections help the network to progress over time even when input is static and each unit is affected by its neighboring units. This feature of RCNN merges the image context information, which is an essential feature for object recognition and detection [18].

RCNN is a kind of neural network where the outcome of the preceding steps is fed to the succeeding layer as input, whereas, in traditional neural networks, every layer's input and output are independent of each other. In some networks, it requires the outputs of previous layers to predict the next layer outcome; thus, the output of previous layers is important in prediction models. Hence, RCNN had been implemented to resolve the traditional network problem. The hidden layers of RCNN, which retain the previous information, help to solve this issue. RCNN has a memory that helps to remember all the previous information and values of the network. It utilizes similar parameters for performing input and output operations of every layer, reducing the parameter complexity, unlike traditional neural networks.

The main difference between a recurrent neuron and a feed-forward neuron is demonstrated in Figure 5.5. The traditional feed-forward neurons have only one connection between the input and output layer, whereas the recurrent network has two connections (i.e., one from input to output) and the other from output to input (thus, it contains three weights). This extra third connection is known as the feed-back connection, and along this activation can move around the loop. When such feed-forward connections and recurrent neurons are concatenated, a RCNN is formed.

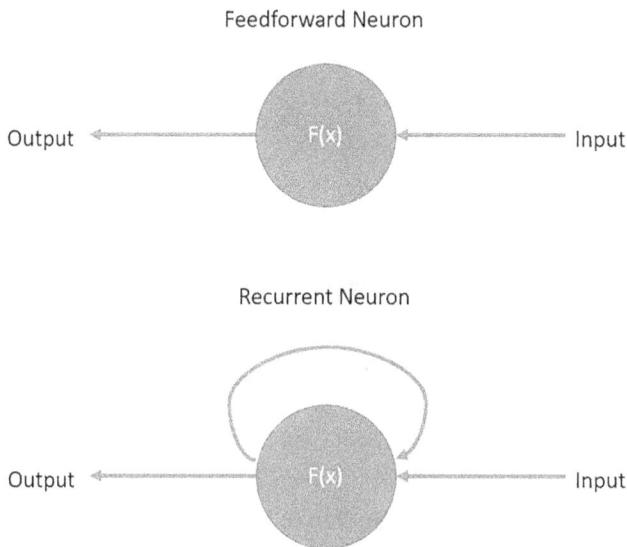

FIGURE 5.5 Recurrent neuron basic structure.

The main advantages of RCNN are the storage of information and the learning of sequential data. Recurrent connections often offer advantages. Every unit makes use of its context information and particularly in image recognition tasks it plays a vital role.

5.4.3   UNET

It is a specific type of CNN that has been developed for segmenting biomedical images. It is developed based on a FCN (fully convolutional network). FCN architecture has been altered and expanded so that it could function with fewer training images and produce accurate segmentation. The main difference between UNet and FCN are as follows:

    a. The UNet model is symmetric, and its architecture is divided into three parts:
- The contracting/down-sampling path: acquires and captures the context of the input image.
- Bottleneck
- The expanding/up-sampling path: is adapted to validate accurate localization through the transposed convolutions method.

    b. The skip connections between down-sampling and the up-sampling employ a concatenation operator substitute for the addition operator. Local to global knowledge about the network is provided by skip connections while up-sampling. Due to its symmetric nature, a wide range of feature maps are provided during up-sampling of the network, this feature map helps to transfer information, whereas the FCN model contains very few feature maps during up-sampling.

The system comprises a contracting and expansive path, and that forms the "U" shaped network. The contracting path is usually a convolutional model that comprises recurrent convolutional layers; exclusively every layer is accompanied by ReLU (rectified linear unit) and a max-pooling layer, as shown in Figure 5.6. While the contraction phase, data related to spatial (dimensional information/data) is decreased, whereas feature information is expanded. During expansion spatial and feature information are merged as a series of up-sampling and concatenations, including contracting path features.

5.4.4   RESNET

After AlexNet architecture based on CNN, all successive architectures employ a large number of layers in deep neural network algorithms to reduce the error rate. These types of networks work well when there are fewer layers, but if they are a significant amount of layers, a common problem arises known as the vanishing/exploding gradient problem, which converts the gradient to zero or very large. The increasing number of layers increases the test and training error rate.

During the back-propagation phase, the error rate is calculated, and gradient values are defined. These gradient values are sent in a backward direction to the

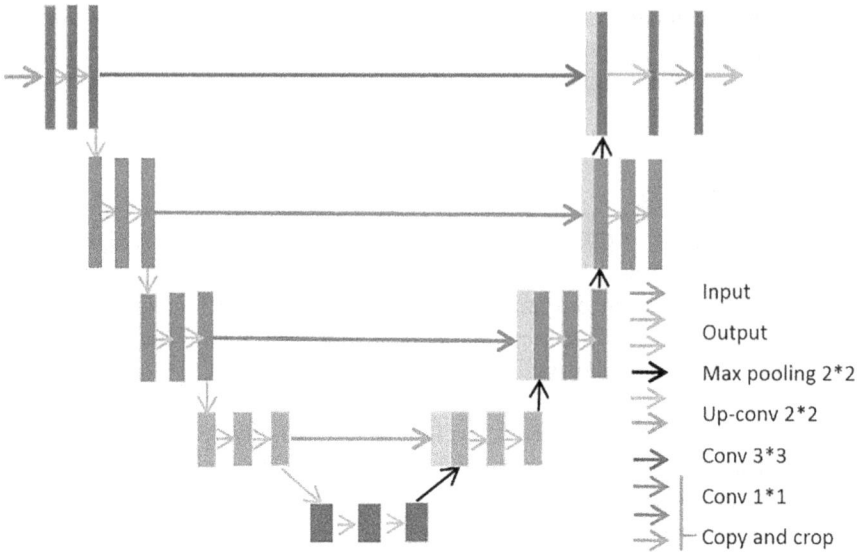

FIGURE 5.6 UNet architecture.

hidden layers, and parallelly weights are updated. This process iterates till the input layer arrives. During this process, the gradient value becomes smaller until it reaches the input layer through the backpropagation method. Thus, the weights of primary layers remain the same in some cases or update very slowly, and due to this, the primary layers won't learn efficiently. Hence, training the deep networks demonstrates low accuracy, and it will either reduce or saturate at a specific value.

Kaiming He [19] developed ResNet in determination to develop ultra-deep architecture so that the vanishing gradient problem can be eradicated.

Deep residual architecture is relatively identical to a network, which possesses convolution layers, activation functions, pooling layers, dense layers, and fully connected layers [20]. The identity connection between these layers transforms the simple network into a residual network. In this network skip, the connections technique is utilized, which skips training from a few layers and connects directly to the output layer. Figure 5.7 demonstrates the residual blocks implemented in

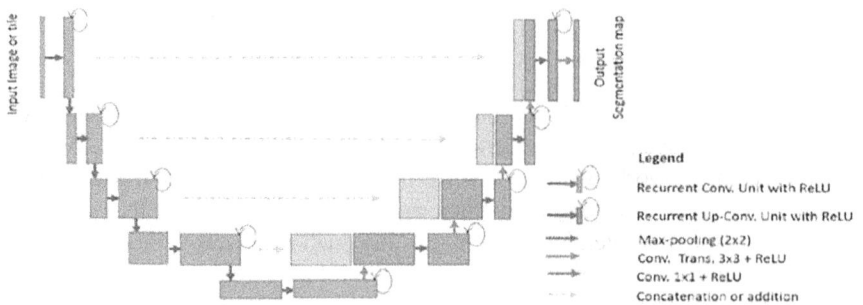

FIGURE 5.7   RU-Net architecture.

networks. The curved arrow from the input pointing to the end of the block is known as the identity connection.

5.5   CASE STUDIES

5.5.1   PRE-PROCESSING

Images obtained from all types of diagnostic imaging modalities need to be pre-processed before training the model. Based on the type of the image various image pre-processing techniques are attainable: background removal, noise removal, resampling, denoising, normalization, registration, and image enhancement. The most widely used pre-processing techniques used for all imaging modalities are normalization and artifact removal. Artifact removal is the primary phase in every pre-processing workflow. For instance, consider colored retinopathy image classification using a DL algorithm. Before training the algorithm for classification, pre-processing the original data is necessary. For example, the colored image should be processed for better visibility. The red and blue channels are removed using a split operation (green channel extractor). Then, the intensity of the image can be enhanced using the contrast limited adaptive histogram equalization algorithm (CLAHE) [21–24].

5.5.2   OBJECT DETECTION

Object detection is an identification object or process of locating and identifying many objects in an image. Object detection techniques have also been applied in medical images to identify and detect regions of interest (ROI) areas that can assist physicians in better and more accurate diagnoses. Object detection using DL is classified into two types depending on the detection methods (i.e., region-based detection) and region-proposal, also known as selective search, which works by extracting the ROI. To accelerate the identification procedure in particular, the regional proposal network was created [25,26]. Object detection was done through employing other methods like one-stage network and regression models. Medical imaging object detection algorithms are dependent on bounding box values and pixel labels.

5.5.3   SEGMENTATION

Literature survey states that several DL applications have been implemented, particularly for segmenting medical images, because these kinds of images face the problem of data insufficiency [27]. Among these algorithms, UNet is one of the widely used algorithms for medical image segmentation. Later on, various UNet versions have been developed. For example, CNN-based UNet model for medical image segmentation had been developed [28]. Researchers had noticed the performance improvement, but they concluded that there is no advantage when features are grouped during the testing phase. But this concept proved that feature summation impacts the performance of a network. The advantage of skipped connections in the field of medical imaging has been experimentally evaluated with the UNet and ResNet [29].

5.5.4 Classification

Transfer learning a DL approach is applied to train the models as CV techniques require and work well when the dataset is large and fails in the case of small datasets. Most of the researchers make use of transfer learning algorithms for several reasons; among them the two main reasons are, pre-trained weights are used for feature extraction, and these weights are also used for training the existing networks [30]. For example, various studies have been conducted where the trained weights are utilized in the training of the networks, and many researchers have proposed that transfer learning is the best and shows the best results for classifying medical images. One more preeminent work is the Google Inception-v3 technique along with transfer learning for classifying skin cancer, which achieved high-level performance similar to the dermatologist for skin cancer detection. DeepCNN techniques, 2D and 3D convolutional kernels are profoundly applied for neuroimages and MRI scans for segmentation and classification of brain tumors and Alzheimer's disease [31–35]. These models achieved the best performance compared to other existing approaches. DL techniques are also applied for X-ray image analysis for chest radiographs. Similar to neuro-imaging, there are distinct several deep CNN models applied for lung nodule segmentation, classification, and detection and achieved excellent performance when compared to traditional ML models.

5.6 CHALLENGES AND ISSUES

Even though DL addresses some specific issues in medical image analysis, such as spontaneous information extraction, there are certain challenges and issues that ought to be addressed by DL in medical imaging like handling high dimensional data, data acquisition, data balancing, and class imbalance data. A large amount of data is required by DL models to train and build the network for producing accurate outcomes. It is further enhanced by attaining DL techniques trained on ImageNet datasets. Still, it is not proven whether DL approaches can successfully work and give better results with smaller datasets. This ambiguity particularly in medical images is induced through the characteristics or properties of an image and the source of an image, for example, intensity, color, texture, edges, angle, and so on. Therefore, huge training parameters and training samples are needed by networks to learn and analyze meaningful representations of images. When medical images are compared to normal images, there are substantially fewer discrepancies in medical images.

DL networks are known to interpret complex structures by adding additional layers, and parameters to understand and analyze complex operations. This is possible when a network with many parameters can perform well in case of enormous data is utilized for training the network because an overfitting problem occurs when limited data is used to train the model. DL networks are therefore incompatible with the models that require enormous data. The benchmark and publicly available medical datasets are not large enough to train the models efficiently; therefore, this issue is addressed by data augmentation or data degeneration techniques, for example, deep generative algorithms.

The major issue faced when dealing with medical images is data balancing. The public datasets usually consist of two types of images, abnormal images (images affected with disease) and normal or healthy images, and according to the survey done, it is observed that the normal healthy images are more compared to abnormal images in the ratio of 70:30, respectively. For example, if we take the cancer dataset, then non-cancerous images are more compared to cancerous images. Another important area of research is developing DL models that can work effectively with imbalanced data. Employing DL networks for medical imaging analysis must be carried out peculiarly as the medical data will be as complex as building large balanced datasets.

5.7   CONCLUSION

DL for medical image analysis has a substantial impact on both healthcare and academic research. Recent advancements in DL have been outspread in the field of healthcare and particularly in medical imaging. Data from clinical images are used to analyze and diagnose diseases by identifying morphological and complex patterns in images. Although DL techniques have outperformed in a variety of medical applications, there are still challenges and potential for advancement. This chapter presents a brief survey of various DL approaches used for analyzing medical images. It highlights the challenges and issues of DL algorithms in medical image analysis. This study also presents the case studies of the medical image analysis process: pre-processing, object detection, segmentation, and classification.

REFERENCES

1. Meyers, Phillip H., Charles M. Nice Jr, Hal C. Becker, Wilson J. Nettleton Jr, James W. Sweeney, and George R. Meckstroth. "Automated computer analysis of radiographic images." Radiology 83, no. 6 (1964): 1029–1034.
2. Kruger, R. P., J. R. Townes, D. L. Hall, S. J. Dwyer, and G. S. Lodwick. "Automated radiographic diagnosis via feature extraction and classification of cardiac size and shape descriptors." IEEE Transactions on Biomedical Engineering BME-19 (1972): 174–186.
3. Sezaki, N., and K. Ukena. "Automatic computation of the cardiothoracic ratio with application to mass screening." IEEE Transactions on Biomedical Engineering BME-20 (1973): 248–253.
4. Doi, Kunio, Heber MacMahon, Shigehiko Katsuragawa, Robert M. Nishikawa, and Yulei Jiang. "Computer-aided diagnosis in radiology: Potential and pitfalls." European journal of Radiology 31, no. 2 (1999): 97–109.
5. Litjens, Geert, Thijs Kooi, Babak Ehteshami Bejnordi, Arnaud Arindra Adiyoso Setio, Francesco Ciompi, Mohsen Ghafoorian, Jeroen A. W. M. van der Laak, Bram van Ginneken, and Clara I. Sánchez. "A survey on deep learning in medical image analysis." Medical image analysis 42 (2017): 60–88.
6. Greenspan, Hayit, Bram van Ginneken, and Ronald M. Summers. "Guest editorial deep learning in medical imaging: Overview and future promise of an exciting new technique." IEEE Transactions on Medical Imaging 35, no. 5 (2016): 1153–1159.
7. Suna, Tao, Jingjing Wanga, Xia Li, Pingxin Lvc, Fen Liua, Yanxia Luoa, Qi Gaoa, Huiping Zhua, and Xiuhua Guo. "Comparative evaluation of support vector machines for computer aided diagnosis of lung cancer in CT based on a multi-dimensional data set." Computer Methods and Programs in Biomedicine 16, no. 3 (2013): 519–524.

8. Al-Tarawneh, M. S. "Lung cancer detection using image processing techniques." Leonardo Electronic Journal of Practices and Technologies 11 (2012): 147–158.

9. Ahmed, Elnakib, Hanan M. Amer, and Fatma E. Z. Abou-Chadi. "Early lung cancer detection using deep learning optimization." International Journal Of Online and Biomedical Engineering (IJOE) 16 (2020): 82–94.

10. Han, Zhongyi, Benzheng Wei, Yuanjie Zheng, Yilong Yin, Kejian Li, and Shuo Li. "Breast cancer multi-classification from histopathological images with structured deep learning model." Scientific reports 7, no. 1 (2017): 4172

11. Jacobs, C., and B. van Ginneken. "Google's lung cancer AI: A promising tool that needs further validation." Nature Reviews Clinical Oncology 1 (2019). 10.1038/s415 71-019-0248-7.

12. El-Regaily, S. A., M. A. Salem, M. H. Abdel Aziz, and M. I. Roushdy. "Survey of computer aided detection systems for lung cancer in computed tomography." Current Medical Imaging Reviews 14, no. 1 (2018): 3–18.

13. Elnakib, A., H. M. Amer, and F. E. Abou-Chadi. "Computer aided detection system for early cancerous pulmonary nodules by optimizing deep learning features." *In Proceedings of the 2019 8th International Conference on Software and Information Engineering* (2019, April), pp. 75–79.

14. Pompe, E., P. A. de Jong, and F. A. M. Hoesein. "Unraveling complexities of the subsolid pulmonary nodule-detection, characterization, natural history, monitoring, and (future) patient management." Journal of Thoracic Disease 11, no. Suppl 9 (2019): S1402.

15. Winkels, M., and T. S. Cohen. "Pulmonary nodule detection in CT scans with equivariant CNNs." Medical image analysis 55 (2019): 15–26.

16. Sarvamangala, D. R., and Raghavendra V. Kulkarni. "Convolutional neural networks in medical image understanding: A survey." Evolutionary Intelligence 15, no. 1 (2022): 1–22.

17. Aytaç, Utku Can, Ali Güneş, and Naim Ajlouni. "A novel adaptive momentum method for medical image classification using convolutional neural network." BMC Medical Imaging 22, no. 1 (2022): 1–12.

18. Vankdothu, Ramdas, and Mohd Abdul Hameed. "Brain tumor MRI images identification and classification based on the recurrent convolutional neural network." Measurement: Sensors 24 (2022): 100412.

19. He, Kaiming, Xiangyu Zhang, Shaoqing Ren, and Jian Sun. "Deep residual learning for image recognition." *In Proceedings of the IEEE conference on computer vision and pattern recognition* (2016), pp. 770–778.

20. Gibson, E., M. R. Robu, S. Thompson, P. E. Edwards, C. Schneider, K. Gurusamy, B. Davidson, D. J. Hawkes, D. C. Barratt, and M. J. Clarkson. "Deep residual networks for automatic segmentation of laparoscopic videos of the liver. SPIE Medical Imaging." International Society for Optics and Photonics 2017 (2017), pp. 101351M-101351M-101356.

21. Abdou, Mohamed A. "Literature review: Efficient deep neural networks techniques for medical image analysis." Neural Computing and Applications 34, no. 8 (2022): 5791–5812.

22. Tariq, Mehreen, Sajid Iqbal, Hareem Ayesha, Ishaq Abbas, Khawaja Tehseen Ahmad, and Muhammad Farooq Khan Niazi. "Medical image based breast cancer diagnosis: State of the art and future directions." Expert Systems with Applications 167 (2021): 114095.

23. Um, Hyemin, Florent Tixier, Dalton Bermudez, Joseph O. Deasy, Robert J. Young, and Harini Veeraraghavan. "Impact of image preprocessing on the scanner dependence of multi-parametric MRI radiomic features and covariate shift in multi-institutional glioblastoma datasets." Physics in Medicine & Biology 64, no. 16 (2019): 165011.

24. Scannell, Cian M., Mitko Veta, Adriana D. M. Villa, Eva C. Sammut, Jack Lee, Marcel Breeuwer, and Amedeo Chiribiri. "Deep-learning-based preprocessing for quantitative myocardial perfusion MRI." Journal of Magnetic Resonance Imaging 51, no. 6 (2020): 1689–1696.
25. Li, Zhuoling, Minghui Dong, Shiping Wen, Xiang Hu, Pan Zhou, and Zhigang Zeng. "CLU-CNNs: Object detection for medical images." Neurocomputing 350 (2019): 53–59.
26. Sahiner, Berkman, Aria Pezeshk, Lubomir M. Hadjiiski, Xiaosong Wang, Karen Drukker, Kenny H. Cha, Ronald M. Summers, and Maryellen L. Giger. "Deep learning in medical imaging and radiation therapy." Medical Physics 46, no. 1 (2019): e1–e36.
27. Zhang, Ling, Xiaosong Wang, Dong Yang, Thomas Sanford, Stephanie Harmon, Baris Turkbey, Bradford J. Wood et al. "Generalizing deep learning for medical image segmentation to unseen domains via deep stacked transformation." IEEE Transactions on Medical Imaging 39, no. 7 (2020): 2531–2540.
28. Huang, Huimin, Lanfen Lin, Ruofeng Tong, Hongjie Hu, Qiaowei Zhang, Yutaro Iwamoto, Xianhua Han, Yen-Wei Chen, and Jian Wu. "Unet 3+: A full-scale connected unet for medical image segmentation." In *ICASSP 2020-2020 IEEE International Conference on Acoustics, Speech and Signal Processing (ICASSP)* (2020), pp. 1055–1059. IEEE.
29. Raoof, Syed Saba, M. A. Jabbar, and Syed Aley Fathima. "Lung cancer prediction using feature selection and recurrent residual convolutional neural network (RRCNN)." In Machine Learning Methods for Signal, Image and Speech Processing, pp. 23–46. River Publishers, (2022).
30. Deepak, S., and P. M. Ameer. "Brain tumor classification using deep CNN features via transfer learning." Computers in biology and medicine 111 (2019): 103345.
31. Rehman, Arshia, Saeeda Naz, Muhammad Imran Razzak, Faiza Akram, and Muhammad Imran. "A deep learning-based framework for automatic brain tumors classification using transfer learning." Circuits, Systems, and Signal Processing 39 (2020): 757–775.
32. Zhang, Jianpeng, Yutong Xie, Qi Wu, and Yong Xia. "Medical image classification using synergic deep learning." Medical image analysis 54 (2019): 10–19.
33. Maier, Andreas, Christopher Syben, Tobias Lasser, and Christian Riess. "A gentle introduction to deep learning in medical image processing." Zeitschrift für Medizinische Physik 29, no. 2 (2019): 86–101.
34. Yadav, Samir S., and Shivajirao M. Jadhav. "Deep convolutional neural network based medical image classification for disease diagnosis." Journal of Big Data 6, no. 1 (2019): 1–18.
35. Sathiyamoorthi, V., A. K. Ilavarasi, K. Murugeswari, Syed Thouheed Ahmed, B. Aruna Devi, and Murali Kalipindi. "A deep convolutional neural network based computer aided diagnosis system for the prediction of Alzheimer's disease in MRI images." Measurement 171 (2021): 108838, ISSN 0263-2241, 10.1016/j.measurement.2020.108838.

6 Deep Learning for Designing Heuristic Methods for Healthcare Data Analytics

J. Joselin
Department of Computer Applications, Sri Krishna Arts and Science College, Coimbatore, Tamil Nadu, India

V.S. Anita Sofia
Department of Computer Applications (MCA), PSG College of Arts & Science, Coimbatore, Tamil Nadu, India

S. Dhanalakshmi
Department of Software Systems, Sri Krishna Arts and Science College, Coimbatore, Tamil Nadu, India

S. Indhumathi
Department of Software Systems, Sri Krishna Arts and Science College, Coimbatore, Tamil Nadu, India

6.1 INTRODUCTION

In the era we currently live in, the phenomenon of healthcare information has been in the news since the early twenty-first century. Healthcare big data in its many forms is currently being analyzed for knowledge discovery and decision making, advanced machine learning (ML) and deep learning (DL), as well as neural net approaches. A great amount of data is created in the healthcare business as new computing technologies are developed, opening up several study topics. The massive volume of data must be managed, but today's primary focus is information extraction for decision-making. Academics are researching big data analytics, DL (advanced ML, known as deep neural nets), predictive analytics, and a range of other approaches to innovate healthcare [1]. In light of all of these achievements, it is not inaccurate to assert that illness prediction with expectation of cure is no longer unrealistic Classification of Healthcare Analytics is depicted in Figure 6.1.

DOI: 10.1201/9781003469605-6

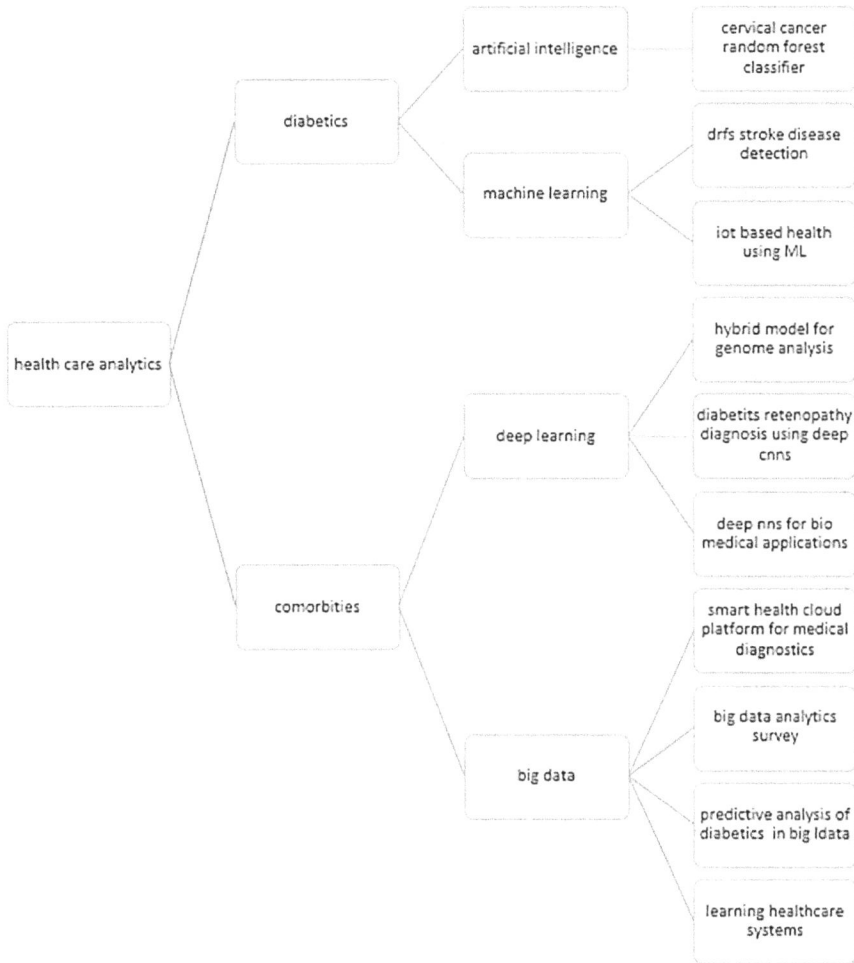

FIGURE 6.1 Classification of healthcare analytics.

Beginning with Dengue Fever (DF) and later COVID-19 are recent outbreaks of infectious conditions that are fatal, and reducing mortality rates requires the early diagnosis of all these infections. Clinicians and specialists are having trouble making an accurate diagnosis of diabetes and calculating the likelihood that underlying disorders may arise. This research uses a mixed DL technique called Louvain Mani-Hierarchical Fold Learning, which is suggested for use in medical diagnosis. It is evaluated and verified using a real-time dataset of 44 Dengue Fever cases provided by Pakistan's Holy Family Hospital and 84 cases discovered regarding the prognosis of infectious disorders such as COVID-19, SARS, ARDS, Pneumocystis, Streptococcus, Chlamydophila, and Klebsiella, as well as applying Louvain Mani-Hierarchical Fold Learning healthcare analytics to 240 instances extracted from comorbidities diagnostic. Laplace rates the accuracy of induced rules as 0.727, 0.701, and 0.203 for 41, 18, and 24 rules, respectively. Shifa International

Hospital in Islamabad, Pakistan, provides information on endocrine diagnostics. Our findings indicate that this method may be evaluated for diagnostics on large-scale healthcare data in the future.

Digital devices have become commonplace, particularly when paired with wireless sensors and mobile devices. Big data is growing in popularity. Technology is needed to handle enormous volumes of increasingly massive and varied heterogeneous health information, such sensor data and electronic health records. To better support the volume and diversity of modern health data, traditional healthcare software and hardware paradigms must be modified. Additionally, new "big data" processing and analysis skills must be added to these paradigms. A means to enhance healthcare while lowering costs, democratizing access, and protecting irreplaceable human lives is possible with the help of healthcare data analytics, which gives researchers the possibility to analyze this vast quantity of data, spot patterns and trends, and provide [2]. In this work, we present a comprehensive study of several big data analytics-integrated healthcare systems and a description of the many healthcare data analytics tools, techniques, and algorithms that may be applied in wireless, cloud, and Internet of Things contexts. Last but not least, the building of a smart health point of convergence for all these platforms is made as a contribution, which might aid in the development of a future unified standard learning healthcare system. Healthcare data analytics is another method that tries to reduce future medical expenditures.

The predictive approach proposed that by obtaining and reviewing past patient facts, information, and records, it is feasible to analyze all potential health risks and forecast future medical treatment in advance diagnostics. Predictive techniques can search via database predictions, saving time and money. Medical care delivery success in the healthcare industry may be achieved by adopting a model that gives algorithms to aid medical therapy for interacting illnesses, which can be reflected in gathering patient behaviors and interactions. Comparison of conventional and advanced traditional analysis, business intelligence, operational research, and data mining are the primary concerns of analytics. Nonetheless, advanced analytics is concerned with the description, prediction, and optimization of data. DL necessitates optimization as a key component [3]. We feel that theoretical research on neural network optimization is interesting for a variety of reasons.

First, the intriguing question of whether a problem can be solved despite non-convexity has the potential to dramatically expand our knowledge of tractable problems. Second, traditional optimization theory cannot adequately describe many situations. As a result, we would want to investigate the existing research in this field and obtain a theoretical grasp of the opportunities and difficulties. Before delving into practical solutions such as cautious initialization, normalization methods, and skip connections, we must first investigate the problem of gradient explosion/vanishing as well as the broader issue of the undesirable spectrum. The second section looks at genetic optimization strategies for neural network training, such as stochastic gradient descent and adaptive gradient.

Because the results of predictive systems allow treatments and actions to be performed when all threats are detected early on, predictive analytics helps healthcare sectors achieve a high level of effective overall care and preventative care, which aids in cost reduction. Conley and colleagues (2008) and Boneshaking (2004) stated that people can contribute to medical care by following up on and updating their medical status so that they can receive the necessary treatment at the appropriate time. Because decision-making systems in healthcare care sectors can be strengthened by focusing on patient diagnoses, behaviors, and prevention to achieve a high level of care and improve healthcare economics, the technology era has added substantial value to the healthcare decision support system (Cannon & Tanner 2007).

6.2 CASE STUDY 1: DEEP LEARNING'S ROLE IN ASSESSING THE IMPACT OF DOSING

DL gives the healthcare business the power to evaluate data at breakneck speed while maintaining accuracy. It's neither ML nor artificial intelligence (AI) but an exquisite combination of the two, using a layered algorithm architecture to sift through data with incredible speed. Pharmaceutical companies are using AI to speed up the discovery of new drugs. The occurrence of dosing means the number of times per day that wastewater is introduced into an absorption system or sand filter [4]. Metering a tank means a closed tank that receives wastewater from a septic tank or other treatment device, equipped with a siphon or a pump used to draw wastewater. ML models can generate new molecules with particular properties that can be combating specific diseases in minutes and could take a human for months to complete manually. DL techniques that take months to finish manually are developing as a burgeoning field of study. DL is commonly employed in medical imaging to determine the presence or absence of illness.

As medical procedures are employed for early detection, monitoring, diagnosis, and treatment, medical imaging plays a significant role in a number of clinical applications. Various medical disorders are assessed for treatment purposes. fundamental understanding of medical image analysis in computer vision necessitates knowledge of the ideas and applications of artificial neural networks and DL. The option selection issue is solved using DL approaches. ML incorporates DL, which can extract needed characteristics from raw input data automatically. AI can help to tackle these challenges. ML is a type of AI application. Without being explicitly programmed, ML learns from data and makes predictions or conclusions based on prior data. There are three types of learning strategies used in ML: supervised learning, unsupervised learning, and semi-supervised learning. A domain expert is required for ML approaches that incorporate feature extraction and feature selection for a specific issue.

Four electronic databases were searched in order to locate relevant studies. The prospective study design was one of the study selection criteria as well as stable chronic disease. The patient population was prescribed drug interventions in each therapy group for at least 6 weeks, with MEMS used to measure compliance. Data on chronic disease treatment and the frequency of drug administration were extracted. The ratio of days to the exact number of doses was used to systematically review the correct data on the effect of daily dosing frequency on medication adherence in chronic disease states, as determined by a medication event monitoring system (MEMS). Twenty studies met the selection criteria. All trials found that patients receiving lower dosages of the medicine had higher adherence rates, and these differences were statistically significant. (P 0.05) at 75% (P 0.05) in 15 of 20 studies [5]. Patients taking once-daily doses had 22% to 41% more days of compliance than patients taking three times a day in 5 of 6 trials comparing once-daily treatment to thrice-daily dosing. Patients receiving once-daily doses had 2% to 44% more days of compliance than patients getting twice-daily dosing in trials comparing the two regimens, with the bulk of studies accounting for roughly 13% with a frequency of 26%.

The term "machine-proven intelligence," commonly known as AI, refers to the ability of a machine to exhibit human-like cognitive abilities, such as learning and problem-solving. AI has revolutionized all fields, including academic and commercial disciplines. In recent years, drugs with intermittent dosing have become increasingly popular, with the assumption that less frequent use would improve patient adherence and the effectiveness of drug therapy while reducing non-compliance costs. However, the impact of adherence to intermittent dosing regimens has yet to be studied.

Drug-target interaction refers to the interaction between chemical compounds and two-molecule drug targets in the human body, which is crucial in drug discovery and development. The limited knowledge of drug-target interactions (DTIs) based on wet laboratory experiments has resulted in a large gap between known and unknown drug-target pairs, which has increased the interest in developing effective methods of predicting DTIs. Traditional DTI prediction methods have faced financial and technical constraints, while computational strategies have been successful in predicting DTIs.

Currently, the primary computational methods used in DTI prediction are ligand-based approaches, docking simulations, gene valence methods, text mining methods, and ML-based methods. DTI prediction methods and drug target binding affinity (DTBA) prediction methods are broadly categorized into computational prediction methods. Structure-based and non-structure-based DTBA methods are further classified. Classical scoring function methods and ML-SF methods are further categorized as structure-based methods, with DL-SF and classical scoring function methods being subdivided into knowledge-based empirical SF-based methods and SF force field-based methods.

6.3 CASE STUDY 2: DEEP LEARNING-BASED SMART HEALTH CARE SYSTEM FOR PATIENTS' DISCOMFORT

To save healthcare costs overall and improve workflows and processes, remote health monitoring technologies are needed in both hospitals and homes. One of the most important remote monitoring indicators for identifying diseases and easing patients' discomfort is pain. Some telehealth research projects have used patient-reported outcomes via surveys administered over the phone, online, or via mobile applications. It is practical and efficient to monitor daily pain conditions using a remote pain monitoring and feedback system.

Automatic pain evaluation has been the focus of certain attempts, either through the use of physiological signal fusion or facial expression detection in face videos.

However, there have only been a few attempts to integrate remote health monitoring systems with automatic pain evaluation. For remote patient monitoring systems, this research proposes an automated pain assessment tool using both cloud and Internet of Things (IoT) technologies

The pain intensity detection technique suggested in this work monitors facial surface electromyography to detect and assess pain from facial expressions (sEMG). A facial mask with surface sensors, which is used to check the movements of facial muscles, may be turned into a wearable device and then linked to a remote monitoring system [6]. The suggested system is capable of signal processing, wireless data transfer, multi-channel bio potential data gathering, and remote data display.

6.3.1 Remote Discomfort Monitoring System

An architecture for an IoT-based remote discomfort monitoring application has been developed to enable real-time central monitoring of inpatients and intensive care patients within the hospital is given in Figure 6.2.

6.3.1.1 Wearable Sensor Mode

The passive sEMG sensor facial mask and the sEMG detecting and processing module make up the sensor node. The material on which the mask is made is supple and flexible. After use, it is replaced [7]. The hardware module in charge of digitization, wireless data transfer, and bio signal conditioning is reusable. The targeted facial muscles dictate where the electrodes should be placed. The electrode position and mask form can be somewhat modified in order to account for individual facial characteristics because the applied mask is soft.

6.3.1.2 Gateway

The gateway serves as the mediator linking sensor nodes, and the cloud and can take the form of a standard router, the mobile phone's personal hotspot, or a smart gateway that supports additional characteristics like heterogeneity, scalability, and

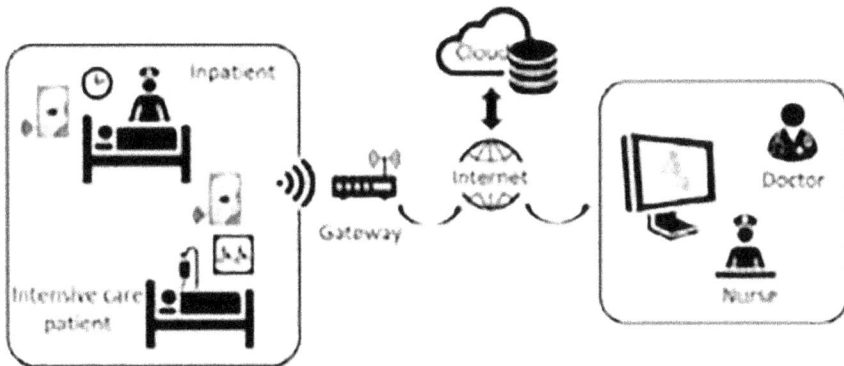

FIGURE 6.2 Discomfort monitoring system.

reliability. Smart gateways can help the system, especially if the total healthcare remote monitoring system uses a variety of data and communication technologies.

6.3.1.3 Cloud Server

The cloud server uses either the UDP or TCP protocol to obtain data from the sensor node [8]. After receiving the data, it transfers it to a data streaming channel that can connect to an HTML5-capable portal and another database server for storage. This server paradigm supports various cloud computing models such as Software as a Service (SaaS) and Platform as a Service (PaaS). This feature could prove advantageous for developing signal processing and data mining techniques while also allowing for adaptable data privacy laws.

6.3.1.4 Mobile Web Application

A multimedia interface between the system and caregivers in this design is provided by a mobile HTML5 application. It has the ability to draw real-time waveforms, run simple algorithms, save information to a database stored within the browser, and go along with external database servers. The web browser-based application, which uses a web browser for its user interface, is a client server program. The web app's ability to be extensively used on a variety of terminal devices is one of its benefits. Generally speaking, this program is cross-platform and works with famous operating systems like Microsoft Windows, Mac OS, and Android. Any terminal device with a portal, including stationary terminals and mobile devices, is able to run the implemented web app.

6.3.2 Devices Used for Discomfort Detection

6.3.2.1 Wearable Sensor Design for Discomfort

The wearable sensor node is initially created to accommodate data gathering and passing needs while taking into account the sEMG data rate. The entire sensor node, including the operational modules, battery power supply, and skin-friendly device packaging, is then combined. A facial mask wearing passive electrode is also included in the design. The wearable sensor monitoring face sEMG is made up of the facial mask and sensor node [9].

6.3.2.2 Wearable Biosensing Facial Mask

In the Facial Action Coding System, the pain behaviors are mainly represented by the muscles involved in one or more facial action units (AU). According to the Fridlund and Cacioppo Guidelines, passive electrodes are positioned on one part of the face to track the activity of certain facial muscles. the soft facial mask and sensor node, which are the two components of the facial mask concept. The sensor node component, as previously noted, is responsible for sEMG signal conditioning, digitalization, and wireless transmission. The purpose of the soft facial mask is to record multiple-channel sEMG.

Along with the electrodes for recording the sEMG signal, the soft facial mask has electrodes that act as a means of connecting the electrodes to the sensor node. The mask uses six bio potential channels in a monopolar arrangement to track six facial

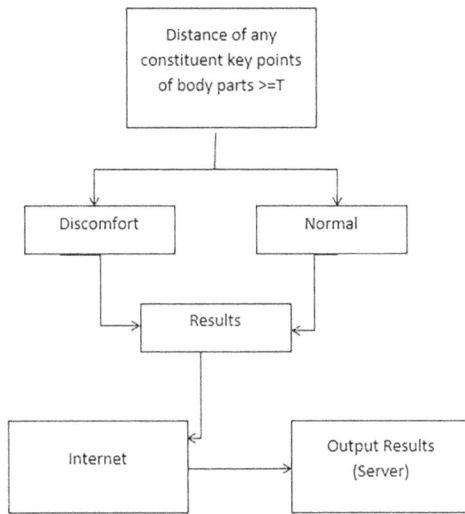

FIGURE 6.3 Discomfort detection system.

locations [10]. Each bio potential channel is recorded in the monopolar configuration in relation to the frequent reference electrode, which is positioned on the bony area behind the ear. In contrast to a bipolar design, in which the two differential input electrodes of an amplifier are located close to one another in the same face region, this reduces the number of electrodes and connecting connections.

The discomfort detection system is given in Figure 6.3, The discomfort detecting electrodes are included into a soft polydimethylsiloxane (PDMS) substrate to create the suggested face mask. Subsequently, the developed mask is simple to use and only requires one step to set up, which can significantly retain caregivers' important time when doing so, especially in the atmosphere of an ICU ward [11].

Finally, the entire pain assessment tool, including the electrode-integrated PDMS face mask, the leads linking these two components, and the combined Wi-Fi sensor node fixed behind the ear. The installed pain assessment instrument weighs 39.08 g in total, which is a little amount and places little strain on the user over time.

6.4   CASE STUDY 3: DEEP LEARNING-BASED CLOUD COMPUTING TECHNIQUE FOR PATIENT DATA

In general, a fitness center affords effective, safe, best, and maximum potential to prioritize the first-class hobby of patients. Currently, numerous fitness care clinics use papers for affected person's clinical information for statistics, which can explain vulnerable facts being misused [12]. This case is because of a fee challenge of the unique health center time and human sources in presenting statistic sources for numerous clinics. The various services involved in Cloud computing are mentioned in Figure 6.4. The Cloud computing era gives an extraordinary ability for a short entry to scientific statistics structures and solves trouble in presenting statistics-era

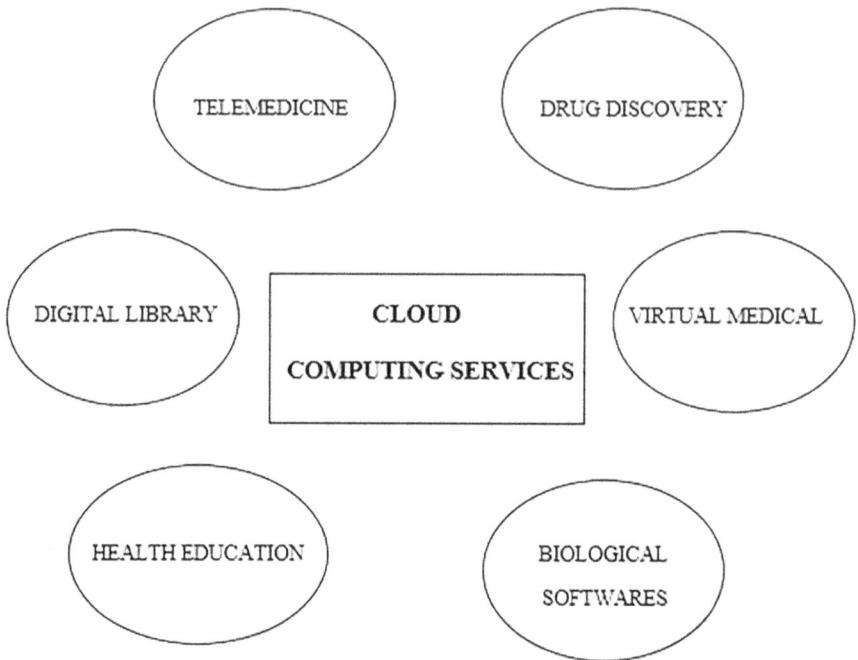

FIGURE 6.4 Cloud computing services.

sources. This paper makes a specialty of the layout of included scientific statistics structures in conjunction with the adoption of cloud computing offerings. The mixture of statistics device improvement and cloud computing adoption techniques is implemented with 4 one-of-a-kind steps such as planning, analysis, layout, and implementation [13].

The result of this look is a scientific statistics device, together with affected person management structures, affected person prognosis offerings, pharmacy structures, laboratory providers, and clinical report control structures that are included in every logo in concomitance with an espousal of the cloud computers era. The good-sized result of the device implementation is decreasing the health center's costs for services, enhancing performance, and the device's clean and flexible use as needed. Cloud computing is a type of net provider that can be accessed everywhere on call, which offers customers consolation and speedy service with minimum control of provider vendors Roadmap for Cloud Computing Adoption Model (ROCCA) for studying and figuring out the ranges of the utility procedure that may be implemented to numerous domains of cloud computing, as properly as organizations, system, and any infrastructure of cloud computing. Thus, it may bring the possibility to make use of the version framework in diverse paperwork of organizations such as fitness offerings in clinics. Cloud computing in the fitness quarter gives the extraordinary ability for quick entry of scientific statistics.

It continues the confidentiality and integrity of statistics saved in all paperwork and affords facts backup and recuperation tactics in extreme cases that are essential in this field. A short entry to an affected person's clinical records in any area can accelerate the prognosis procedure and best treatment, avoid complications, enhance the performance, and improve human life [14]. A health center is certainly considered one of the fitness provider vendors that covers prognosis, pharmacy, laboratory offerings, and patient clinical information. The growing call for fitness offerings influences enhancing clinics' offerings.

There are many clinics with limited fees, time, and human sources in presenting statistics-era sources to connect to all current clinics; for this reason, the use of cloud computing is an essential requirement in presenting the supply of statistics-era sources. Past studies have finished scientific control statistics structures with clinical information such as drug control devices, clinical information, examinations, and offerings fees, even as advanced applications that may be published on web-primarily based affected person's clinical information so it may back up facts while the laptop reports any damages. Research and improvement of cloud computing and interoperability in fitness statistics structures and bank utility improve the use of cloud computing offerings. Cloud computing has been adopted for small to medium sized enterprises (SMEs) and the implementation of the non-public cloud for training institutions.

Drawing on preceding studies, the improvement of statistics devices makes use of a fast utility improvement approach, but there are few studies on scientific clinical report statistics that utilize cloud computing. In this regard, researchers performed studies and improvements of scientific statistics devices primarily based totally on cloud computing with a mixture of the Rapid Application Development (RAD) approach and the way for cloud computing adoption (ROCCA). ROCCA is used as a cloud computing espousal roadmap and advanced right into the framework referred to as the RAF (ROCCA Achievement Framework). The programming language with which the duration of the device improvement applied is PHP, JavaScript, HTML, and Cascading Style Sheet (CSS), and MySQL is used as a database control device.

The motive of this review is to lay out a scientific statistics device in conjunction with the adoption of cloud computing offerings that can create a higher control device with excessive velocity for clinical tactics and can improve a health center. At the end of this review, a statistics device for health centers is produced that includes affected person management devices, nurse offerings, the prognosis of docs or midwives, laboratory offerings, and scientific pharmacies that are included in every department in conjunction with the adoption of the cloud computing era. Thus, it's predicted that scientific control will be higher with an excessive velocity for the statistics integration to enhance the best of scientific offerings. The ROCCA adoption version has been selected primarily based totally on device layout necessities and implementation into cloud computing.

6.4.1 METHODS

During the development of this device, RAD is employed, which comprises four distinct stages: planning, analysis, design, and implementation. However, in the transition from design to implementation, ROCCA is incorporated as a roadmap to assist in the adoption of cloud computing technology. The healthcare facility's data system utilizes a Platform as a Service (PaaS) service model with a private cloud deployment model. The adoption of the ROCCA model was chosen based on the device's design requirements and its implementation into cloud computing.

6.4.1.1 Planning Phase

A widespread description of the agency is the primary learning stage and a typical view of the agency, such as a profile, each imaginative and prescient, and mission, structure, and challenge initiation. A challenge initiation within the agency summarizes a choice statistics device wanted via way of means of a clinic.

6.4.1.2 Analysis Phase

The evaluation phase is the stage where the exam questions are answered. For example, the stakeholders, individuals who will use the device, and details on time and region where the device can be implemented. In this stage, researchers recognize the needs of consumers, the prevailing culture, and the preparedness of agencies to undertake the cloud computing technology [15].

It additionally brings out a dedication requirement that gives an outline of the necessities of the device design method, possible weaknesses, and threats. A SWOT evaluation is used to investigate the strength, weaknesses, possibilities, and impediments of the implementation agency of cloud computing-based clinic statistics.

6.4.1.3 Design Phase

The result of the preceding section produces the proposed device's necessities and specifications. Those statistics are defined by the use of the Unified Modelling Language (UML) diagrammatic reference for commercial enterprise methods and purposeful modeling. The layout section additionally produces a database structure as database layout and record specification and produces an interface photograph of the device.

6.4.1.4 Implementation Phase

This stage produces device construction, the desire for cloud infrastructure, and the adoption and migration plan. At the gadget construction level, the black-field trying-out approach is used to check the code in the course of the improvement method. The desire for cloud infrastructure is used in the course of this section alongside the backing and planning of migration. The software and information incorporation section constructs the method of transferring to cloud computing via means of integrating and adapting programs and information to be transferred with the goal of cloud platform and infrastructure. The very last step in this section is the gadget consumer assessment which entails consumer software trying out and the crowning glory of satisfaction assessment via way of means users. The assessment is in the shape of a questionnaire deployed via means of researchers wherein the responses have analyzed the use of a percent calculation to retrieve assessment results.

6.5 CASE STUDY: CHALLENGES AND BENEFITS OF DEEP LEARNING IN ADVANCEMENTS OF THE CLINICAL TRIAL

DL, also known as hierarchical or deep structured learning, is a subset of ML that employs multi-layered algorithmic architectures to analyze data. In DL models, data are processed through a series of successive layers, with each layer utilizing the output of the previous layer to inform its results. This approach is more thorough in accessing important data and improving connections and correlations for future use. DL is based on the biological connections of neurons in the animal brain for processing information, with subsequent layers of nodes activated by stimuli from neighboring neurons. Artificial neural networks (ANNs) underlie DL models, where each layer is assigned a specific part of the transformation task, and data can be passed through the layers multiple times to refine and optimize the final output. Hidden layers are designed to perform mathematical transformation tasks that convert unstructured inputs into meaningful outputs, which is depicted in Figure 6.5.

As per a 2015 *Nature* article authored by engineers from Meta, Google, the University of Toronto, and the University of Montreal, a DL approach is a representation learning method that consists of multiple levels of representation. Simple yet nonlinear modules make up each level of the representation, with each module transforming one level of depiction (initial from the raw key in) into a slightly more abstract level of illustration. By assembling these levels, complex functions can be learned, and higher-level representations can enhance the significance of input while limiting irrelevant variability. The multi-layered structure of DL models enables them to perform classification tasks such as identifying anomalies in medical images, grouping patients with similar characteristics into risk-based cohorts, or highlighting symptom-outcome relationships in vast amounts of unstructured data. Unlike other ML methods, DL requires less intervention from a human trainer to make decisions, as the multi-layered structure of the models allows the programmer to assess the correctness of the answer themselves. Basic ML approaches only indicate

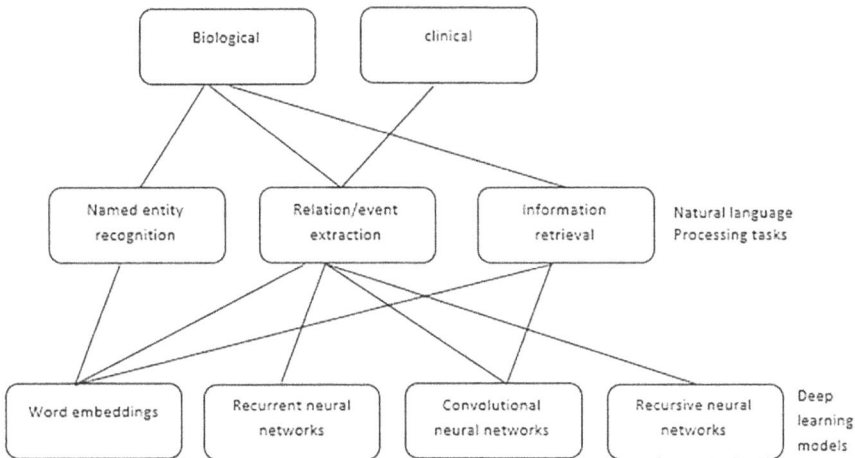

FIGURE 6.5 Biological and clinical process.

whether the output is correct or incorrect, whereas DL's multi-layered structure empowers the programmer to determine correctness.

According to a *Nature* article, DL techniques require less pre-processing of data, as the network can handle many of the normalization and straining tasks that human programmers must perform when using other ML methods. Traditional ML techniques have limitations in processing raw, natural data, and for decades, designing feature extractors that transform raw data into feature vectors for the appropriate internal representation or learning subsystem was necessary. This process required expertise and careful engineering, and only then could an organization recognize or classify patterns in the input. However, DL "automatically discovers the representations needed for detection or classification," reducing the need for oversight and accelerating the process of mining valuable insights from extensive, uncured data.

6.5.1 Deep Learning Use Cases

While many headlines in the DL industry today are about small pilots or experiments in the pre-commercial stage, DL is making its way into innovative tools with high-value applications in real-world clinical settings. This technology is particularly useful for patient-centric applications and improving the usability of healthcare IT. While the current pilots and projects are exciting, they are just the beginning of the potential for DL in health analytics and patient care. The Office of the National Coordinator is optimistic about the future of DL and has recognized developers for their exceptional results. According to a recent report on the state of AI in healthcare, some DL algorithms have already achieved "revolutionary" results.

Management of clinical trial participants includes a preference of the points of the patient or suffering population, patient recruitment, and participant retention. Unfortunately, patient dropouts and non-compliance often lead to studies becoming unacceptable despite the typically significant resources expended in managing participants, including the time, planning, and effort of study coordinators. It often exceeds time, and costs, or fails to produce usable data. In fact, 33.6% to 52.4% of Phase 1–3 clinical cases bear development of the drug, which does not progress to the next stage, and overall there is a 13.8% chance that a Phase 1 study drug will be approved. The ML approach allows us to identify, recruit and retain participants more efficiently and equitably [16].

The usage of ML in scientific ease can alternate the facts series, and evaluation strategies required. Consequently, ML strategies can assist in dealing with a number of problems related to lacking facts and accumulating real-global facts. Patient-generated fitness facts from wearable and different cell/digital devices can complement or maybe update a look at visits and their related conventional reality series in certain situations. Wearables and different devices might also additionally allow the use of new, sufferer-focused. Expansion of new "virtual bio-markers" from the facts amassed with the aid of using a cell device's numerous sensors (which comprise cameras, audio recorders, accelerometers, and photoplethysmography) frequently calls for ML processing to procure applicable insights due to the fact the facts capitulate from those devices may be sparse in addition to variable in quality, ease of access and simultaneity.

By using the exceedingly big and complicated facts, climbing down with the aid of using wearables and different gadgets for studies functions consequently calls for specialized facts series, storage, validation, and evaluation strategies. To illustrate that, a deep neural community was used for procedure entry from a cell single-lead electrocardiogram platform, a random wooded area version was used for procedure audio output from sufferers with Parkinson's disease, and a recurrent neural community was used for procedure accelerometer facts from sufferers with atopic dermatitis.

The virtual bio-markers might also additionally ease the green behavior and patient-centeredness of scientific evaluation. However, this method consists of ability pitfalls. As has been proven to improve with the electrical-diagram type version, ML accessing of wearable sensor output to derive studies end points finds the new opportunity for deceitful effects besides the ML version is brought down with the aid of using deliberately or accidentally changed sensor facts (even though this chance exists with any facts irrespective of processing methods). In view of the fact that of the high risk used, software program supposed to the pronouncement, monitor, or deal with scientific situations is regulated with the aid of using the FDA, and the FDA had strategies and also steerage associated with biomarker validation and also qualification to be used in regulatory evaluation [17].

Further, the increase of new digital biomarkers and other device-centric patient-centric opportunities adds the ability to send data and analysis to participants to utilize education and insight [18]. Major blocks to implementing ML processing of data in devices include defining how before approved clinical endpoints and patient-centric digital bio-markers intersect, and sharing. This includes understanding participants' privacy feelings related to their use. FDA approval of new biomarkers will also be required. Researchers interested in harnessing the power of these devices should explain the advantages and disadvantages to their patients for ethical and private reasons [19].

6.6 CASE STUDY: APPLICATION OF DEEP LEARNING TO NEUROIMAGING

Magnetic resonance imaging (MRI) has been a crucial tool in recognizing brain function and disorders for over a decade. With the assistance of powerful computational tools and novel ML techniques, neuroimaging has opened up unprecedented opportunities for neurological disease identification. However, accurately identifying neurological diseases from neuroimaging data is extremely challenging due to the similarity of disease phenotypes. This article discusses existing DL methods for identifying neurological disorders and compares their performance [20]. The analysis suggests that convolutional neural networks (CNNs) outperform other methods in detecting neurological disorders from different diseases and imaging modalities. The article also highlights recent research questions and suggests future directions of research.

Neuroimaging is an imaging technology that analyzes the structure and function of the nervous system, including the brain [21]. With the increasing prevalence of neurological diseases, there is a growing demand for neuroimaging technology and subsequent data analysis. Various imaging techniques and DL-based analysis methods have been developed to diagnose neurological disorders for early detection and appropriate therapeutic strategies [22].

In recent years, DL algorithms have been applied to various domains, including image analysis, anomaly detection, disease detection, and natural language processing. Neuroimaging researchers have attempted to use deep structured learning approaches, such as CNNs, to detect neurological disorders from MRI scans. Cross-media approaches, like data fusion, are also employed in various domains, including personalized services and diagnosing neurological disorders. Among the diverse architectures in DL, researchers are mainly leaning on CNN-based approaches to extract MRI data.

This NLD has been generated from deep neural networks (DNN), and autoencoders (AE). Moreover, from 2015 to 2019, the diagnosis of AD compared with PD or SZ received more attention in the published literature [23].

As there is a growing concern in this domain and the increase in reported approaches for analyzing MRI scans, we summarize that there are subsistent articles to expedite the selection process of suitable techniques, from different perspectives for specific tasks and datasets. There are several reviews summarizing the progress from various approaches. One of these targets is to integrate the application of big data and ML into mental health research [24]. Various ML-based tasks are being studied to improve the diagnosis of neurological disorders. They have also investigated the applications of DL for better understanding and diagnosis of PD.

An elaborate review of DL enforced with the analysis of several medical images such as neurological, pathological, and pulmonary is available [25]. However, data selection and pre-processing is not explained easily in any available review articles. To fill this hiatus, this work focuses on providing a general outlook of the application of DL in the detection of NLDs (i.e., Alzheimer's disease, AD; Parkinson's disease, PD; schizophrenia, SZ) from MRI scans, and further with the common open-access datasets and pre-processing methods [26].

Therefore, the supreme purposes of this work are:

- The content describes several aspects of DL approaches to analyzing MRI scans to detect neurological disorders (NLDs). It includes a preface with references to various DL architectures and pre-processing techniques that are used for identifying anomalies from MRI scans. The purpose of this preface is to help newcomers understand the framework and serve as a reference for the future.
- The content also includes a detailed review of existing studies that have used DL in MRI scans for the diagnosis and classification of three main NLD variants: AD, PD, and SZ. The review attempts to validate a DL-based categorization approach for these three disorders.
- Furthermore, the content reviews popular open-access datasets and provides information on subjects, including age, gender, and MRI scan modalities. This facilitates the verification and comparison of the performance of new methods using open-access benchmark datasets.

- Finally, the content includes a focused discussion on current research issues faced and future research analysis ideas that can help beginners for effective development. It briefly describes different DL architectures currently used in the analysis of MRI scans to detect AD, PD, and SZ. The section also describes common pre-treatment techniques and provides detailed reports on the detection of these three NLDs.

This section dispenses existing open-access datasets that are available for exploration. The section contains a performance evaluation of the techniques and sections reviewed. It offers challenges and future perspectives in seconds to complete the work.

6.7 CONCLUSION

The main goal of DL is to enhance with each piece of data. This includes the ability to adapt its underlying structure to evaluate the data exactly. Once entirely built using test data, this network enables greater ease of use through customer analytics.

Similar to streaming service, which suggests what you should watch next, the data of the shows you watch are processed and decisions are made to recommend what you might like too. The DL model focuses on cognitive computing and mimicking a human-like structure of thought.

As a part of ML, DL works with neural networks to mimic how the brain responds to inputs and makes decisions. Neural networks have nodes that link from the input to the hidden layers of the network and then to the output. DL attempts to enhance the decision-making process; the longer the model runs, the more precise and expressive it becomes. Later, AI adopted DL to enhance its analyzing process. So, with breakthroughs, AI can become intelligent in terms of accuracy and speed. As DL drives our future, big data has made this model intuitive.

REFERENCES

1. Jiménez J., Skalic M., Martinez-Rosell G., De Fabritiis G. K deep: Protein-ligand absolute binding affinity prediction via 3d-convolutional neural networks. J ChemInf Model. 2018;58(2):287–296.
2. Jha A., Gazzara M. R., Barash Y. Integrative deep models for alternative splicing. Bioinformatics. 2017;33(14):i274–i282.
3. Jung E., Kim J., Kim M., Jung D. H., Rhee H., Shin J-M, Choi K., Kang S-K, Kim M-K, Yun C-H, et al. Artificial neural network models for prediction of intestinal permeability of oligopeptides. BMC Bioinform. 2007;8(1):245.
4. Zhang J., Chen K., Wang D., Gao F., Zheng Y., Yang M. Editorial: Advances of neuroimaging and data analysis. Front Neurol. 2020;11:257. doi: 4.3389/fneur.2020.00257
5. Jeon J., Nim S., Teyra J., Datti A., Wrana J. L., Sidhu S. S., Moffat J., Kim P. M. A systematic approach to identify novel cancer drug targets using machine learning, inhibitor design and high-throughput screening. Genome Med. 2014;6(7):1–18.
6. Kadurin A., Aliper A., Kazennov A., Mamoshina P., Vanhaelen Q., Khrabrov K., Zhavoronkov A. The cornucopia of meaningful leads: Applying deep adversarial autoencoders for new molecule development in oncology. Oncotarget. 2017;8(7): 10883.

7. Kandoi G., Acencio M. L., Lemke N. Prediction of druggable proteins using machine learning and systems biology: a mini-review. Front Physiol. 2015;6:366.
8. Kearnes S., Goldman B., Pande V. Modeling industrial ADMET data with multitask networks. arXiv: Machine Learning:2016;1606.08793
9. Finnegan A., Song J. S. Maximum entropy methods for extracting the learned features of deep neural networks. PLoS Comput Biol. 2017;13(10):e1005836.
10. Free S. M., Wilson J. W. A mathematical contribution to structure-activity studies. J Med Chem. 1964;7(4):395–399.
11. Kapoor R., Haganb M., Paltab J., Ghosha P. Artificial intelligence methods in computer-aided diagnostic tools and decision support analytics for clinical informatics. ArtifIntellPrec Health FromConcAppl. 2020;31:31–59.
12. Etzold T., Ulyanov A., Argos P. SRS: Information retrieval system for molecular biology data banks. Methods Enzymol. 1996;266:114–128.
13. Falchi F., Caporuscio F., Recanatini M. Structure-based design of small-molecule protein-protein interaction modulators: The story so far. Future Med Chem. 2014; 6(3):343–357.
14. Zsoldos Z., Reid D., Simon A., Sadjad S. B., Johnson A. P. eHiTS: A new fast, exhaustive flexible ligand docking system. J Mol Graph Model. 2007;26(1):198–212
15. Esposito E. X., Hopfinger A. J., Madura J. D. Methods for applying the quantitative structure-activity relationship paradigm. In Chemoinformatics. Springer, 2004, pp. 131–213.
16. Ferrero E., Dunham I., Sanseau P. In silico prediction of novel therapeutic targets using gene-disease association data. J Transl Med. 2017;15(1):182.
17. Friedman J., Hastie T., Tibshirani R. The elements of statistical learning, volume 1. 1. New York: Springer Series in Statistics; 2001.
18. Friesner R. A., Banks J. L., Murphy R. B., Halgren T. A., Klicic J. J., Mainz D. T., Repasky M. P., Knoll E. H., Shelley M., Perry J. K., et al. Glide: A new approach for rapid, accurate docking and scoring. 1. method and assessment of docking accuracy. J Med Chem. 2004;47(7):1739–1749.
19. Asher M. The drug-maker's guide to the galaxy. Nature News. 2017;549(7673):445.
20. Bai F., Morcos F., Cheng R. R., Jiang H., Onuchic J. N. Elucidating the druggable interface of protein-protein interactions using fragment docking and coevolutionary analysis. Proc Natl Acad Sci. 2016;113(50): E8051–E8058.
21. Bakheet T. M., Doig A. J. Properties and identification of human protein drug targets. Bioinformatics. 2009;25(4):451–457.
22. Bengio Y., Lamblin P., Popovici D., Larochelle H. Greedy layer-wise training of deep networks advances in neural information processing systems. Cambridge, MA: MIT Press; 2007.
23. Boyiadzis M. M., Kirkwood J. M., Marshall J. L., Pritchard C. C., Azad N. S., Gulley J. L. Significance and implications of FDA approval of pembrolizumab for biomarker-defined disease. J Immunother Cancer. 2018;6(1):1–7.
24. Beck A. H., Sangoi A. R., Leung S., Marinelli R. J., Nielsen T. O., Van De Vijver M. J., West R. B., Van De Rijn M., Koller D. Systematic analysis of breast cancer morphology uncovers stromal features associated with survival. Sci Trans Med. 2011;3(108):108ra113–108ra113.
25. Sathiyamoorthi V., Ilavarasi A. K., Murugeswari K., Thouheed Ahmed S., Aruna Devi B., Kalipindi M. A deep convolutional neural network based computer aided diagnosis system for the prediction of Alzheimer's disease in MRI images. Measurement. 2021;171:108838, ISSN 0263-2241, 10.1016/j.measurement.2020.108838
26. Bengio Y. Learning deep architectures for AI. Norwell: Now Publishers Inc; 2009.

7 Deep Learning-Based Smart Healthcare System for Patient's Discomfort Detection

J. Antony Vijay
Department of Computer Science and Engineering,
Karpagam College of Engineering

B. Gomathi
Department of Computer Science and Engineering,
PSG Institute of Technology and Applied Research

M. Mythily
Department of Computer Science and Engineering, Karunya
Institute of Technology and Sciences

Beaulah David
Department of Information Technology, Hindusthan
College of Engineering and Technology

7.1 INTRODUCTION

The evolution of the Internet of Things (IoT) revamped almost all fields, namely the education, agriculture, transportation, and healthcare sectors, as smart sectors by interconnecting the entities to communicate, capture, share, and store information. The development of IoT, high-speed networks, and deep learning algorithms transformed and expedited the capability of smart healthcare. IoT has had a major influence on the medical field and is enabling more reliable outcomes at reduced costs through connecting necessary parameters in the healthcare system, which controls the devices by an [1,2] IoT-based patient monitoring system that observes patient mistakes and highly efficient check-ups to predict the diseases immediately. The Internet of Medical Things (IoMT) refers to healthcare devices for communication processes that take place in highly secured devices that have the ability to convey data over a secured network [3,4].

Based on the capacity of the built-in functions inserted to the patient's body and the regular charging or battery replacement, traditional remote monitoring systems [5–7] are uncomfortable for patients. The IoMT innovation addresses the aforementioned problems by creating extremely small-capacity IoT devices and streamlined communicative channels [8]. The compatible patient observation zone at the patient's house or in the ambulance is the major component of the remote health monitoring system [9–11]. Patients suffering from long-term diseases can be remotely monitored according to IoMT systems. As a result, it can offer patients prompt diagnostics that can save their lives in emergencies. In IoMT, the sensors and devices are interconnected to support the exchange of data through wireless communication and enable the acquisition and process of a large amount of data that provides insights into healthcare data to specialists in healthcare [12–14].

According to survey results, some elderly people's dependence levels have steadily risen. The loneliness of elderly individuals living alone in their houses can mostly be attributed to the modern lifestyle. There are instances in which they are frequently ignored and do not receive prompt care, which could be harmful to their life. Nowadays, the monitoring of depression, blood pressure, sleep, heart function, and pain is all done through various computer-based patient monitoring techniques [15–17]. When a medical team is not available, these automated systems are mostly employed to observe patients and elderly people continuously. By monitoring health-related factors like breathing, heart rate, blood sugar level, etc., the patient's movements and activities are observed [18]. In addition, automated systems provide a comfortable environment to patients by avoiding their personal visits and also enhance their experiences, improve therapeutic outcomes, provide a better caregiver experience, and reduce costs [19].

In the smart healthcare sector, object detection and localization are important disciplines in medical imaging analysis that can be done in the modern world by using computer vision. In this field, various neural network algorithms [20,21] and deep reinforcement learning techniques [22,23] will provide a way for researchers to do the development activities in localization and object detection methods to identify the images in the medical field. Sustainable smart cities greatly benefit from IoT-based smart healthcare systems [24]. A real-time healthcare system demonstrates the value of IoT, computer vision, and machine learning algorithms in improving healthcare facilities. Digital technology is used to enable remote surveillance of patients when the clinical team is not available.

On the hardware side of the patient monitoring system, sensors and specialized hardware are used for patient behavior monitoring, posture monitoring [25], and pain detection, while on the software end, machine learning and computer vision algorithms are employed. In order to monitor their health, patients are not showing any enthusiasm for having sensors connected to their bodies. Face expressions were thus employed as a method of pain detection. However, only when patients face the camera directly can the facial emotion be captured [26,27]. Similar to this, posture-based monitoring strategies focus on the patient using numerous cameras.

The suggested non-invasive discomfort detection [28–30] based on the AX-YOLOV5 (Arbitrary Extra-Large You Only Look Once Version 5) algorithm, can overcome these shortcomings. Different sensors and line-of-sight devices are not necessary for the suggested model. In order to locate the patient in the video input, the AX-YOLOV5 algorithm is applied. Additionally, the patient's body's 17 critical locations are detected using the AlphaPose Library [31,32], and an IP camera consistently records the patient's motions. To determine where the human body is located in real-time photos, the AX-YOLOV5 algorithm is used. Using the rule of mining associations, the key points are correlated to the five most crucial key point coordinates of the human body. These distinguishing characteristics are utilized to determine whether a patient is seated or lying in bed. With the help of the temporal threshold technique, healthcare problems can be identified by tracking how frequently the coordinates of the body's major points change over time. Finally, the diseases from the patient's body are categorized using the distance between important locations and the temporal threshold. Additionally, the critical points' coordinates are accessible in order to pinpoint the correct ailment within the human body.

The research covered in this chapter is arranged consequently: The detailed review of the literature survey is well-equipped in Section 7.2. The patient's discomfort detection process is covered in Section 7.3. The summary of datasets and system configuration for the machine training process is represented in Section 7.4. The implementation for the patient discomfort detection algorithm is described in Section 7.5. AX-YOLOV5 model training phase is discussed in Section 7.6. The various performance metrics calculations are represented in Section 7.7. The comparative results of various performance metrics based on neural networks are presented in Section 7.8. The conclusion of the research paper is discussed in Section 7.9. References are presented in the final section.

7.2   RELATED WORK

In the domain of healthcare controlling, significant efforts have been made recently. Diverse fields, including computer vision, machine learning, and deep learning, have achieved significant advancements. The systems and methods that have just lately been developed will be briefly described in this part. For applications involving patient monitoring, the researcher proposed various fall detection and surveillance systems [33]. It is also acknowledged as a vital procedure due to the essential stage for numerous fatal injuries, especially in tracking the elders. Electroencephalography [34] accustomed to assess the injury of a patient while they are walking, and support vector machines are used to analyze the data using the radial basis functional kernel. Here, a non-invasive device has been used to track the patient's pain levels when the patient moves around. The major goal of this research is to identify pain intensity early in order to lessen depression brought on by pain. The support vector machine (SVM) is proposed to classify the pain–no pain expressions [35,36] by using the facial indicators of the pain of the patients. The parameters and shapes of the digitized face images are decoupled using active appearance models [37].

The systems for tracking sleep are considered to be an important sign of patient health. In a typical sleep monitoring system, sleeping habits are recorded, including wake/sleep time, body part mobility habits, fluctuations in heartbeat and breathing rate, and sleep postures. The development of a depth analysis approach [38,39] allowed for the non-contact monitoring of a user's respiration rate, sleep posture, and body movement while they were asleep. Eight volunteers were requested to switch between supine and side-lying sleep postures on the bed every 15 breaths during the experiment. The findings indicated that the suggested technique is likely to be successful in detecting the head and torso in a variety of sleeping positions and body types. For persistent recognition of the sleep status, including on-bed mobility, bed exit, and respiration section, the Sleep Sense [40] monitors the motion and sound activity to track sleeping status effectively and based on the effect of Doppler the sleeping movements and noise can be captured effectively, which has three components of Sleep Sense. For the framework of sleep recognition, many TD and FD attributes are released from this work. For the medical treatment, healthcare, and fitness industries, it is crucial to be able to track one of the key signs, the respiration rate. The monitoring of respiration [41] is proposed using a novel and reliable method that can accurately bring out the respective attributes such as heart pumping count and body temperature that are extremely dynamic, which also considers the oxygen intake and continuous body movements made easy to protect the patient's health effectively. By assessing during controlled respiration exercises in highly heat-dynamic settings, the system's extraordinary endurance to monitor the nose region is established, and the breathing rate is recorded.

The multiple signals classification (MUSIC) approach [42], depending on a subspace-based approach, is used to help determine the rate of respiration by the radio frequency-based system that is introduced. The authors of this study monitored breathing or respiration using infrared vision sensors. A number of researchers created methods for monitoring sleep that are comparable to breathing monitoring systems. For tracking respiration rates, they tracked the mobility of the chest and abdominal muscles and employed infrared scanning of the nasal region. The creation and deployment of a wireless sensor-based healthcare system that is adaptable, scalable, and affordable for remote patient monitoring of several critical physiological parameters is covered in the following research paper. The suggested healthcare process has been created to incorporate various innovative methodologies to help patients with neuromotor impairments and their carers communicate more effectively. The presented system has the capacity to simultaneously collect, store, and process a small number of essential patient physiological parameters. As a result, it can be used to continuously monitor neuromotor handicapped individuals who have a chronic illness or are at high medical risk from a distance in real time for an extended length of time at home or in specialized facilities.

Electroencephalogram (EEG) monitoring [43] is possible outside of clinical settings with cordless EEG equipment, which allows patients to go about their normal lives without restriction. However, using such a device to collect, encrypt, and transport the EEG data to the backend consumes a lot of energy. Currently, EEG has various models for patient monitoring.

Facet-based analysis has been used to handle pain detection and depression monitoring. This work [44–46] uses a feature-based approach to make use of facial expressions for pain detection. Prkachin and Solomon pain intensity metrics are used to evaluate the various levels of pain intensity in order to identify and study pain. In addition to closing eyelids, this matrix considers many facial expression-related aspects such as brow lifting, brow lowering, and tightening. The people who undergo research all the time concentrate on patient by patient, as well as various healthcare systems were created to monitor the patients' health efficiently, in all systems and procedures as previously indicated. In order to read and record various metrics, these created systems call for attaching sensors or gadgets in a human's bed or body, which is costly as well as not liked by patients. Few scientists have experimented with vision-based techniques; instead, they have mostly used infrared or depth cameras to track breathing, identify falls, and track sleep [47–49]. Facial expression-based systems have also been created; however, the system requires a camera with an open eye. Researchers used movement and posture data to determine the sleeping status and key points of body parts using blob detection and feature-based approaches.

In this work, based on Internet of Healthcare Things (IoHT), the system can handle and monitor multiple patients at once and may function in the current layout of wards. Our system's independence from specialist gear, fancy beds, or wearable tech other than a single top-view camera is one of its key advantages. One of the drawbacks is, the patients never show their attention to all the steps of the healthcare treatment process.

7.3 PROPOSED SYSTEM

The AX-YOLOV5 is a deep learning-based algorithm, which identifies the position of the human body in real-time images. The step-by-step process involved is mentioned in Figure 7.1. Initially, the IP camera continuously captures the movements of the patient's human body in hospital, which extracts the input images from the video. In the pre-processing stage, the patient image is kept as an input, which removes the noises from an input image. Image dataset is created from the surveillance video from the hospital. This image dataset is applied to the AX-YOLOV5 model to train the deep learning model properly to avoid overfitting. Alpha pose library detects the 17 key points of a patient's body and the concatenate of key points formed organs, which is performed with mining association rules. This helps to detect the important organs of a patient's human body.

The Euclidean distance between the key points of two consecutive image frames can be calculated and then evaluated with T value. If the distance is higher than threshold value, then the patient is considered in discomfort. Otherwise, the patient is in the comfort stage. Figure 7.2 graphically represents the AX-YOLOV5-based patient discomfort approach.

In this approach the input images are extracted from NTU RGB+D video dataset. These images were applied to the AX-YOLOV5 model to bring out the feature regions of the patient to recognize the body parts. The processing of color images decreases the performance and storage of the model so that the system needs to reduce the dimensionality of the input images with the Maxout technique, which minimizes the burden from heavy processing time and storage.

The image regions are filled with bounding boxes, from which we need to pick the correct bounding boxes for patient organ monitoring. To select the right bounding boxes from the patient image non-maximum suppression technique

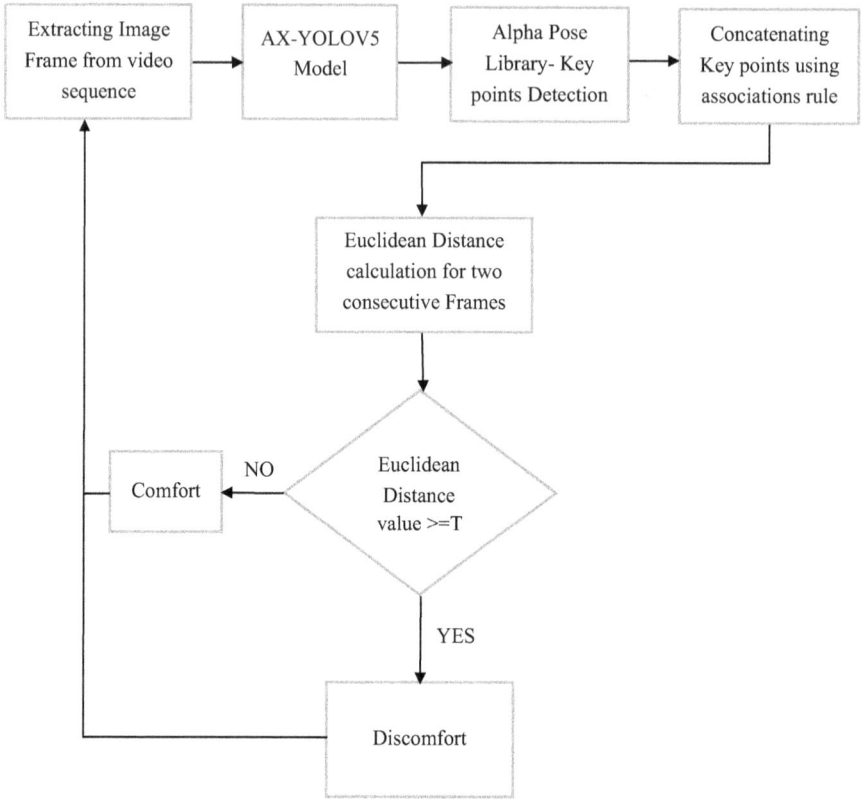

FIGURE 7.1   Step-by-step process of discomfort detection system.

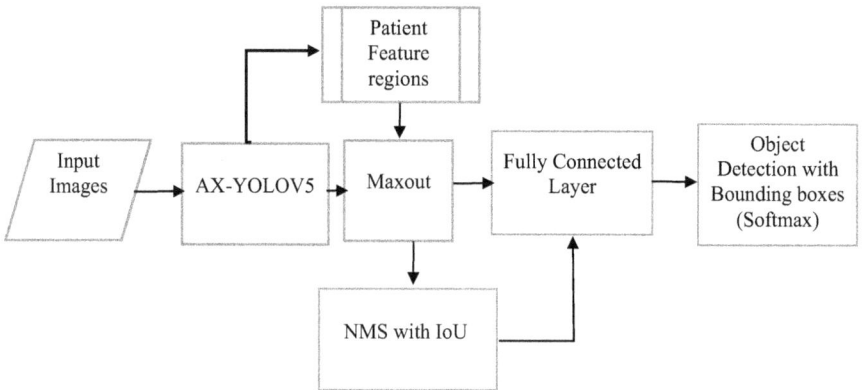

FIGURE 7.2   AX-YOLOV5-based patient discomfort approach.

(NMS) with confidence score is the best choice. This technique produces the confidence score for each bounding box based on the comparison of intersection over union (IoU), which produces various resolutions of bounding boxes for most of the organs. AX-YOLO V5 can handle different sizes of bounding boxes and feature extraction from an image parallelly. Due to this concurrent process some loss may occur in detecting the bounding boxes effectively. To evaluate the loss function by

$$B(l) = B(l)_{cl} + B(l)_r + B(l)_m \qquad (7.1)$$

In Eq. 7.1., B(l) represents the loss function evaluated from bounding boxes, $B(l)_{cl}$ denotes the categorization loss during classification process, $B(l)_r$ represents the regression loss and $B(l)_m$ loss function in masking the image. $B(l)_{cl}$ can be calculate by the formula

$$B(l)_{cl}(prob, T) = -loglog\ prob_T \qquad (7.2)$$

In Eq. 7.2., T represents the trueness of bounding boxes detection and *prob* denotes probability values of various bounding boxes represented as prob $= (p_i, p_{i+1}, p_{i+2}, \cdots p_{i+n})$. The regress loss can be calculated as

$$B(l)_r(R^T, G) = \sum_{a\epsilon\{a,c,b,h\}} L1(R - G) \qquad (7.3)$$

Where R={b,h,a,c}is the actual bounding boxes and $G^T = \{G_a^T, G_c^T, G_b^T, G_h^T\}$ green boundary boxes for the set *T*.
    In Eq. 7.3., $L1$ is represented as

$$L1 = \{0.5x^2,\ if|x| < 1|x| - 05,\ otherwise \qquad (7.4)$$

In Eq. (7.1), $B(l)_m$ denotes the overall losses of masking process, which produces the output is n_k^2 for all feature regions. In this, n represents a softmax mask with predefined width and height (w x h). $B(l)_m$ is calculated as follows

$$B(l)_m = \frac{1}{k^2}\sum_{xy}\left[S_{xy}logQ_{x,y}^T + \left(1 - S_{xy}log\left(1 - Q_{x,y}^T\right)\right)\right] \qquad (7.5)$$

In Eq. 7.5., S represents actual evaluated mask, which is represented by red color bounding boxes with only binary option {0,1}, and Q^T represents the predicted bounding boxes, which is denoted by green color.
    The deep learning model masks the 17 key points of the patience body that are available in MS-COCO dataset, which are right and left shoulder joints, knee joints, ankle joints, etc., which are listed in Table 7.1. Key point positions are continuously monitored to detect the discomforts of the patient from the video

TABLE 7.1

Recognized Key Points and Body Parts with ID

Index	Recognized Key Points	Body Parts with ID
0	Nose	Head
1	Left-Eye	(1)
2	Right-Eye	
3	Left-Ear	
4	Right-Ear	
5	Left-Shoulder	Left Arm
6	Left Elbow	(2)
7	Left-Wrist	
8	Right Elbow	Right Arm
9	Right-Shoulder	(3)
10	Right-Wrist	
11	Left-Hip	Left Leg
12	Left-Knee	(4)
13	Left-Ankle	
14	Right-Hip	Right Leg
15	Right-Knee	(5)
16	Right-Ankle	

sequences. In some cases, we predefined some of the actions of the patients to be considered as:

- If any rashes or pain happened in any of the places in the body at which point the patient continuously rubbed their respective places, which can be continuously monitored.
- When the patient shakes their hands, legs on both sides due to its pain, and sometimes massages their head repeatedly due to headache.

Those above constraints will vary based on the different diseases. To avoid such a situation, a generalized platform is created to identify the discomfort that can effectively monitor the patient's body movement for a long time. The body parts can be analyzed and tracked by their key points. To detect the movement of organs in the image frames, the Euclidean distance formula is applied in image frames. In Eq. 7.6, the Euclidean distance formula to detect the closest points nearby to the predefined boundary.

$$E = \sqrt{(j_{xj} - j_{xj-1})2 + (j_{xj} - j_{xj-1})2} \qquad (7.6)$$

The threshold value is set as default, which is compared with distance key points so that two different image frames were selected easily. The threshold value (T) conditions were monitored regularly by the following in Eq. 7.7:

$$T = \{1, \quad D > d_p \ 0, \quad Otherwise \tag{7.7}$$

The Eq. 7.8 identifies the distance between two consecutives image frames for ensuring the body movements. The patient's body is analyzed regularly through the various datasets.

$$Body = \{1, \ if \ \ V_{i=1}^n = 1 \ 0, \ Otherwise \tag{7.8}$$

The patient conditions were regularly followed by Eq. 7.9

$$ICon_{Patient} = \{Discomfort, \ body \rightarrow T_t \ Comfort, \ otherwise \tag{7.9}$$

$ICon_{Patient}$ represents the condition of a patient, which identifies the difference of comfort and discomfort. Once the model has trained with the image dataset, the prediction rate of the algorithm drastically improves to achieve approximately 99.25% result.

7.4 DATASET

The NTU RGB+D 125 dataset demonstrates how the created method locates key points of the human body at various locations. The important elements have been further organized into a bodily skeleton and six organs. After the key points have been found, the pairwise distance is examined using the related data for the key points. The patient's level of difficulty has been identified in accordance with time regulations.

The suggested experiments were carried out using a Radeon RX 5500 XT 8GB GPU, 32GB of DDR3 memory, and an Intel Core i7-7700 processor. The proposed model for object detection's training time can be reduced by using the graphical processing unit. With millions of video samples and 62 motion captures, NTU RGB +D 125 is a sizable dataset that contains RGB+D human action recognition. It is gathered. For each sample in this dataset, there are death map sequences, IR movies, RGB videos, and 3D skeletal data. Each frame of an RGB video has a resolution of 2560×1440 pixels, while an IR video frame has a resolution of 640×480 pixels. The proposed system comprises 3-D color pictures from the dataset to determine the health issue of patients.

7.5 IMPLEMENTATION OF AX-YOLOV5 ALGORITHM FOR DISCOMFORT DETECTION

1. Take the input from the NTU RGB+D dataset.
2. Maxout technique applied for pre-processing the input image to reduce the dimensionality.
3. Propose the effective region (i.e., ROI in an input image using AX-YOLOv5).
4. This step is continuously applied to non-maximum suppression techniques (NMS) to detect the single object from overlapping objects.

5. This is combined with IoU technique to calculate the confidence score for detecting the best bounding boxes.
6. Steps 3,4, and 5 are repeated until detecting the right bounding boxes.
7. Image frames are compared continuously for patient discomfort detection using Euclidean distance formula.
8. When Euclidean distance value is greater than or equal to threshold (Distance>=T), it is considered as discomfort, or else comfort.

7.6 MODEL TRAINING PHASE

The deep learning model AX-YOLOV5 was applied for the training process with a certain ratio of dataset in Radeon RX 5500 XT 8GB GPU, 32GB of DDR3 memory, and an Intel Core i7-7700 processor. The dataset was forwarded to a fully connected layer, which contains various hidden layers to analyze the content of images pixel by pixel. The training process takes place of 95 hours' time to understand the dataset properly, which helps to avoid overfitting issues. The correct proposition of training and testing process will perfectly work for any dataset easily.

We have used the TensorFlow framework to provide a better implementation of the YOLOv5 model. The proposed model attained enhanced performance with an average precision of 97.2%. To achieve more precise detection by the proposed model, ADAM optimization algorithm is used along with 0.0003 learning rate. The convergence rate is achieved at the 60th epoch.

7.7 PERFORMANCE METRICS

It is categorized in two metrics, which are regression and classification metrics. Regression metrics usually deal with continuous values in the relationship between predicted and actual. Likewise, classification metrics only consider the discrete values. These two categorized metrics are only applicable for supervised deep learning models. From these metrics, patient discomfort errors can be easily identified.

7.7.1 REGRESSION METRICS

7.7.1.1 Mean Absolute Error (MAE)
This metric finds the absolute error from the predicted and actual value of value. In this metric comparison of values between predicted and actual image frames calculated for predicting the discomfort, which is measured by the Eq. 7.10

$$MAE = \frac{1}{M} \sum_{j=1}^{M} \left| x_j - \hat{x}_j \right| \tag{7.10}$$

7.7.1.2 Mean Squared Deviation (MSD)
This metric finds the relationship between actual and predicted values. It removes the negative values automatically using the squaring function. If the model has errors in prediction, then the outcome abruptly shows an error. This is another form

of error spotting technique in patient health discomfort identification, which is measured by the Eq. 7.11

$$MSD = \frac{\Sigma(x_j - \hat{x}_j)^2}{M} \qquad (7.11)$$

7.7.1.3 Root Mean Squared Error (RMSE)

This metric predicts the error using Euclidean distance, which is the square root of mean square deviation. Mobility of the organs can be easily monitored by the Euclidean distance formula. This is calculated by the Eq. 7.12

$$RMSE = \sqrt{(MSD)} \qquad (7.12)$$

7.7.2 CLASSIFICATION METRICS

Classification metrics yield only discrete output in the form of True or False. There are various metrics under classification to evaluate the performance of a model.

7.7.2.1 Accuracy

Accuracy (A) is a metric categorized under classification, which accurately predicts the correct location of discomfort that can be implemented by predicting the true predictions from the total observations. This is represented by the Eq. 7.13

$$A = \frac{True\ Predictions}{Total\ Observations} \qquad (7.13)$$

Where True Predictions=TN+TP, Total Observations= TP+TN+FP+FN

Based on metrics of all of the input images, ground truth is manually created in order to assess the program's results. Each image's results from the approach were contrasted with the actual data. The following are the confusion matrices and corresponding performance measures:

- TP: Mobility is both observed and occurs in a specific body organ.
- TN: Mobility is neither observed nor experienced in a specific body organ.
- FP: Mobility is identified but it does not actually take place in a specific body organ.
- FN: Mobility takes place in a certain body organ but is not noticed.

From the aforementioned factors, many performance targets are derived, including TP, FP, accuracy, precision, and recall. Figures 7.3 and 7.4 display the typical TP, FP, as well as the loss rate for each body organ.

It recognizes several body organs in the collection of posture photographs with amazing accuracy. The average TP and FP are shown on the y-axis in Figures 7.3 and 7.4, while the x-axis shows various body parts. It can be shown that the average

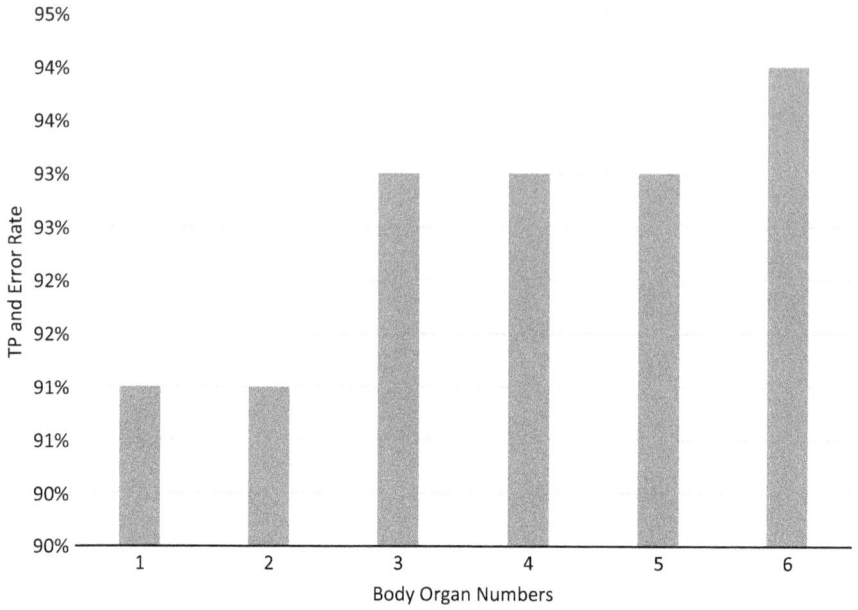

FIGURE 7.3   TP and error rate for different body organs.

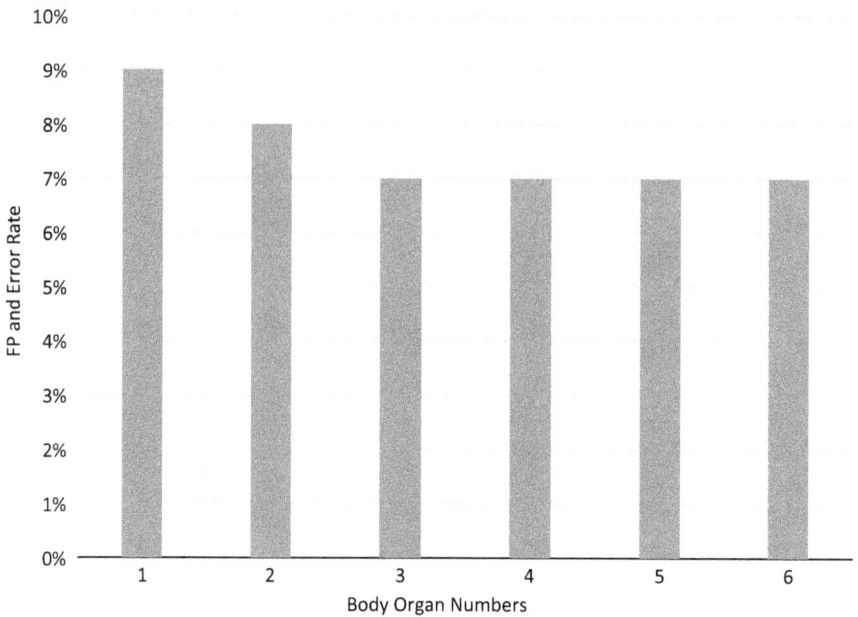

FIGURE 7.4   FP and error rate for different body organs.

TP for various body organs is more than 92%. The FPR fluctuates between 9% and 7% at the same period. We also provide the TP and FP error rates for various body organs, as shown in Figure 7.3 and 7.4. The standard deviation method was used to determine the error rate. As shown in Figures 7.3 to 7.8, we also determine the typical precision, TPR, accuracy, and PPV for various body parts.

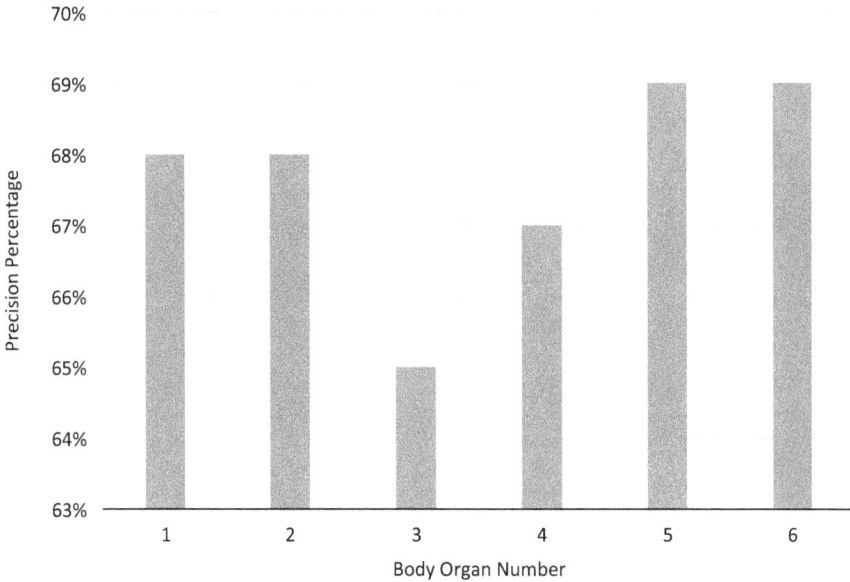

FIGURE 7.5 Average precision for different body organs.

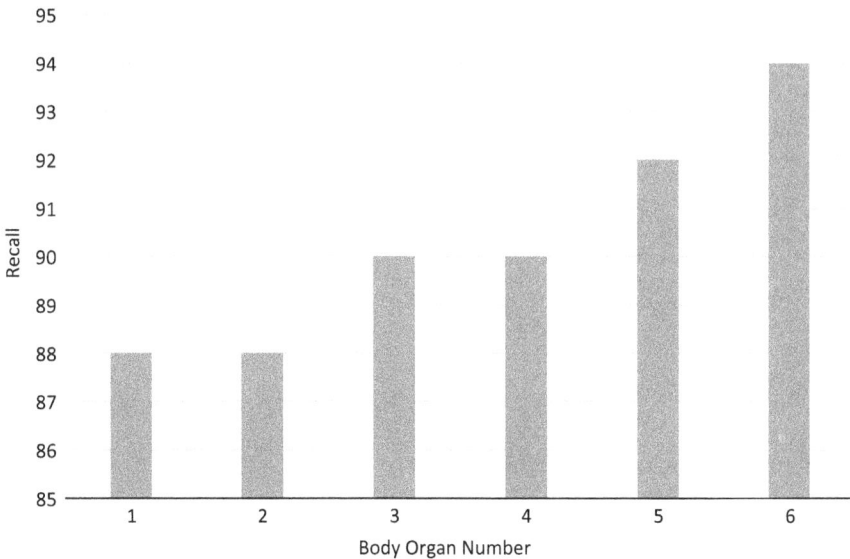

FIGURE 7.6 Recall for different body organs.

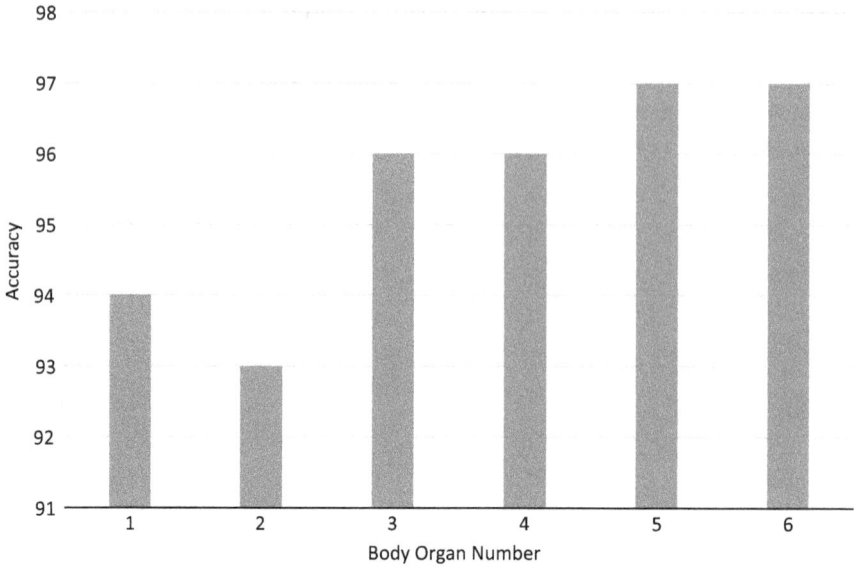

FIGURE 7.7   Accuracy for different body organs.

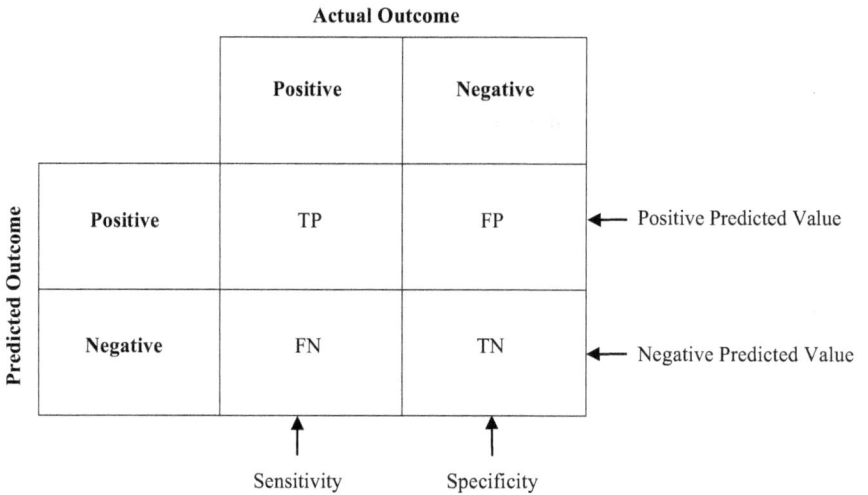

FIGURE 7.8   Error matrix.

7.7.2.2   Intersection Over Union (IoU)

IoU is an evaluation metric used to measure the accuracy in predicting object detection, which is measured by dividing the area of intersection of boxes and the area of union boxes. This method is widely used in object detection. It is measured by the following Eq. 7.14

$$IoU = \frac{Area\ of\ Intersection\ of\ boxes}{Area\ of\ Union\ Boxes} \tag{7.14}$$

Threshold (T) is set to be 0.5 and IoU =1 is the maximum value

if the value of IoU>=T, then the prediction is correct

or else the prediction is incorrect (i.e., the patient is not identified efficiently).

The y-axis in the figures display the AP, PPV, TPR, and accuracy values for the developed system, while the x-axis in the figures display the various body organs. Precision, recall, and accuracy values trade along with each body and organ movement. By detecting patient movement, key points, and bodily organs, it can be seen that the system produces accurate findings. All testing video sequences had accuracy rates that are higher than 91%. In a similar vein, the system's PPV rate is high, demonstrating that the majority of the detected key points and bodily organ movement values match the coordinate values of the ground truth. The same outcomes are produced at precision settings that roughly equal 70% and characterize the overall system performance in most cases.

7.7.2.3 Positive Predictive Value (PPV)

Usually the positive predicted value can be determined by the error matrix, which is represented in Figure 7.8

PPV, also known as precision, is used to classify only the positive observations from the dataset. This metric helps to identify the patient's health issues correctly, which can be measured by the following Eq. 7.15

$$PPV = \frac{True\ Positive}{Predicted\ Positive} \tag{7.15}$$

Where True Positive=TP, Predicted Positive=TP+FP

Performance evaluated based on mean average precision (mAP) with various values of IoU ranges between 0.55 and 0.97 with the fixed step size of 0.06. In 95 hours of training, AX-YOLOV5 trained with 15k step sizes with various ranges of IoU values.

Positive predicted value of the model had various sizes of mAP values in the form of bounding boxes such as mAP(s), mAP(m), mAP(l), and mAP(xl). Here, small, medium, large, and extra-large classified IoU values ranged between 0.5 and 1.0, which is mentioned in Table 7.2.

TABLE 7.2
PPV Values of VGG NET-19–Based AX-YOLOV5 with Various IoU

S.No	Parameters Evaluation Metrics	mAP Score
1	Bounding Box PPV-mAP(s)	0.674412755
2	Bounding Box PPV-mAP(m)	0.674412755
3	Bounding Box PPV-mAP(l)	1.0
4	Bounding Box PPV-mAP(xl)	0.87124484

TABLE 7.3
mAP Metrics vs Step Size

Metrics	520	2.5k	5k	7.5k	10k	12.5k	15k
mAP(s)	0.5015	0.5976	0.7256	0.7566	0.7587	0.7887	0.7987
mAP(m)	0.5015	0.5977	0.6792	0.7092	0.7556	0.7890	0.7987
mAP(l)	0.8915	0.8999	0.9204	0.9489	0.9845	0.9967	1.0
mAP(xl)	0.4957	0.5967	0.8233	0.8345	0.8768	0.9180	0.9456

The comparison of mAP metric values with step size is represented in Table 7.3.
The mAP metrics with number of iterations start with 520 to 15k with step size of 0.06. This table clearly reveals that the large parameter produced by the IoU values ranges from 0.8915 to 1.0. The conclusion from the table is that mAP(l) predicts the region effectively at the step of 15k.

7.7.2.4 Prevalence

Prevalence is one of the metrics of error matrix, which covers only the portion of positive outcome by the total outcomes. This metric only takes the positive prediction from the human body, which can be measured by the Eq. 7.16

$$P = \frac{Actual\ Positive}{Total\ Observations} \qquad (7.16)$$

Where Actual Positive= FN+TP, Total Observations= TP+TN+FP+FN

7.7.2.5 Sensitivity

Sensitivity is also called as true positive rate or recall. This metric is suitable for analyzing the positive test cases correctly, making it is easy to predict the diagnosis of body organs issues perfectly. It can be measured by the Eq. 7.17

$$S = \frac{True\ Positives}{Actual\ True} \qquad (7.17)$$

Where True Positives= TP, Actual True= TP+FN.
In this, it focuses only on sensitive areas with different sizes of pixels such as small, medium, large and extra-large. The iteration process starts from 520 to 15k steps. True positive rate of the model with various sizes of mAP values in the form of bounding boxes such as mAP(s), mAP(m), mAP(l), mAP(xl). Here small, medium, large, and extra-large classified based IoU values range between 0.5 and 1.0, which is mentioned in Table 7.4.
The comparison of TPR metric values with step size is represented in Table 7.5.

7.7.2.6 False Negative Rate (FNR)

The FNR metric only calculates the false negative (i.e., wrongly predicted cases). Usually, in the body organ diagnosis process, some percentage of flaws

TABLE 7.4
TPR Values of VGG NET-19–Based AX-YOLOV5 with Various IoU

S.No	Parameters Evaluation Metrics	mAP Score
1	Bounding Box TPR -mAP(s)	0.7991085
2	Bounding Box TPR -mAP(m)	0.7991085
3	Bounding Box TPR -mAP(l)	0.7991085
4	Bounding Box TPR -mAP(xl)	0.7991085

TABLE 7.5
TPR Metrics vs Step Size

Metrics	520	2.5k	5k	7.5k	10k	12.5k	15k
TPR(s)	0.7838	0.7957	0.8230	0.8828	0.8891	0.8962	0.9228
TPR(m)	0.7838	0.7957	0.8230	0.8828	0.8891	0.8962	0.9228
TPR(l)	0.7838	0.7957	0.8230	0.8828	0.8891	0.8962	0.9228
TPR(xl)	0.7838	0.7957	0.8230	0.8828	0.8768	0.8962	0.9228

or errors happen that can be identified by FNR, which can be measured by the Eq. 7.18

$$FNR = \frac{False\ Negatives}{Actual\ True} \qquad (7.18)$$

Where False Negatives=FN, Actual True = TP + FN

7.7.2.7 False Positive Rate (FPR)

The FPR metric is also called the miss rate. It is used to predict the outcome wrongly (e.g., pregnant instead of not pregnant). This will calculate the error rate of the AX-YOLOV5 model, which can be calculated by the Eq. 7.19

$$FPR = \frac{False\ Positive}{Actual\ False} \qquad (7.19)$$

Where False Positive=FP, Actual False = TN + FP

7.7.2.8 Specificity

Specificity is a metric for predicting the negative cases correctly. This metric is very useful in predicting negative issues of the body organ effectively, which can be measured by the Eq. 7.20

$$SP = \frac{True\ Negatives}{Actual\ False} \qquad (7.20)$$

Where True Negatives = TN, Actual False = TN + FP

7.7.2.9 F1-Score

F1-score metric is the combination of positive predictive value (PPV) and sensitivity (S). This metric can be used instead of accuracy when the data are uneven. It is represented by the harmonic mean of the above two metrics. This can be effective in predicting the discomfort of a patient's body organs even if the values are uneven, which can be measured by the Eq. 7.21

$$F1 - Score = \frac{PPV_*S}{PPV + S} \qquad (7.21)$$

The AX-YOLOV5 model based VGGNET-19 shows better performance in detecting patient's discomfort than other neural networks.

7.8 COMPARATIVE RESULTS

Surveying the results of various deep learning models from the various research papers, the following result is consolidated, which is represented in Table 7.6.

Comparison of training time and number of steps with various neural networks is discussed in Table 7.7. Comparison of mean average precision metric with the present work is discussed in Table 7.8.

TABLE 7.6
Comparison of CNN, PPV, TPR and F1-Score

Model	Neural Network	PPV	TPR	F1-Score
AX-YOLOV5	VGG NET-19	84.1%	89.2%	89.7%
	Darknet53	79.5%	77.4%	79.82%
	ResNet-50	82.5%	81.4%	80.06%

TABLE 7.7
Performance Evaluation of Various Neural Networks

Model	Neural Network	Training Time (hrs)	No. of Steps
AX-YOLOV5	VGG NET-19	95	15 K
	Darknet53	40	9 K
	ResNet-50	62	13 K

TABLE 7.8

Performance Evaluation of mAP Metric Various Neural Networks

Model	Neural Network	mAP
AX-YOLOV5	VGG NET-19	82.3%
	Darknet53	74.2%
	ResNet-50	76.1%

7.9 CONCLUSION

Arbitrary Extra-large You Only Look Once version 5 (AX-YOLOV5) is one of the best object detection variants of the Yolo family. This version works better for detecting extra-large objects effectively in an image frame. The proposed system continuously monitors the movements of patient's organs effectively from the IP camera. This methodology is applied with various performance metrics in terms of regression and classification. In this system, three neural networks, such as VGG NET-19, Darknet53, and ResNet-50, accompanied separately with the AX-YOLOV5 model to identify the performance of the neural network based on four metrics (PPV, TPR, F1-Score, mAP). Based on experimental results, AX-YOLOV5 with VGGNET-19 produces the highest PPV (84.1%), TPR (89.2%), F1-Score (89.7%), and mAP (82.3%). When VGGNET-19 is compared with the other two neural networks, it performs well in detecting the patient's body organ key points.

REFERENCES

1. Ahmed, I., Camacho, D., Jeon, G., & Piccialli, F. (2022). Internet of health things driven deep learning-based systems for non-invasive patient discomfort detection using time frame rules and pairwise keypoints distance feature. *Sustainable Cities and Society*, *79*, 103672.
2. Liz, H., Sánchez-Montañés, M., Tagarro, A., Domínguez-Rodríguez, S., Dagan, R., & Camacho, D. (2021). Ensembles of convolutional neural network models for pediatric pneumonia diagnosis. *Future Generation Computer Systems*, *122*, 220–233.
3. Ahmed, I., Jeon, G., & Piccialli, F. (2021). A deep-learning-based smart healthcare system for patient's discomfort detection at the edge of internet of things. *IEEE Internet of Things Journal*, *8*(13), 10318–10326.
4. Rootjes, P. A., Nubé, M. J., de Roij van Zuijdewijn, C. L., Wijngaarden, G., & Grooteman, M. P. (2021). Effect of various dialysis modalities on intradialytic hemodynamics, tissue injury and patient discomfort in chronic dialysis patients: Design of a randomized cross-over study (HOLLANT). *BMC Nephrology*, *22*(1), 1–10.
5. Kimura, A., Mitsukura, Y., Oya, A., Matsumoto, M., Nakamura, M., Kanaji, A., & Miyamoto, T. (2021). Objective characterization of hip pain levels during walking by combining quantitative electroencephalography with machine learning. *Scientific Reports*, *11*(1), 1–10.
6. Sun, Y., Hu, J., Wang, W., He, M., & de With, P. H. (2021). Camera-based discomfort detection using multi-channel attention 3D-CNN for hospitalized infants. *Quantitative Imaging in Medicine and Surgery*, 11(7), 3059.

7. Elevado, A. Z., Sagao, E., Sales, A. F., Ibarra, J. B., & Valiente, L. (2021, June). Discomfort monitoring system using IoT applied to a wheelchair. In 2021 IEEE International Conference on Automatic Control & Intelligent Systems (I2CACIS) (pp. 120–125). IEEE.

8. Shu, F., & Shu, J. (2021). An eight-camera fall detection system using human fall pattern recognition via machine learning by a low-cost android box. *Scientific Reports*, *11*(1), 2471.

9. Leng, J., Lin, Z., & Wang, P. (2020). Poster abstract: An implementation of an Internet of Things system for smart hospitals. In 2020 IEEE/ACM Fifth International Conference on Internet-of-Things Design and Implementation (IoTDI), Australia (pp. 254–255). doi: 10.1109/ IoTDI49375.2020.00034.

10. Wang, X., & Jia, K. (2020, July). Human fall detection algorithm based on YOLOv3. In 2020 IEEE 5th International Conference on Image, Vision and Computing (ICIVC) (pp. 50–54). IEEE.

11. Hussein, R., & Ward, R. (2020). Energy-efficient EEG monitoring systems for wireless epileptic seizure detection. *Energy efficiency of medical devices and healthcare applications*, Elsevier, pp. 69–85, 2020.

12. Marchenko, A., & Temeljotov-Salaj, A. (2020). A systematic literature review of non-invasive indoor thermal discomfort detection. *Applied Sciences*, *10*(12), 4085.

13. Li, C., Pourtaherian, A., Van Onzenoort, L., a Ten, W. E. T., & de With, P. H. (2020). Infant monitoring system for real-time and remote discomfort detection. *IEEE Transactions on Consumer Electronics*, *66*(4), 336–345.

14. Yang, B., Li, X., Hou, Y., Meier, A., Cheng, X., Choi, J. H., … & Li, H. (2020). Non-invasive (non-contact) measurements of human thermal physiology signals and thermal comfort/discomfort poses-a review. *Energy and Buildings*, *224*, 110261.

15. Ding, Y., Cao, Y., Duffy, V. G., & Zhang, X. (2020). It is time to have rest: How do break types affect muscular activity and perceived discomfort during prolonged sitting work. *Safety and Health at Work*, *11*(2), 207–214.

16. Kwak, G. H., Kwak, E. J., Song, J. M., Park, H. R., Jung, Y. H., Cho, B. H., … & Hwang, J. J. (2020). Automatic mandibular canal detection using a deep convolutional neural network. *Scientific Reports*, *10*(1), 5711.

17. Marchenko, A., Temeljotov-Salaj, A., Rizzardi, V., & Oksavik, O. (2020). The study of facial muscle movements for non-invasive thermal discomfort detection via bio-sensing technology. Part I: Development of the experimental design and description of the collected data. *Applied Sciences*, *10*(20), 7315.

18. Piccialli, F., Casolla, G., Cuomo, S., Giampaolo, F., & Di Cola, V. S. (2019). Decision making in IoT environment through unsupervised learning. *IEEE Intelligent Systems*, *35*(1), 27–35.

19. Liu, J., Shahroudy, A., & Perez, M. (2019). NTU RGB+D 120: A large-scale benchmark for 3D human activity understanding. *IEEE Transactions on Pattern Analysis and Machine Intelligence*, *42*, 2684–2701.

20. Sun, Y., Shan, C., Tan, T., Long, X., Pourtaherian, A., Zinger, S., & de With, P. H. (2019). Video-based discomfort detection for infants. *Machine Vision and Applications*, *30*, 933–944.

21. Sun, Y., Shan, C., Tan, T., Tong, T., Wang, W., & Pourtaherian, A. (2019). Detecting discomfort in infants through facial expressions. *Physiological Measurement*, *40*(11), 115006.

22. Rajamhoana, S. P., Devi, C. A., Umamaheswari, K., Kiruba, R., Karunya, K., & Deepika, R. (2018, July). Analysis of neural networks based heart disease prediction system. In 2018 11th International Conference on Human System Interaction (HSI) (pp. 233–239). IEEE.

23. Fang, H.-S., Xie, S., Tai, Y.-W., & Lu, C. (2017). Rmpe: Regional multi-person pose estimation. In Proceedings of the IEEE International Conference on Computer Vision (pp. 2334–2343).

24. Cho, Y., Julier, S. J., Marquardt, N., & Bianchi-Berthouze, N. (2017). Robust tracking of respiratory rate in high-dynamic range scenes using mobile thermal imaging. *Biomed Opt Express*, *13* (8), 4480–4503. 10.1364/BOE.8.004480.

25. Rotariu, C., Bozomitu, R. G., Pasarica, A., Arotaritei, D., & Costin, H. (2017). Medical system based on wireless sensors for real time remote monitoring of people with disabilities. 2017 E-Health and Bioengineering Conference *(EHB)*, Sinaia, Romania (pp. 753–756). 10.1109/EHB.2017.7995533.

26. Lin, F., Zhuang, Y., Song, C., Wang, A., Li, Y., Gu, C., Li, C., & Xu, W. (2017). SleepSense: A noncontact and cost-effective sleep monitoring system. *IEEE Transactions on Biomedical Circuits and Systems*, *11*(1), 189–202. 10.1109/TBCAS.2016.2541680.

27. Lin, T. Y., Dollár, P., Girshick, R., He, K., Hariharan, B., & Belongie, S. (2017). Feature pyramid networks for object detection. In Proceedings of the IEEE Conference on Computer Vision and Pattern Recognition (pp. 2117–2125).

28. Liu, S., & Ostadabbas, S. (2017). A vision-based system for in-bed posture tracking. In Proceedings of the IEEE International Conference on Computer Vision Workshops (pp. 1373–1382).

29. Shahroudy, A., Liu, J., Ng, T-T, & Wang, G. (2016). NTU RGB+D: A large-scale dataset for 3D human activity analysis. IEEE Conference on Computer Vision and Pattern Recognition (pp. 1010–1019).

30. Merrouche, F., & Baha, N. (2016, August). Depth camera based fall detection using human shape and movement. In 2016 IEEE International Conference on Signal and Image Processing (ICSIP) (pp. 586–590). IEEE.

31. Zhang, C., Kjellström, H., Ek, C. H., & Bertilson, B. (2016, December). Diagnostic prediction using discomfort drawings with IBTM. In Machine Learning for Healthcare Conference (pp. 226–238). PMLR.

32. Ren, S., He, K., Girshick, R., & Sun, J. (2015). Faster R-CNN: Towards real-time object detection with region proposal networks. *Advances in Neural Information Processing Systems*, *28*.

33. Khan, R. A., Meyer, A., Konik, H., & Bouakaz, S. Pain detection through shape and appearance features. In 2013 IEEE International Conference on Multimedia and Expo (ICME) (pp. 1–6). IEEE, 2013.

34. Sokolova, M. V., Serrano-Cuerda, J., Castillo, J. C., & Fernández-Caballero, A. (2013). A fuzzy model for human fall detection in infrared video. *Journal of Intelligent & Fuzzy Systems*, *24*(2), 215–228.

35. Yu, M. C., Wu, H., Liou, J. L., Lee, M. S., & Hung, Y. P. (2012). Multiparameter sleep monitoring using a depth camera. International Joint Conference on Biomedical Engineering Systems and Technologies, Springer, Vol. 357, pp. 311–325. 10.1007/978-3-642-38256-7_21

36. Rougier, C., Meunier, J., St-Arnaud, A., & Rousseau, J. (2011). Robust video surveillance for fall detection based on human shape deformation. *IEEE Transactions on Circuits and Systems for Video Technology*, *21*(5), 611–622.

37. Fu, Y., Li, S., Yin, M., & Bian, Y. (2009). Simulation-based discomfort prediction of the lower limb handicapped with prosthesis in the climbing tasks. In Digital Human Modeling: Second International Conference, ICDHM 2009, Held as Part of HCI International 2009, San Diego, CA, USA, July 19-24, 2009. Proceedings 2 (pp. 512–520). Springer Berlin Heidelberg.

38. Leung, F. W. (2008). Methods of reducing discomfort during colonoscopy. *Digestive Diseases and Sciences*, *53*, 1462–1467.

39. Christiansen, R., Kirkevang, L. L., Hørsted-Bindslev, P., & Wenzel, A. (2008). Patient discomfort following periapical surgery. *Oral Surgery, Oral Medicine, Oral Pathology, Oral Radiology, and Endodontology, 105*(2), 245–250.
40. Polat, Ö. (2007, December). Pain and discomfort after orthodontic appointments. In *Seminars in orthodontics* (Vol. 13, No. 4, pp. 292–300). WB Saunders.
41. Marcus, G. M., Cohen, J., Varosy, P. D., Vessey, J., Rose, E., Massie, B. M., … & Waters, D. (2007). The utility of gestures in patients with chest discomfort. *The American Journal of Medicine, 120*(1), 83–89.
42. A. B. Ashraf, S. Lucey, J. F. Cohn, T. Chen, Z. Ambadar et al. (2009). The painful face-pain expression recognition using active appearance models. *Image and Vision Computing, 27* (12), 1788–1796.
43. Mitsumune, T., Senoh, E., & Adachi, M. (2005). Prediction of patient discomfort during fibreoptic bronchoscopy. *Respirology, 10*(1), 92–96.
44. van de Leur, J. P., van der Schans, C. P., Loef, B. G., Deelman, B. G., Geertzen, J. H., & Zwaveling, J. H. (2004). Discomfort and factual recollection in intensive care unit patients. *Critical Care, 8*, 1–7.
45. MacGougan, C. K., Christenson, J. M., Innes, G. D., & Raboud, J. (2001). Emergency physicians' attitudes toward a clinical prediction rule for the identification and early discharge of low risk patients with chest discomfort. *Canadian Journal of Emergency Medicine, 3*(2), 89–94.
46. Kim, W. H., Cho, Y. J., Park, J. Y., Min, P. K., Kang, J. K., & Park, I. S. (2000). Factors affecting insertion time and patient discomfort during colonoscopy. *Gastrointestinal Endoscopy, 52*(5), 600–605.
47. Hurley, A. C., Volicer, B. J., Hanrahan, P. A., Houde, S., & Volicer, L. (1992). Assessment of discomfort in advanced Alzheimer patients. *Research in Nursing & Health, 15*(5), 369–377.
48. Gills, J. P., Cherchio, M., & Raanan, M. G. (1997). Unpreserved lidocaine to control discomfort during cataract surgery using topical anesthesia. *Journal of Cataract & Refractive Surgery, 23*(4), 545–550.
49. Sathiyamoorthi, V., Ilavarasi, A. K., Murugeswari, K., Thouheed Ahmed, S., Aruna Devi, B., & Kalipindi, M. (2021). A deep convolutional neural network based computer aided diagnosis system for the prediction of Alzheimer's disease in MRI images. *Measurement, 171*, 108838, ISSN 0263-2241, 10.1016/j.measurement.2020.108838.

8 Gesture Identification for Hearing-Impaired through Deep Learning

M. Maragatharajan

School of Computing Science and Engineering, VIT Bhopal University, Kothrikalan, Bhopal, Madhya Pradesh, India

S.P. Balakannan

Department of Information Technology, Kalasalingam Academy of Research and Education, Krishnankoil, Tamil Nadu, India

C. Balasubramanian

Department of Computer Science and Engineering, Kalasalingam Academy of Research and Education, Krishnankoil, Tamil Nadu, India

P. Naveen

Department of Electrical and Electronics Engineering, KPR Institute of Engineering and Technology, Coimbatore, Tamil Nadu, India

8.1 INTRODUCTION

According to the report propagated by the World Health Organization (WHO), it is estimated that around the world there could be more than a billion disabled people. Among this group, the report further mentioned, there are 360 million people handicapped by hearing impairment. People affected by this hearing impairment undergo a large number of unpleasant experiences in their daily life. They face challenging situations in education, jobs, professions, and personal lives, thereby being unable to lead a comfortable and happy life [1].

It is high time that this sort of grievance among the hearing-impaired category of people should be provided with a technological solution. Hence, efforts can be made to offer them advanced assistive technologies and access to their needs. Nevertheless, such technologies should be affordable and as per their core needs. This work focuses on a concept of assistive technologies that can help them lead somewhat normal lives in order to meet their needs [2,3]. Furthermore, they will be

DOI: 10.1201/9781003469605-8

free of the difficulties that come with hearing loss. Having analyzed all these factors, this work devised the prime objective of developing a cost-effective and easy-to-access communication means for deaf-dumb people [4]. It is presumed that this approach will ease them from making use of sign language or any other non-verbal communication. During the research analysis, it was found that this category of deaf-dumb employed some visual media other than sign language. As a result, the primary goal of this effort would be to develop an improved communication platform that deaf and mute people may readily utilize.

Hearing sounds and words, according to the American Speech Language Hearing Association, aids in learning, communication, and comprehension. Those with hearing loss cannot hear these sounds. This can lead to difficulties with speaking, reading, academic achievement, and social skills. If you suspect that a person has trouble hearing, it is essential to test them. Hearing loss can result in delayed speech development, learning difficulties, etc.

The difficulty of discerning speech from background noise is a common issue among people with hearing loss. Despite significant efforts to develop hearing technology, this issue remains fairly disabling. Sensorineural hearing loss of cochlear origin is characterized by an increase in audiometric thresholds and a subsequent decrease in audibility. Because they commonly detect powerful sounds at ordinary loudness, these listeners demonstrate a rapid increase in loudness as signal strength increases, limiting their dynamic range. Reduced audibility is one of the challenges that hearing-impaired listeners confront. Speech recognition in silence can be acceptable for many hearing-impaired people since current hearing aids do a decent job of amplifying sounds in a way that is appropriate for each ear. Hearing impaired listeners have difficulty understanding speech in noisy situations as a result of these restrictions, and finding a solution to this problem is equally difficult. Modern hearing technology uses microphone arrays to improve speech comprehension in noisy environments. Beamforming, also known as spatial filtering, dampens sound from one direction while enhancing sound from another. The most basic method (delay-and-sum) assumes that the noise is generated elsewhere and that the signal of interest is at zero azimuth. In adaptive beamforming, a main microphone that takes up both the target speech and the noise is utilized to subtract the noise from the target speech in order to cancel out the noise source.

In practice, as mentioned earlier, deaf-dumb people make use of several visual references in communication, apart from common sign language. Recent years have witnessed a remarkable volume of research done on hand gestures [5]. The following basic steps in hand gesture have been observed, based upon a literature review.

- Data acquisition
- Data pre-processing
- Feature extraction
- Gesture classification

The remaining part of the paper is organized as follows: Section II deals with the existing work and Section III deals with the proposed work. Section IV discusses the conclusion.

8.2 EXISTING WORK

This work involves the basic idea of employing a normal camera, aided by the tasks carried out with the aid of a machine learning algorithm. This algorithm can recognize the patterns found on the hand in addition to providing real-time text output [6]. The plan of the entire work is spread across processes in a single system: a study on Image Classification Using Deep Learning and TensorFlow [7] and Gesture Recognition Method Based on Computer Vision. Several speech augmentation algorithms were tested on a variety of speech datasets by Zhuohuang Zhang et al., with an emphasis on hearing loss simulation settings [8]. For listeners with normal hearing, the recurrent neural network (RNN)-based techniques produce noticeably higher PESQ and HASQI scores. The BLSTM technique delivers the best results for hearing-impaired listeners of all ages and genders. They also found that mel-frequency domain processing frequently leads to higher PESQ scores and lower HASQI scores for both DNN-based and RNN-based techniques. The inability of hearing-impaired listeners to comprehend speech while another talker is present was demonstrated by Eric W. Healy et al. [9], who also showed how well hearing listeners are able to do this. A deep neural network (DNN)-based algorithm was created to solve this problem after the probable reasons for it were looked into. A special set of properties gleaned from the voice signals were used to train the DNN. The advantages of the proposed approach enabled young listeners who are not deaf to function on par with listeners who are deaf under identical background noise interference settings (in the absence of the algorithm). To our knowledge, this is the first monaural (single-microphone) algorithm that significantly improves hearing-impaired listeners' comprehension of speech when it is competing with other speech.

8.2.1 DATA ACQUISITION

The common methods applied in gathering data on hand gestures are listed below [10]:

1. **Sensory instruments:** Electromechanical instruments are employed to provide hand configuration and positioning in a precise manner. Alternatively, various glove-based methods are available to extract any sort of information.
2. **Vision-based approach:** This approach makes use of an input device in the form of a computer camera to observe and record information from hands or fingers. The vision-based methods employ just a camera by which natural interactions between humans and computers can be facilitated. In this method, no other equipment is necessary for communication.

However, the challenging task in vision-based hand detection is to manage and cope with the increased variables found in the appearance of human hands. This is chiefly due to the occurrence of varied movements and the reflection of different skin shades on humans. Differentials in viewpoints, scales, and the capture speed rate of the camera also contribute to this challenge. We have formed exclusive datasets to arrive at comparative elements of this algorithm's performance efficiency. As per the literature survey, several algorithms have been in practice, leading us to choose the best one. Thus, our study engaged in the performance analysis of a few worthy algorithms related to the proposed concept.

8.2.2 DATA PREPROCESSING

In this research work, trials were conducted on segmenting the hand by making use of an image with the aid of segmentation techniques. Still, as mentioned in the previous context, the outputs for the inputs fed in the trials were not up to the mark of greatness. This is due to the variations in skin color, lighting conditions, and scaling during the segmentation process. Further, the task involved the application of a huge volume of symbols having similarities, which challenged the training of gestures, for example, the alphabet "V" and the numerical "2". Based on this observation, we planned the approach to achieve better accuracies for the voluminous input symbols. As a result, the hand segmentation was replaced by the background of a stable skin hand. This saved segmentation of the hand on skin color.

8.2.3 FEATURE EXTRACTION

Feature extraction is an ideal process for hand detection in which the combination of threshold-based color detection with background subtraction is applied. The differentiation between faces and hands based on skin is done by using an Ad Boost face detector. Furthermore, the necessary image to be trained can be extracted by applying Gaussian blur filters. The filter is easy to apply by using open computer vision, which is also known as OpenCV and is described in Figure 8.1, which shows the grayscale image of a hand gesture. After applying Gaussian algorithms, the gray color of the image will disappear, and the resultant image is shown in Figure 8.2.

8.2.4 GESTURE CLASSIFICATION

Hidden Markov Models (HMMs) were used to classify motions, allowing for the evaluation of numerous characteristics of a gesture. Gestures are frequently retrieved from a set or collection of video images. In this case, the skin-color blobs from the hand are mapped into the body-facial space of the user's face. The primary goal of

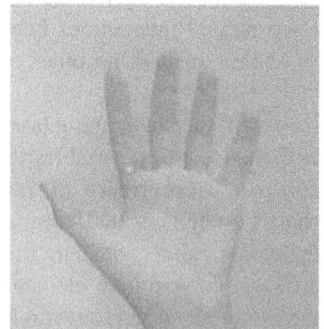

FIGURE 8.1 Gray scale image.

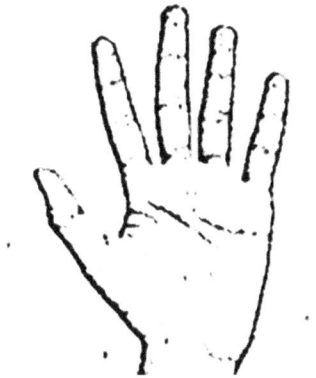

FIGURE 8.2   After applying Gaussian algorithm.

this technique is to differentiate between deictic and symbolic movements. To filter the photographs in this operation, an indexing database for quick look-ups is used. Skin-color pixels combine to form blobs during post-filtering.

Blobs are typically thought of as statistical objects used to identify homogenous areas. The location (x,y) and color vertices (Y,U,V) of skin color pixels are used to make this determination. The Naive Bayes classifier was utilized in the proposed investigation to enable effectiveness and a quick method in the recognition of static hand movements. When segmentation is complete, various motions are categorized based on the extraction of geometric invariants from the visual input. One method that is unaffected by a person's skin tone is this one. By using a static background, it is possible to get gestures from each frame of the film. In the initial stage of the retrieval, segmentation, labeling, and extraction of geometric invariants from the objects of interest are done [11].

The sequence of the process consists of constructing a skin model for extracting the handout of an image, followed by the application of the binary threshold to the whole image [12]. Once the threshold image is obtained, the calibration about the principal axis to center the image occurs. This image is fed as an input to a convolutional neural network model for training and predicting the outputs. The model was trained over seven hand gestures, and the use of this model yielded an accuracy of about 95% for those seven gestures.

8.3   PROPOSED WORK

In the proposed work, research methodology included primary capturing of the hand's signs through the camera. These images were extracted in the form of frames, preferably in large volumes for better results. However, it is true that the extraction of many frames may incur additional time. These frames are collected by the processing unit, which in turn will examine the exact inference of each frame. In this regard, the process is highly enabled by image processing and deep learning. Though the method may appear simple, the constraints involved in real terms take many forms, including configuration of the analyzing processor, specification of hand gestures, and application of an exclusive algorithm for individual frames. All these tasks prove to be challenging as well as complex. Though several algorithms exist for this purpose, choosing the most appropriate to suit the proposed objective is the major task. This choice requires more time and physical effort since many of them are patented with specified applications. Based on these reservations and constraints, we finalized two specific algorithms, which are Canny edge Detection and SURF (Speeded Up Robust Features).

8.3.1 DEEP LEARNING ALGORITHMS

Machine learning offers huge promise for solving a wide range of everyday problems. It frequently performs tasks such as categorization, naming, detection, and forecasting. The automation of data-driven procedures is also incredibly efficient. The primary idea is to use data to create a model that can produce results. If a new input is provided, the outcome may provide an appropriate response or may offer predictions for previously accessible data.

This paper's objective is to train a deep learning system that can recognize photos of various hand motions, including a fist, palm, showing the thumb, and others. For example, gesture navigation can benefit from solving this specific classification challenge. Convolutional neural networks built with the aid of deep learning and based on TensorFlow and Kera's will be used in the procedure.

Deep learning is built on the utilization of layers that process the input data, extract features from it, and create a mathematical model.

This makes use of the Kaggle-hosted Hand Gesture Recognition Database. It includes 20,000 pictures of various hands and hand gestures. The data set contains a total of 10 hand motions made by 10 different individuals. There are 5 male and 5 female participants. The Leap Motion hand tracking device was used to take the pictures.

With that, we need to get the photos ready for algorithm training. Both the labels and the photos must be loaded into separate arrays, X and Y, respectively.

We will employ the idea of linear regression to make the model's construction concept more understandable. We can make a simple model and use the equation to describe it. This is called "linear regression."

In the equation $y = axe + b$, where a and b are slope and intercept, respectively, we can forecast y by determining the optimal parameters for any given value of x. The use of convolutional neural networks makes the same concept considerably more intricate.

A convolutional neural network (ConvNet or CNN) is a deep learning technique capable of taking in an input image, assigning importance (learnable weights and biases) to various traits and objects in the image, and differentiating between them. In comparison to other classification methods, a ConvNet requires significantly less pre-processing.

Using the information from Figure 8.3 and the linear regression model equation we discussed, we can assume that the input layer is represented by x and the output layer is represented by y. Different models have different hidden layers, but they are all used to "learn" the parameters for our model. Although they each serve a different purpose, they all strive to get the best "slope and intercept."

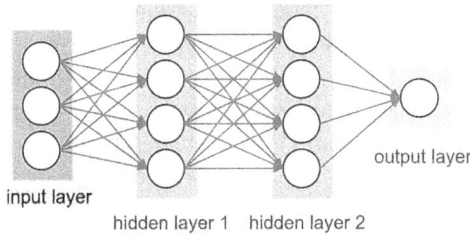

input layer

hidden layer 1   hidden layer 2

output layer

FIGURE 8.3 Example of convolutional neural network.

To extract and learn higher-level properties from the raw pixel data of an image, CNNs apply a series of filters. The model can then use these properties for categorization. CNN consists of three sections.

- Convolutional layers, which apply a preset number of convolution filters to an image. Each subregion is subjected to a series of calculations by the layer, which results in a single value for the output feature map. Convolutional layers frequently use a ReLU activation function to the output to inject nonlinearities into the model.
- Pooling layers, which reduce the dimensionality of the feature map to down sample the image data generated by the convolutional layers and accelerate processing. The "max pooling" pooling process takes areas of the feature map (such as 2×2 pixel tiles), keeps the maximum value of those portions, and discards all other values.
- Denser (fully connected) layers that classify the features down sampled by the convolutional and pooling layers.

We may infer from the findings in the preceding section that our system correctly categorizes various hand gesture photographs with sufficient confidence based on a deep learning model.

A few elements of our situation directly affect how accurate our model is. The gestures displayed are rather distinct, and the visuals are without a background. Furthermore, there are a respectable number of photos, which strengthens our model. The disadvantage is that we would probably need additional data for various challenges to move the model's parameters in the right direction. A deep learning model's abstractions make it extremely challenging to understand. Although this method eliminates the need to take feature engineering into account, it makes it much simpler to begin working on the actual problem. This means that CNN automatically extracts the key features from the photos without us having to pre-process them using edge or blob detectors. Additionally, it performs well overall and can be quickly modified to solve new issues.

8.3.2 CANNY EDGE DETECTION ALGORITHMS (CEDA)

The multi-stage edge detection technique used by the canny edge detection algorithm can identify many different types of image edges. Edge tracking with hysteresis, noise detection, gradient computation, non-maximum suppression, double threshold, and maximum suppression are the main parts of this method [13].

The results of edge detection are quite sensitive to image noise because mathematics is mostly reliant on derivatives. Image noise can be eliminated in one way by smoothing the image with Gaussian blur. The image convolution method using a Gaussian kernel (3×3, 5×5, 7×7, etc.) is used to accomplish this. The desired blurring effect determines the kernel's size. In general, as the kernel size shrinks, the blur is less noticeable. A 5 ×5 Gaussian kernel will be used in this example. Given by is the equation for a Gaussian filter kernel of size (2k+1) (2k+1) [14].

$$H_{ij} = \frac{1}{2\pi\sigma^2}\left(-\frac{(i - (k + 1)) + (j - (k + 1))}{2\sigma^2}\right); \ 1 \leq i, j \leq (2k + 1) \qquad (8.1)$$

In the step of computing the gradient, edge detection operators are used to identify the strength and direction of edges to determine the gradient of the image. Changes in pixel intensity are reflected by edges. The simplest way to detect it is to use filters that emphasize this intensity change in both directions. The distribution of the gradient intensity level, which ranges from 0 to 255, is also uneven. The product's edges need to have the same intensity throughout.

Sharp edges are ideal in the final image. Non-maximum suppression is necessary to reduce the edges. The algorithm goes through each point in the gradient intensity matrix and looks for the pixels on the edges that have the highest values.

The two threshold steps aim to separate the three kinds of pixels—strong, weak, and unimportant. Strong pixels are those whose intensity is great enough to guarantee that they will shape the edge. Pixels with an intensity value that is neither high enough to be classified as strong nor low enough to be regarded as irrelevant for edge detection are referred to as "weak pixels." Additional pixels are omitted because they have nothing to do with the edge. The threshold results show that hysteresis only occurs when at least one strong neighboring pixel is present, and only then does it result in the transformation of weak pixels into strong pixels.

8.3.3 SPEEDED UP ROBUST FEATURE ALGORITHM (SURF)

A patent has been granted for the local feature detector and descriptor SURF in computer vision. Object identification, image registration, categorization, and 3D reconstruction are just a few of its many applications [14]. It is connected to the SIFT (scale-invariant feature transform) descriptor. According to the developers of SURF, the basic version is much faster than SIFT and can handle more image changes.

SURF can produce an approximate integer representation of the determinant of the Hessian blob detector, which is used to discover interesting things, using a previously computed integral picture and three integer operations. The sum of the local Haar wavelet responses acts as the location of interest's distinguishing feature. These can also be computed using the integral image. SURF descriptors have been used to locate and identify things, individuals, and faces, in addition to generating 3D scenes, tracking objects, and identifying points of interest.

To produce an image with the same size but less bandwidth, the image is translated into coordinates and then reconstructed with a pyramidal Gaussian or Laplacian pyramid shape using the multi-resolution pyramid technique. As a result, the original image is given a one-of-a-kind blurring effect known as Scale-Space, which ensures that the points of interest are independent of scale. This strategy's three primary components are matching, locating interesting sites, and locating nearby neighbors.

SURF uses square-shaped filters to approximate Gaussian smoothing. Filtering the squared image with the integral image is much quicker.

$$S(x, y) = \sum_{i=0}^{x} \sum_{j=0}^{y} I(i, j) \qquad (8.2)$$

The integral image permits speedy evaluation of the whole original picture contained within a rectangle by requiring just four evaluations. SURF uses a blob detector based on Hessian theory to find interesting locations. The determinant of the Hessian matrix, which reveals how much the region surrounding the location has changed, is maximized to select points.

Finding points of interest at different sizes is achievable, thanks to the fact that you must compare the images you see at different sizes to hunt for relationships. Other feature recognition techniques often depict scale space as a pyramidal image. The next level of the pyramid is built by subsampling images that have been constantly filtered with a Gaussian filter. As a result, many floors or staircases with varying mask proportions are created.

$$\sigma_{approx} = current\ \ filter\ \ size\ \ X\ \ \frac{base\ \ filter\ \ scale}{base\ \ filter\ \ size} \qquad (8.3)$$

Each of the scale space's octaves, which represent scale doublings, is made up of a collection of response maps. The output of the 99 filters in SURF determines the lowest level of the scale space. In contrast to previous approaches, SURF scales spaces by employing a variety of box filters of varying sizes. Rather than constantly lowering the image size, the scale space is examined by increasing the filter size. According to the previous explanation, the 99-filter output is the initial scale layer with scale s = 1.2, which is comparable to Gaussian derivatives with scale s = 1.2. To create the subsequent layers, the image is filtered with progressively larger masks while accounting for the discrete nature of integral images and the filter structure. Filters with dimensions of 99, 1515, 2121, 2727, and so on are generated as a result. In a 333 neighborhood, non-maximal suppression is employed to localize points of interest in the image and across scales.

The maxima of the Hessian matrix's determinant are then interpolated in scale and image space using the method proposed by Brown et al. The beginning layers of each octave have a significant scale difference, demanding scale–space interpolation. The responsibility of a descriptor is to provide a detailed and clear description of an image characteristic, such as the intensity distribution of pixels surrounding the object of interest. Because many descriptors are computed locally, each previously specified place of interest receives a description. The computational cost of the descriptor, as well as the accuracy and resilience of its point-matching, are directly influenced by its dimensionality. A brief description might be more resistant to aesthetic alterations, but it might not be sufficiently distinguishing, leading to an excess of false positives. Establishing a repeatable orientation using information from a sphere that includes the point of interest is the first stage. Then, using a square section aligned with the preferred orientation, the SURF descriptor is extracted. Corresponding pairs can be found by comparing the descriptors extracted from various images.

8.3.4 EXPERIMENTAL SETUP AND RESULTS

The experimental model for the proposed methodology is illustrated in the Figure 8.4.

The hand gestures will be converted into frames. We have to apply the algorithms to the frames to make them identifiable. This study employed the proposed algorithm

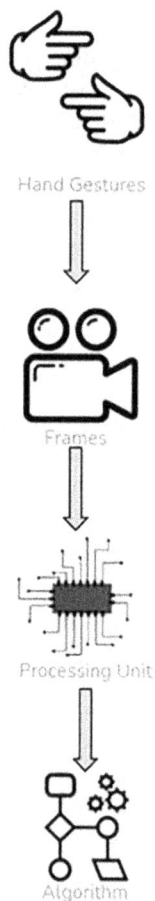

FIGURE 8.4 Methodology.

to defend and justify the performance level, with some modifications to yield better results. We focused on deriving excellent outputs on the number of datasets produced or obtained. By using the said algorithm, the performance analysis of the proposed method is shown in the form of cycles. The performance cycles are very accurate and produce the results that were expected. Here we are going to investigate the performance of CEDA and SURF algorithms. We have taken a real-time data set (hand signs), and we have tested the algorithms. We have also done the experiment with 2000 and 5000 cycles. The fact that the current algorithm can produce intelligibility for hard-of-hearing listeners that is superior to that obtained when those listeners are exposed to loud stimuli is highly encouraging and shows that the current method might be simplified in several ways to decrease processing load while still offering appropriate levels of benefit. This could be crucial because the goal is to incorporate it into hearing equipment, such as hearing aids and cochlear implants.

The processed gestures initially undergo the edge detection algorithms. As we have already explained, SURF and CEDA are the two algorithms used for detecting edges of the gestures. Then the deep learning algorithm was applied. We have taken the CNN algorithm to detect the gesture image. We stress that the current approach is not yet ready for implementation and that this is a long-term goal. The current technique, however, has properties that imply its potential implementation may be viable. The algorithm's monaural nature, as opposed to microphone array methods, makes implementation easier in the first place. Second, a significant amount of labor is transferred to the training phase by the classification-based architecture. The algorithm's operational phase merely calls for feature extraction and binary labeling with trained classifiers, both of which may be completed quickly.

8.3.5 ABOUT DATASETS

Dynamic hand gesture recognition has a variety of applications which includes gaming, automation, AR & VR etc. This dataset has been collected from the students who are really speech and impaired. We have clearly observed the videos which are captured for the hearing-impaired students, in such a way we ensure that there are no plain videos. Each movement is performed 3 times. So, we have 204120 HD video frames collected. Starting frame time, ending frame time, total mean, and standard deviation time of all the frames have been verified (Figure 8.5).

In the process, the cycles were doubled to derive maximum accuracy from the datasets. It was found that doubling of the cycles yielded better results and justified the objective of this proposed study. Also, the CEDA and SURF algorithms can facilitate average estimation of the datasets since the accuracy depends upon the number of datasets. The outputs also rely upon the datasets [15] (Figure 8.6).

The graph found above exhibits the results when the cycles were increased to 5,000, which yielded tremendous output. This led to the assumption of the performance level, which, in turn, ended up with a definite conclusion on accuracy derived from the CEDA and SURF.

From the graph, it is obvious that there has been a difference in terms of performance level in accordance with the number of datasets. The desired result with remarkable accuracy was observed with 10 datasets and 2000 and 5000 cycles.

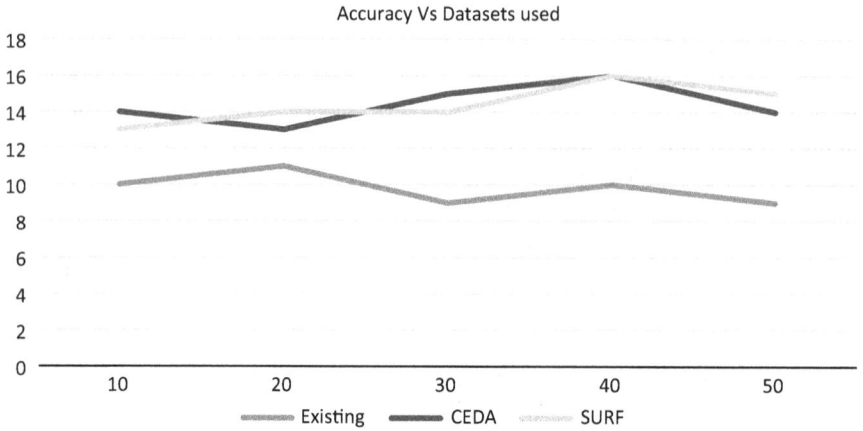

FIGURE 8.5 Accuracy vs datasets used (2000 cycles).

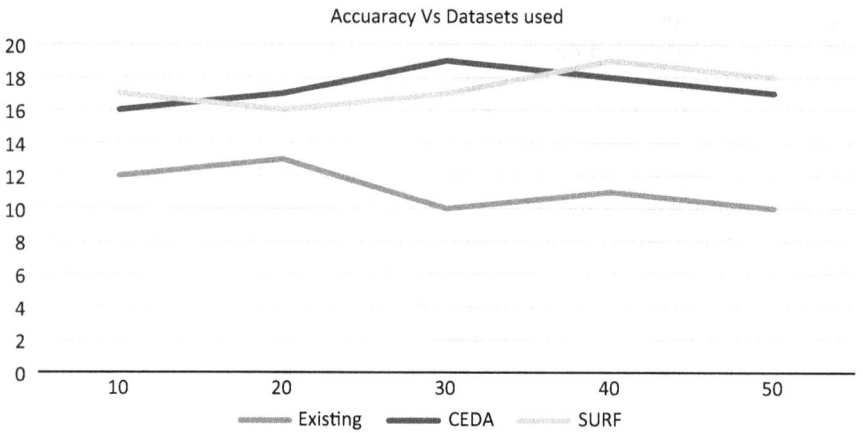

FIGURE 8.6 Accuracy vs datasets used (5000 cycles).

When these features were inserted into the proposed model, the derived score was around 20% improved. This is the level which we anticipated, and it paved the way for future scope to derive even better results and to prove the efficiency of the proposed model.

8.4 CONCLUSION

The comparative analysis of the performances leads to the following conclusion: This research study employed a set of five datasets to train and try the model. From the initial five sets, 2000 cycles were allotted, from which the resultant score of 15 was derived. The next five datasets had a total of 5000 cycles by which the resultant score of 25 could be derived. When the number of datasets and the number of cycles were increased to 10 and 5,000, respectively, the score yielded 15% improvement. Based on these variables, it is assumed that if the datasets were increased to 50 and the cycles were 80000–1000000, the score could be at the level of 85 or above. Hence, it is again stressed that the accuracy of the hand gestures will be in accordance or in proportion with the increase in the number of datasets and cycles. This study, therefore, examined the performance level to prove the efficiency of the proposed algorithm and the model. In every term, the algorithm and the consequent model proved their worth. The proposed study increased the scope of deriving better and higher accuracy levels amidst complexities by adopting several of the background subtraction algorithms. Equally, there is a proposal to try and enhance the preprocessing stage for gesture detection under low lighting conditions, thereby extracting the maximum possible accuracy. Furthermore, the algorithm is applicable to a variety of hearing impairments, including conductive hearing loss, sensorineural hearing loss, mixed hearing loss, and central hearing loss.

REFERENCES

1. Qiya Niua, Yunlai Teng, Lin Chen, "Design of gesture recognition system based on deep learning", International School, Beijing University of Posts and Telecommunications, Beijing 100876, China.
2. Xianghan Wang, Jie Jiang, Yingmei Wei，Lai Kang，Yingying Gao, "Research on gesture recognition method based on computer vision", Department of Systems Engineering, National University of Defense Technology, Changsha 410000, China.
3. X. Jiang, L. Maiolo, A. Pecora, L. Colace, Carlo Menon, Andrea Ferrone, "A fabric-based wearable band for hand gesture recognition based on filament strain sensors: a preliminary investigation", EMBS Student Member, IEEE Member.
4. Paulo Trigueiros, Fernando Ribeiro, Luís Paulo Reis, "Hand gesture recognition for human computer interaction: a comparative study of different image features", Departamento de Electrónica Industrial da Universidade do Minho, Campus de Azurém 4800–05, Guimarães, Portugal 3EEUM – Escola de Engenharia da Universidade do Minho.
5. Hanwen Huang, Yanwen Chong, Congchong Nie, Shaoming Pan, "Hand gesture recognition with skin detection and deep learning method", College of Remote Sensing and Information Engineering, Wuhan University, 129 Luoyu Road, Wuhan 430079, China.
6. Okan Kopuklu et al., "Real-time hand gesture detection and classification convolutional neural networks", 14th IEEE International Conference on Automatic Face and Gesture Recognition, 2019.
7. Hind Ibrahim Mohammed, "An inclusive survey of machine learning based hand gesture recognition systems in recent applications", IOP Conference Series: Material Science and Engineering, 2021.
8. Zhuohuang Zhang, "Objective comparison of speech enhancement algorithms with hearing loss simulations", IEEE Conference on ICASSP, 2019.
9. Eric. W. Healy et al. "An algorithm to increase intelligibility for hearing-impaired listeners in the presence of a competing talkers", Acoustical Society of America, 2017, 141 (6), 4230–4239.
10. S. Bourennane, C. Fossati, "Comparison of shape descriptors for hand posture recognition in video", Signal, Image and Video Processing, 2021, 6(1), 147–157.

11. Hsien-I Lin, Ming-Hsiang Hsu, Wei-Kai Chen, "Human hand gesture recognition using a convolution neural network", Graduates of Institute of Automation Technology National Taipei University of Technology Taipei, Taiwan.
12. Sakthidasan Krishnan, Vaithiyasubramanian S, Maragatharajan, "SAED: self-adaptive error detection automation for leveraging computational efficiency of HCI Systems", Wireless Personal Communications, 2021.
13. Kewen Liu, Kang Xiao and Hongxia, "An image edge detection algorithm based on Improved canny" 5th International Conference on Machinery, Materials, and Computing Technology, 2017.
14. V. Sathiyamoorthi, A.K. Ilavarasi, K. Murugeswari, Syed Thouheed Ahmed, B. Aruna Devi, Murali Kalipindi, "A deep convolutional neural network based computer aided diagnosis system for the prediction of Alzheimer's disease in MRI images", Measurement, 2021, 171, 108838, ISSN 0263-2241, 10.1016/j.measurement.2020.108838.
15. Herbert Bay et. al, " SURF: speeded up robust features", European Conference on Computer Vision, 2016, 404–417.

9 Deep Learning-Based Cloud Computing Technique for Patient Data Management

K.E. Hemapriya
Department of Information Technology, Sri Krishna Arts and Science College, Coimbatore, India

S. Saraswathi
Dean, Academic Affairs, Nehru Arts and Science College, Coimbatore, India

9.1 INTRODUCTION

It is essential to use cloud computing for data storage. The main concern is the class documentation and the kind of data that has already been put in the cloud storage. Data security and privacy are additional problems. In all facets of consumption, the usage of cloud computing resources and services is essential. When deciding on a prospective way to preserve system data, a precise data protection plan for distributed computing may be employed both before and after understanding the data security demands.

The notion of cloud computing allows for a shared pool of programmable computer resources that can be swiftly built and released with minimum administrative labor or service provider contact [1]. Cloud infrastructure includes both the hardware and software components required for the proper implementation of a cloud computing architecture. Other titles for cloud computing include utility computing and on-demand computing. To show how cloud computing works, client devices may access data and cloud applications from faraway physical servers, databases, and workstations through the network.

9.2 CLOUD COMPUTING

Cloud computing is an evolving technology that is both a technical and social reality. One can only guess at this point as to develop the infrastructure for the new paradigm and which apps can switch over. This technological transition for users, which is dependent upon services offered through massive store data, collecting

DOI: 10.1201/9781003469605-9

private data, and software on systems over which they have no authority, is expected to have substantial economic, social, ethical, and legal ramifications [2].

The client can store data at the back end with the help of a web and application server. Resource multiplexing makes cloud computing affordable. As a result, cloud consumers pay less for the service provider. The app data are retained close to where they will be needed in a specific and device-independent manner; this data storage strategy may improve security and reliability while also lowering transmission costs.

A model for widespread, practical, on-demand network access to a pool of configurable computing resources (e.g., connections, data centers, collection systems) that can be quickly provisioned and released with little management work or service provider interaction is known as cloud computing. Three service models, four deployment methods, and five key criteria make up this cloud model, which encourages availability [3].

9.2.1 CHALLENGES IN CLOUD COMPUTING

- Installing and running the current cloud platform's apps on some other infrastructure can lead in maintenance challenges, setup hassles, and more expenditures [4].
- Apps that consume a considerable amount of information in the cloud require a large amount of network capacity, which is costly. Poor throughput falls way short of the desired computational performance of the cloud application.
- Data safety is an essential consideration while working in cloud settings. One of the most significant concerns with cloud services is that customers must be accountable for their data, while not all providers of cloud computing services can ensure total data privacy. A loss of transparency and control methods, a loss of identity management, data abuse, and cloud misconfiguration are all common causes of cloud privacy leaks.
- Compatibility problems between cloud services and on-premise infrastructure might appear as you move your workload from on-site to the cloud.
- The end-user should expect good service quality, which is one of their top priorities. Since the entire cloud computing ecosystem is displayed in virtual environments, the CSP must fulfill its service commitments, whether they relate to computer resources or client satisfaction.
- The reliability of cloud computing is still not always 24 hours a day. In some circumstances, disruptions of a few hours occurred with cloud computing services [5].

9.2.2 DEEP LEARNING

Supervised learning is a sort of machine learning that enables computers to comprehend the environment in terms of a concept hierarchy and acquire knowledge through experience. Because the computer acquires via experience, it's not necessary for a computer interaction operator to clearly provide all of the information that the computer requires. The idea hierarchy allows a machine to learn big concepts by building them up from simpler ones; a graph depicting these structures would have several layers [6]. Deep learning makes use of a complex collection of algorithms modeled just after the human brain. This enables the processing of unstructured data such as text, images, and documents. Machine learning is a subset of artificial intelligence (AI). Deep learning is a particularly difficult element of machine learning.

9.2.3 HEALTH CARE

Machine learning is swiftly becoming a crucial diagnostic and prognostic tool for a range of medical diseases. Deep learning, which is based on a machine learning approach, deals with complex input-output mappings. Deep neural networks are a popular technique of processing and analyzing medical data because of their effectiveness and resemblance to how the human brain functions. Deep learning is utilized, in addition to diagnosing, to track the development of disease, create a personalized treatment plan, and manage patients as a whole. The capacity to save tremendous volumes of data about specific patients is revolutionizing the healthcare industry, but the sheer amount of data being collected is too large for humans to analyze. Precision medicine, which involves providing patients with individualized care, is made possible by machine learning, which gives computers the ability to automatically identify patterns and make inferences from data.

Machine learning has a widespread series of potential submissions trendy in the healthcare industry, all of which are dependent on having access to sufficient data and authorization to use it.

Prior to this, a medical practice's software included hard-coded alerts and suggestions that were based on outside studies. The reliability of those data may be constrained by the fact that they may come from various demographics and surroundings. On the contrary, machine learning can be improved by utilizing data that are readily available in that specific setting. As an illustration, anonymized patients record data from a clinic and the region it serves [7].

9.2.4 CHALLENGES IN HEALTH CARE

Machine learning is used in many industries, including automotive, manufacturing, and retail. The advancement of both deep learning and machine learning algorithms has enabled a plethora of useful forecasts, notably estimations of stock prices, housing values, and loan defaults. Additionally, there are data available in a variety of formats that can be used to make predictions using machine learning. Machine learning has a lot of room for advancement as data volumes increase, and future forecasts will become increasingly accurate as a result.

- Dealing with healthcare data presents a number of difficulties, one of which is that the data may be causal for machine learning models. When there are data where one trait contributes to the occurrence of another, the relationship is said to have a high causality. This is what is meant by the term "causation."

- The majority of machine learning algorithms operate under the assumption that each feature is independent of the others, with neither causing the other to occur nor vice versa. When there is strong causation between traits, this premise would therefore be challenged.
- Although there is a great deal of potential for machine learning algorithms to be used, the area of medicine still needs a lot of data to fully benefit from it. The amount of data in the form of medical photographs is fairly little, making it difficult to examine them extensively.
- Furthermore, the available data are not labeled in a way that would allow for their application in machine learning. To classify massive amounts of data for machine learning, it actually takes a while.

9.2.5 APPLICATIONS OF MACHINE LEARNING IN HEALTH ATTENTION

- Individualized therapies are one of the most important uses of learning algorithms in the healthcare business. It helps healthcare organizations to deliver customized patient care by assessing people's patient records, symptoms, and test findings. Using machine learning in healthcare and medical research, doctors may develop specialized therapies and give pharmaceuticals that target specific diseases in individual patients.
- The use of machine learning can improve healthcare efficiency, perhaps resulting in cost savings. Machine learning in health care, for example, might be used to develop better programming or clinical record management algorithms. As a result, the time and money that are wasted on repetitive tasks inside this healthcare system may be reduced.
- Both deep learning and machine learning enable the ground-breaking area of computer vision. This has been accepted by the Microsoft Inner Eye Initiative, which creates picture assessment methods for image analysis.
- Personalized therapies are not only likely to be more successful if individual health is combined with predictive analytics, but they are also ripe for additional research and enhanced illness evaluation.

9.2.6 PATIENT DATA MAINTENANCE

Given the rapid progress of information, many hospitals are going towards the numerical storage of permanent data in addition to archives. Surgeons' time-constrained, complicated, ambiguous, and high-stakes judgments have a significant influence on patient outcomes. Heuristics, personal preference, and hypothetical deductive reasoning generally dominate clinical judgments. Conventional decision-support systems and predictive analysis encounter a variety of challenges, resulting in less-than-ideal accuracy and time-consuming human information handling [8].

This might lead to bias, error, or harm that could have been prevented. The use of AI-powered models that leverage machine learning, in which the outputs of telemedicine devices may be fed to cloud-based medical records as an alternate interpretation of clinical information, can overcome the constraints of the traditional methods. Decision-making in these systems includes the human instinct, the preservation of baseline judgments, thorough control and operation, model interpretability, data consistency, and moral considerations such as algorithm bias and mistake accounting.

9.2.7 CLOUD COMPUTING TECHNIQUES

Cloud computing is the capacity to keep and receive data and applications through the Internet rather than a hard disc. Any kind of organization may employ strong development and information technology to develop, become leaner and more flexible, and compete with much bigger organizations. Cloud technology, as opposed to traditional hardware and software, allows businesses to stay on the cutting edge of advances in technology without making large financial investments when it comes to equipment purchases, maintenance, and service.

The furthermost fundamental function of cloud computing technologies is to provide users with online access to particular software, data, and programs. Data are saved on remote servers, independent of the user, rather than on the local network or the device's actual hard drive when cloud computing technologies are employed. By simply signing into a website or portal using legitimate credentials, individuals can access their data, paid applications, and cloud storage over the Internet.

9.2.8 CLOUD-BASED COMPUTING ENVIRONMENT ARCHITECTURE

In Figure 9.1, client infrastructure which is the front end process, communicates with the back end through the application layer. Clients can install and run their software programs in the cloud on sophisticated infrastructure owned and operated by a cloud company (e.g., Amazon Web Services, Microsoft Azure, and Google CloudPlatform). Consumers of the cloud can purchase resources for their

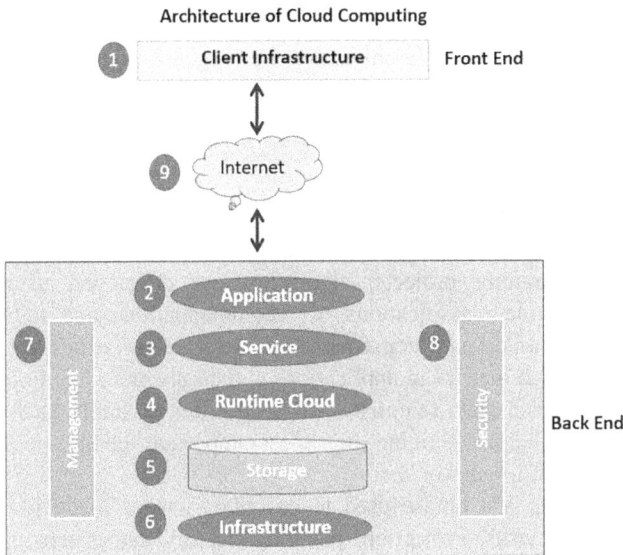

FIGURE 9.1 Cloud computing architecture.

applications on demand, and they only pay for the resources that are actually used. To stay ahead of this cloud computing benefit, a user must determine if the infrastructure as a service can quickly change the kind and number of resources assigned to a cloud implementation based on the application's demand [9].

The cloud's elasticity is really what offers it this property. Microsoft Azure should ideally be totally elastic, ensuring that the resources provided to an application properly match the needs. This allocation should occur as the site's workload increases, without compromising the platform's system performance, and a user should pay only for the capabilities that such an application actually utilizes. Clouds, in reality, are not fully elastic. One argument to this is that it is difficult to anticipate the workload and flexibility needs associated with an application in advance in order to effectively match resources with all of those requirements.

9.2.9 BASELINE CLOUD COMPUTING ARCHITECTURE

Cloud computing, one of today's most popular technologies, is giving every company a new look by providing virtualized services as well as assets on demand. Every business, from small to large, employs services that use cloud computing to transfer data and provide access to them at whatever point in time from anywhere over the Internet. In this post, we will learn more regarding the structural organization of cloud computing.

In Figure 9.2, the baseline is DNS technology to use for load balancing to the cloud storage. Transparency represents one of the furthermost important constraints that any cloud architecture should face. Capacity, confidentiality, and cognitive monitoring are also important restrictions. Ongoing research on extra important restrictions is supporting systems using cloud computing in the development of new features and methodologies that have the potential to offer more complex cloud solutions [10].

Event-driven architecture (EDA) and service-oriented architecture (SOA) are combined in cloud computing architecture. For organization, likewise, programs, functions, real-time clouds, memories, capacities, governance, and privacy are all components of a computing architecture for cloud computing.

9.3 MACHINE LEARNING

Machine learning is an important component of the rapidly increasing study of data science. In data mining projects, algorithms are developed using statistical approaches to provide classifications or recommendations and to uncover key insights. Decisions made as a consequence of these observations should have an impact on key growth metrics in applications and companies. As big data continue to emerge and flourish, data scientists will become increasingly in demand. They will be asked to help determine the most important client queries and the information required to answer them.

Machine learning is a phrase used to describe changes made to systems that perform AI-related tasks. Projection, planning, factory automation, analysis, and detection are examples of such operations. The "upgrade" might be either adjustments to existing systems or the building of new ones from the ground up [11].

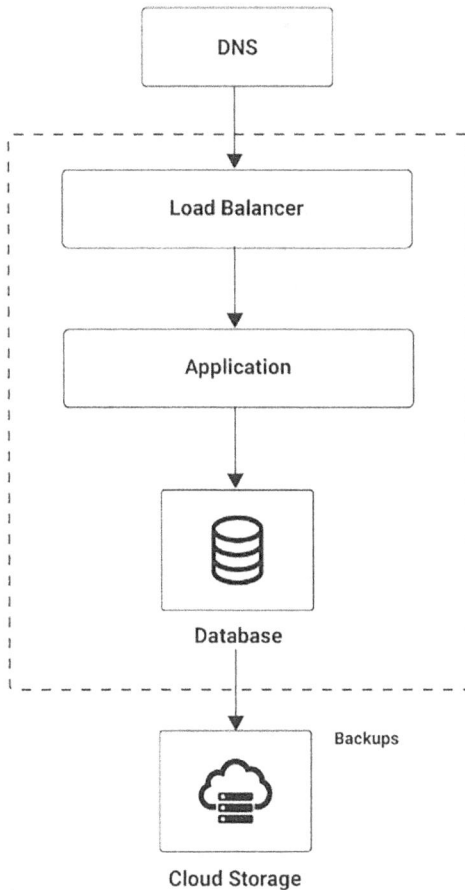

FIGURE 9.2 Baseline cloud computing architecture.

9.3.1 DATA CLASSIFICATION IN MACHINE LEARNING

Classification is a supervised algorithm for machine learning that asks the model to estimate the proper label for particular input data. While doing categorization, the algorithm is fully developed using training data, tested with test data, but then just employed to generate predictions on new, unused data. A given data collection may need to be divided into two or more categories for classification in machine learning. As a result, it creates a likelihood score to classify the data as spam or not, yes or no, sickness or no sickness, red or blue, male or female, and so on. An algorithm, for instance, can be trained to determine if a specific email is spam or not spam.

9.3.2 NETWORK

A data center, also described as a communications system, is made from inter-dependent nodes that can transmit, receive, and exchange data, audio, and video traffic. Network nodes include things like servers and modems. Computer networks are extensively used by endpoint users for regional cooperation and communication. They are common in areas such as homes, companies, and government organizations. Through the application of computer networks, geographical barriers may be erased and information exchange made feasible.

A network comprises two, maybe more, computers connected by a cable (or, in some cases, a wireless network) so that they may interact and exchange information [12]. The majority of us have utilized what computer geeks refer to as the sneaker net. It entails copying a file to a diskette before bringing the disc over to another person's computer.

9.3.3 NETWORK SECURITY

Network security refers to the use of both software and hardware technologies by any company or organization to safeguard its electronic network and data. This aims to ensure the secrecy and accessibility of the network and data. All business organizations that engage with a large amount of data do have a form of cyber defense in place.

Password protection that stands selected by the network user themselves is the most fundamental kind of network security.

Computer networks are no more secure than the machines they connect since networking is all about connecting computers together. A single vulnerable host can pose major problems for your entire network since, if it's in the hands of an enemy, might serve as a powerful base of assault or a tool for reconnaissance. Advanced security solutions like firewalls, intrusion detection systems, and other similar tools are useless if your servers provide services that are vulnerable to attack. Make sure the machines you are in charge of are as safe as feasible before focusing on the network portion of network security [13].

9.3.4 MAINTENANCE IN NETWORKING

Network maintenance means doing whatever is required to keep a network functioning and includes the following tasks: troubleshooting network faults, installing and configuring software and hardware, monitoring and improving network performance, planning for prospective network growth, and so on. Developing and monitoring network documentation, ensuring business regulations are followed, ensuring compliance with legal standards, and safeguarding the network from any risks.

9.3.5 ROUTING

The term "router" is the most accurate description of what the contemporary iterations of these devices do. Information is sent along a route—a path—between two networks by a router. This route may pass through one router or several. Modern routers also utilize a set of procedures to find and use the optimum route in networks where there are several paths to the same destination. In the event that particular route is no longer ideal or completely unsuitable, the router chooses the next-best way.

Network routing is the process of selecting a path across two or more networks. The routing concepts may be applied to any network, including public transportation and telephone networks. In packet-switching networks such as the Internet, routing specifies the paths individual Internet protocol (IP) units travel from their origin to their destination. Routers are specialized network gear that manage Internet routing. Ampere routing protocol refers to the steps taken by the router to determine and choose the best route and to communicate with other routers about the reachability and state of the network [14].

9.3.6 CLUSTERING

Clustering divides a crowd or set of data elements into units in order to ensure that the datasets in every cluster are much closer to each other and more dissimilar from the pieces of information that compose the other groups. It is simply a classification of items based on how related and dissimilar they are in comparison to one another. Image segmentation, knowledge discovery, pattern identification, classification techniques, analysis methods, and other system learning and data mining activities benefit from clustering. It can be viewed as either a preparation phase or an exploration task. If the goal is to study and disclose hidden patterns in the data, clustering would become a stand-alone exploratory effort in and of itself. If the produced clusters are to be utilized to support further data analysis or advanced analytics activity, clustering will constitute a pre-processing step [15].

9.3.6.1 Clustering Methods Types

Clustering methods are widely classified as hard clustering (each datapoint belongs to just one category) and soft clustering (data points may possibly belong to another category); however, more ways to cluster exist. The following are the most common clustering approaches used in machine learning:

1. **Partitioning Clustering:** It is a kind of grouping that creates non-hierarchical groupings out of the data. It's also referred to as the centroid-based approach. The K-means clustering method is the most popular illustration of partitioning clustering. In this kind, the dataset is split into a collection of K pre-defined groups, where K refers to the number of groups. The cluster center is designed so that there is a minimal distance between the information points in one cluster and the center of another cluster.
2. **Density-Based Clustering:** As long as the dense area can be linked, the density-based clustering approach joins the extremely dense areas into clusters, resulting in distributions of any shape. This program accomplishes that by finding several clusters in the information set and joining the regions with dense population into clusters. The sparser portions in data space separate the dense sections from one another. If the dataset is large and contains many dimensions, these techniques may have trouble grouping the data points.
3. **Distribution Model-Based Clustering:** The distribution model-based categorization approach divides data based on the chance that a dataset

corresponds to a specific distribution. The grouping is accomplished by assuming specific distributions, most notably the Gaussian distribution.

4. **The Expectation Maximization Clustering method:** Gaussian mixture models (GMM) is an example of this kind.
5. **Hierarchical Clustering:** Because there is no need to specify the number of clusters to be created, hierarchical clustering can be used as an alternative to partitioned clustering. The dataset is separated into clusters in this approach to form a tree-like structure known as a dendrogram. By pruning the tree at the appropriate level, the observations or any number of clusters may be picked. The Agglomerative hierarchical algorithm is the most typical example of this strategy.
6. **Fuzzy Clustering:** Fuzzy clustering is a soft approach in which a data point can be assigned to a number rather than one category or cluster. Every collection of data has a number of membership coefficients that are proportional to the degree of membership in a cluster. The fuzzy C-means method is an example of this form of clustering; it is additionally referred to as the fuzzy k-means approach at times.

9.3.6.2   Clustering Algorithms

Based on their models, which were previously described, the clustering methods may be separated. There are several clustering methods available, yet only a few of them are widely utilized. The technique for clustering is determined by the type of data being used. Some algorithms, for example, must predict the number of clusters in the supplied dataset, whilst others must discover the shortest distance between the dataset's observations.

1. **K-Means Algorithm:** One of the most often used clustering techniques is k-means. By grouping the samples into several clusters with similar variances, it classifies the dataset. In this algorithm, the quantity of clusters has to be specified. With an $O(n)$ linear complexity, it is quick and requires less calculations.
2. **Mean-Shift Algorithm:** The mean-shift technique looks for dense spots within a smooth distribution of data points. It serves as an illustration of a centroid-based approach that updates the potential centroid candidates to serve as the geographic center of the points inside a particular region.
3. **DBSCAN Algorithm:** Spatial clustering based on the density of programs with noise is what this algorithm stands for. It serves as an illustration of a density-based paradigm that is comparable to the mean-shift but has several notable benefits. The algorithm divides the low-density areas into the high-density zones. The clusters can therefore be produced in any arbitrary form.
4. **Expectation-Maximization Clustering using GMM:** This method can be used in situations when the K-means algorithm fails or as a replacement. It is assumed that the data points in GMM have a Gaussian distribution.
5. **Agglomerative Hierarchical Algorithm:** The bottom-up hierarchical clustering is carried out via the Agglomerative hierarchical method. In this, every

data point is first regarded as an individual cluster and is subsequently merged. A tree structure may be used to illustrate the cluster hierarchy.

6. **Affinity Propagation:** This method differs from previous clustering methods in that it does not call for a certain number of clusters to be specified. Each data point communicates with the other until the pair of points of information converge. The fundamental flaw with this method is that it takes a lot of time—O(N2T).

9.4   BLOCKCHAIN

Blockchain network is an unchangeable database that simplifies asset tracking and transaction recording in a business network. Blockchain is a decentralized, unchangeable network that simplifies the management of resources and the processing of data in a business network. A specific advantage is that it can manage anything that can be touched, such as a house, vehicle, cash, or a plot of land. It can also manage intangible assets, which include intellectual property such as patents, copyrights, and brand awareness. Almost everything of value may be logged and sold on a blockchain network, minimizing risk, and enhancing efficiency for all parties [16,17].

9.4.1   BLOCKCHAIN-BASED CLOUD COMPUTING APPLICATIONS

Cloud services, with their various benefits, have swept the software business. Businesses all across the world utilize cloud computing for data backup and storage, software development and evaluation, data recovery, and other uses. Cloud computing is being used in numerous areas other than information technology and software, including healthcare, automobile, and retail, to generate novel solutions. Cloud computing, on the other hand, carries a distinct set of limits.

Figure 9.3 shows blockchain technology servers with several benefits in cloud computing. Blockchain technology is employed by millions of organizations for a range of industrial applications because of its accessibility, security, and autonomous nature. Combining blockchain and cloud, on the other hand, has the potential to further alter businesses.

Although blockchain enhances network security, data confidentiality, and decentralization, cloud computing provides higher scalability and adaptability. As a result, the marriage of cloud with blockchain seems to have the potential to produce unique solutions, especially when using a decentralized cloud like Ridge Cloud.

9.4.2   THE NEED FOR BLOCKCHAIN CLOUD

Cloud technology and Cloud of Things (CoT) infrastructures have various dangers and limits that blockchain can assist to alleviate. Among the threats and limits are as follows:

• Once uploaded to cloud servers, users have little control over their information, operations, and code.

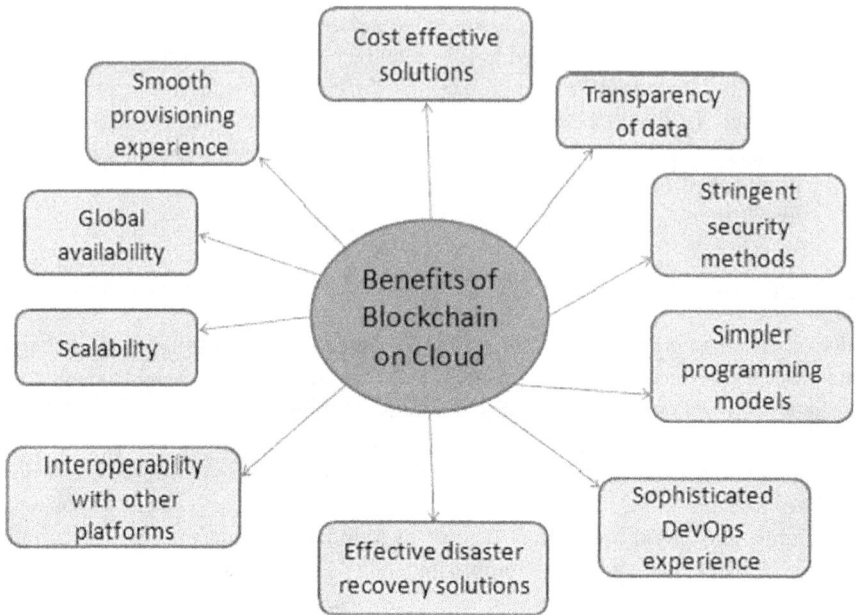

FIGURE 9.3 Benefits of blockchain-based cloud computing.

- Customers are unfamiliar with the underlying workings of cloud-based solutions, which means they have to rely on cloud service providers for information extraction, which might cause security and privacy issues.
- Since CoT uses centralized communication models, growing help desk and expanding Internet of Things (IoT) networks to a bigger deployment is challenging. Centralized network architecture increases communication overhead and power efficiency for IoT devices due to huge data flows.

9.4.3 How Does the Blockchain Cloud Work?

By putting the chain of blocks as Blockchain as a Service (BaaS) together in a cloud environment, blockchain may be utilized for secure computer management in smart contracts cloud computing.

By delivering smart contract services such as smarter companies in return, capacity to conduct monitoring, and cloud blockchain storage, BaaS allows IoT applications.

9.4.4 Decentralization

The reliance on a centralized attendant for data management and decision making is a significant issue with CoT. If the central server fails, it might destabilize the system and result in data loss. Hackers can potentially compromise the central server, trying to make it less secure.

In Figure 9.4, centralized and decentralized nodes are defined. In centralized access data will be organized in the central point. Nevertheless, smart contracts

Centralized   Decentralized

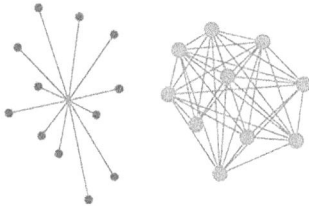

FIGURE 9.4   Centralized and decentralized.

distributed cloud computing can overcome these difficulties. With blockchain-based decentralized cloud computing, several copies of the same data reside on various computer nodes.

Because of this, if one server fails, the entire system won't crash. Distributed cloud computing powered by blockchain also reduces the risk of data loss. In light of this, cloud-based blockchain services provide quicker disaster management.

Improved chasing of belongings and amenities is another benefit of a decentralized cloud computing blockchain network. The logistics sector, which regularly tracks inventory, vehicles, and other items, will especially benefit greatly from this.

9.4.5   Improved Cloud Services and Security

Issues regarding keeping CoT files in the database are relevant since these data usually contain personally identifiable information, such as videos and audio recordings. Such data breaches can be quite harmful. Yet, several blockchain cloud storage services provide extremely secure cryptographic cloud storage choices.

The data user can be divided into many encrypted segments by a decentralized cloud storage blockchain solution, and these segments are connected by a hashing occupation. Each segment is kept in a separate place. These segments are distributed across the network and given an additional layer of security thanks to the cloud storage blockchain solution.

Only manipulators through the encryption significantly can contact or recite the statistics using blockchain in cloud storage. Distributed cloud storage blockchain's robust security features make sure that hackers cannot interpret the information in the data. Blockchain refuge in the cloud computation thus increases the dependability of cloud solutions.

Block chain technology for cloud storage protects against data manipulation as well. To avoid data manipulation, crypto currency storage cloud solutions can trace backup and storage history. Blockchain-powered cloud storage systems are also quicker, lowering expenses, and increasing productivity.

As you can see, the convergence of Ethereum technology and cloud storage provides a safe and effective storage space with infinite storage space.

9.4.6   Database Management

Healthcare data is becoming more computerized, and data in regards to speed, quantity, and value are rising, as they are in most other businesses. Health data management is the practice of generating the most of this information and administering it for the profit of healthcare providers and, ideally, patient well-being and health.

It is necessary to investigate the many forms of data maintained in health data management in order to better comprehend the intricacies and subtleties of managing healthcare data. Electronic health records (EHRs), patient-generated health data (PGHD), claims data, clinical study data, and genomic data are all examples of this. Each form of data poses its own set of obstacles, including such interoperability and data standards issues, privacy concerns, and guaranteeing the data's quality and completeness.

The potential to deliver improved care to patients through enhanced decision-making and higher efficiency in patient care is one of the key benefits of excellent healthcare data management. This, however, entails the obligation of guaranteeing privacy and security of information. Healthcare data is very valuable and sensitive to attackers, making it a potential target for privacy violations. As a result, strong security safeguards must be implemented to prevent access, theft, or damage of patient data.

Encrypting data at their source and during transit, detailed integrated user access and access control, regularly monitoring as well as independent audit view logs, and ensuring that you comply with applicable regulatory requirements, including the Health Care Portability and Accountability Act (HIPAA), are all initiatives to circumvent data breaches when storing health information. Furthermore, healthcare institutions should undertake frequent risk assessments in order to recognize vulnerabilities and put in place necessary controls to limit possible hazards.

Overall, healthcare data management is a complicated and ever-changing sector that needs a thorough grasp of data security issues and solutions. Organizations that manage healthcare data successfully may improve patient outcomes, increase operational efficiency, and preserve the confidentiality and safety of patient information.

Health data management refers to the systematic structuring of wellness data in digital form. This can include everything from electronic medical records (EMR) created during medical visits to electronic health records (EHR) or handwritten hospital records digitized into a digital repository. Health data management takes on the responsibility of not only arranging medical data, but also integrating and supporting its analysis throughout in order to enhance patient care and draw insights that might promote medical outcomes, while also maintaining the privacy and security of the data.

According to an Accenture investigation,

- The majority of health care organizations capture EMR abstracts, claims data, enrollment, and medical program information, and only the most sophisticated organizations also collect computerized EMR inputs and disease management program data.
- Very few organizations complement official medical data with non-health data sources such as consumer lifestyle information, telemonitoring and wearable tech, and survey data regarding patient experience.

9.4.7   ADVANTAGES OF HEALTH DATA STORAGE

Health data management may benefit healthcare organizations, medical personnel, and patients alike:

- **Provide a comprehensive image of the patients, homes, and patient groupings:** Composite ratings that provide a progress report and enable predictions.
- **Increase patient involvement:** Target patients with appropriate warnings and care recommendations using predictive modeling.
- **Improve health outcomes:** Monitor health-related behaviors in specific locations or populations, forecast future patterns, and provide preventative remedies to rising health concerns.
- **Making commercial judgments:** Help healthcare practitioners in producing quality data-driven judgments, such as which sorts of medical staff to recruit, what technologies to participate in, or which psychosocial interventions to sell to.
- **Monitor physician behaviors:** Analyze data about doctor performance, including their success rates, the amount of time they spend on various treatments and medical choices, and how well they fit with the organization's objectives.

9.4.8   HEALTH DATA MANAGEMENT CHALLENGES

- **Data Destabilization**
  Medical data can be kept in workbooks or databases, pictures or streaming video, digital papers, scanned paper documentation, or specialized formats like the DICOM standard for MRI scans. Medical professionals, global health institutions, health insurers, pharmacies, and individuals regularly duplicate data, gather it many times, and store it in multiple forms. There isn't one reliable source for information about patient well-being.
- **Data Modifications**
  In Figure 9.5, security architecture design is built to secure data from external threads and risk management. Healthcare information, as well as patient and physician names, occupations, locations, and ailments, are continually changing. Patients are treated to a range of investigations and treatments throughout time, and the therapies and drugs themselves change. New sorts of data are generated by emerging medically necessary methods, such as telehealth programs.
- **Compliance and Standards**
  Medical data are sensitive and must adhere to government laws such as HIPAA. Data discovery issues and poor data quality make performing mandatory audits and meeting regulatory standards considerably more difficult, as well as limiting the range of data that healthcare practitioners may utilize to benefit patients.

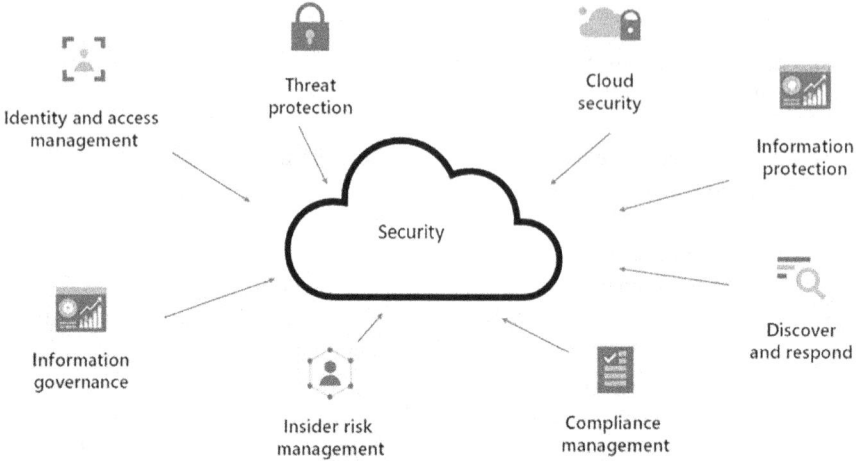

FIGURE 9.5   Health data management security architecture design.

9.4.9 HEALTHCARE DATA STORAGE CONSIDERATIONS

According to IDC research, the quantity of data created by patient data and imaging systems is predicted to increase from 153 petabytes of data in 2013 to 2,300 petabytes of data in 2020.

Apart from the problems described above, healthcare practitioners must decide how they will keep all of that data:

- **Extensibility**
  The fastest-growing sector of healthcare data is unstructured data, which includes MRI scans, computed tomography, X-rays, and PET scans. When these data expand to petabytes, healthcare organizations seek a scalable, low-cost storage solution.
- **Adherence**
  Regulations must be followed when storing items. Data must be safeguarded via role-based access controls (RBAC), independent auditor recording, and encryption keys at rest and in transit, as well as adequately reviewed key management methods, according to HIPAA and other healthcare sector laws.
- **Vendor-Neutral Archive (VNA)**
  A vendor-neutral archive (VNA) serves as an increasing access for numerous healthcare information systems. It enables the consolidation of multiple forms of patient data into a single hub, resulting in a system that categorizes patient records. Storage platforms should support VNA integration.
- **Data Robustness and Protection**
  Health data are a frequent target for hackers, and if they are unintentionally lost or deleted, this poses a major danger to providers. To spread data pieces over several nodes, storage systems should provide resilience, mirroring, incremental backups, and erasure coding.

9.5   CLOUDING PROVIDES SECURE, REDUCED HEALTH DATA HOSTING

Cloudian provides Hyperstore, an exabyte-scale, low-cost on-premise storage solutions for healthcare facilities. It allows the healthcare companies to store, transport, and safeguard information across various places for upwards to 70% less than disk-based storage costs.

The following Hyperstore features help healthcare organizations:

- **Cloud Adaptability**
  Deployments may start small and build as required, ranging from three nodes to hundreds of thousands of them. Each node could represent a virtual or physical appliance running on standard hardware.
- **Numerous Integrations**
  Hyperstore connects with a variety of healthcare apps and archiving services, allowing it to function as a centralized database with a full view of patient information.
- **Compliance and Cybersecurity**
  HIPAA-compliant encryption process and transparency access agreement, AES-256 virtual machine encrypted for stored data, SSL for transmitted information, RBAC with predefined access privileges, audit trail recording, with WORM (Write-Once-Read-Multiple) enabling permanent data storage are all features of Hyperstore.
- **Extensive Metadata**
  Data scientists may use HyperStore's sophisticated metadata tagging tools to identify new insights and trends in healthcare data.
- **Data Security**
  HyperStore delivers data persistence of 99.99% by spreading data via replication or erasure coding. The number of copies and erasure code technique may be customized to fulfill the SLA.

9.5.1   Retention of Medical Records

Medical records are essential for in-patient treatment as well as the day-to-day activities of healthcare information administration. They include a complete timeline of a patient's condition, including diagnosis, treatments, prescriptions, and other pertinent information. Several standards, rules, and laws control medical records to preserve client privacy, privacy, and accessibility.

Figure 9.6 shows how data are stored in Cloudian. The Health Insurance Portability and Accountability Act (HIPAA) of the United States mandates healthcare providers to keep medical records for at least six years, while other states may have longer retention periods. Furthermore, some medical disciplines, such as maternity and pediatrics, may have extended retention periods because of the possibility of future medical complications.

Maintaining medical records may be difficult, especially when they must be kept for years, if not decades. To efficiently maintain and store medical records, a thorough

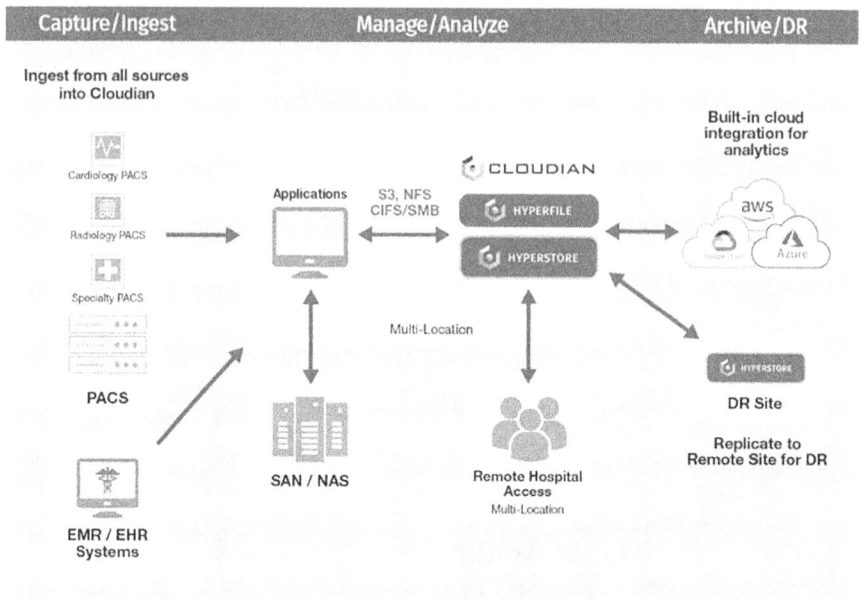

FIGURE 9.6   Data storage with Cloudian.

and structured system must be in place. This involves ensuring that medical records are properly indexed, labeled, and tracked, as well as employing adequate security measures to safeguard confidentiality laws and prevent illegal access.

Electronic health records (EHRs) have transformed medical record management by allowing healthcare practitioners to digitally store and retrieve patient information. EHRs provide various benefits compared to conventional journal article health records, including faster information access, increased accuracy, and simpler information exchange among healthcare practitioners.

Finally, medical records are an important component of medical administration and patient care. Understanding the standards, laws, and rules governing medical records is critical, as is implementing a successful procedure for handling and preserving them. EHRs have the potential to significantly improve medical record administration, but it is critical to ensure that adequate precautions have been taken to safeguard patient privacy and prevent unauthorized visits.

9.5.2   What Exactly Are Medical Records?

Indeed, practically everyone in the industrialized world has a medical record including a lot of useful and sensitive information on their health, medical issues, and treatments. Medical records give a detailed history of a patient's condition, allowing healthcare practitioners to make educated decisions regarding diagnosis, treatment, and follow-up care.

Identifying data such as a reference number, birth date, their Social Security number, contact info, and medical records, in addition to confidential material such as mental health disorders, infectious illnesses, and reproductive health, may be included in medical records. To preserve patients' security and prevent illegal access or exposure of personal information, medical records must be maintained confidential and secure.

Apart from the benefits for personal patient care, medical records also play an important role in community health administration and medical research. Medical records may be used to track disease outbreaks, determine health trends, and evaluate the efficacy of medical interventions and therapies.

As technology advances, a greater focus is being placed on how to utilize EHRs to store and manage medical information. EHRs provide various benefits compared to conventional journal article systems, such as faster information access, increased accuracy, and simpler information exchange among healthcare practitioners. But, as with any technology, adequate security measures must be in place to preserve patient confidentiality and avoid data breaches.

Ultimately, medical records are an important part of healthcare since they give vital information to healthcare professionals, researchers, and policymakers. To safeguard patient privacy and provide the greatest feasible patient care, medical records must be maintained discreet, secure, and correct.

9.5.3 Personal Identification Information

PII, often referred to as private health information, or PHI, is information such as Social Security numbers, residential addresses, and healthcare provider identification.

- **Medical Background**
  Even if the patient is unaware of it, a medical record is kept. For example, if a person wasn't recently immunized, his or her medical records may show this. The medical history includes any diagnostic, previous and existing health issues, and potentially vital life data such as sensitivities or medication intolerance.
- **Medical History of the Family**
  Close family members' medical records may also include important medical issues that are hereditary or have an influence on their relatives in some manner.
- **Medications Log**
  What chemicals a person has ingested, such as prescription pharmaceuticals, over-the-counter medicines, herbal therapies, and even illicit drugs.
- **Medical History**
  The medical procedures the client has received and the way they've addressed problems.
- **Medical Directives**
  Health records may also include a "living will," or recommendations the individual intends to transmit to medical workers should someone be unable to speak.

9.5.4 THREE DIFFERENT TYPES OF DIGITAL MEDICAL RECORDS

Thirty years ago, almost everything about patient history was written on paper and stored in practitioners' book shelves or hospital archive rooms. Several medical practices still maintain paper patient records. Medical records, on the other hand, are progressively being computerized, and the healthcare sector now controls three key forms of digital health records.

- **Electronic Medical Record**
  Simply explained, electronic medical records (EMRs) are a device that enables practitioners to track the location of their patients' appointments. The EMR contains a plethora of information regarding patient diseases or complaints, therapies they have undergone and the consequences of all those medications, and account statements for medical services performed.
- **Electronic Health Record**
  An EHR represents a more complete system that integrates data from many medical facilities. It supplements EMRs with data from wearable tech, accessible clinical science, mental well-being resources, and socio-economic or survey data, which can give insight on patient well-being. An EHR is intended to involve patients and aid them in contributing additional information about their behaviors and circumstances, resulting in better therapy for themselves and others with similar situations.
- **Personal Health Record**
  A personal health record (PHR) is a system that enables people to monitor their healthcare information and is often administered and given by insurance companies. It is often in the shape of an application with which users may engage in order to save and utilize medical data. This includes personal data acquired via wearable technology or user information entry, medical papers that the user provides, and info someone enters in from EMR systems.

9.5.5 HOW LONG DO MEDICAL RECORDS REMAIN ON FILE?

Medical records must be kept for a specific amount of time by medical providers as well as specific practitioners by law. As an example,

- **In the United States**
  HIPAA requires healthcare organizations and other covered entities to keep medical records for six years from the date the record was produced or when it was last enforced, whichever is later.
- **In the United Kingdom**
  According to the Recordkeeping Standards of Practice for the Health and Social Care Sector, 2016, anybody wanting to work with or through the NationalHealthService (NHS) is obligated to preserve health history for a maximum of 20 years just after the person's last interaction with the patient, a maximum of eight years after their own dying, or up to 25 years after the birth of their last child for maternity records.

9.5.6 Other Factors Influencing the Retention Period of Medical Records

Many other variables may impact the necessity to retain medical records in the United States:

- **Visit Frequency**
  Patients who see their carers less frequently may be obliged to preserve records for a longer period of time.
- **Health Plans**
  Third-party payers may be required by contract to preserve medical records. Insurance firms and government healthcare programs, for example, may have contractual requirements to maintain medical data as part of the reimbursement process. These records aid in documenting the patient's diagnosis and suitability of the treatments performed, as well as ensuring that the payer only reimburses for covered services.
- **Limitation of Liability**
  There is a date in the United States when a client may bring an action, as well as the person's records must be retained until then. There are statutes of restrictions in the United States that specify dates by which a person must file a lawsuit connected to medical care. The particular date varies depending on the state and the kind of claim being made. The limitation period for medical malpractice lawsuits, for example, may differ from the deadline for bringing a claim for personal injury.
- **State Legislation**
  Medical retention regulations from one or more states may apply to physicians practicing in different states.

9.5.7 Medical Records Management

Throughout many contemporary medical institutions, the continual monitoring of medical records is a specialty that needs committed employees and experience. Medical records management entails the following tasks:

- Increasing the accessibility, safety, and security of medical records
- Managing digitization activities and assuring compliance with organizational goals, appropriate industry standards, and regulatory requirements
- Provide medical record resilience via diversity, replication, and disaster recovery
- Administering information technology systems, such as EMR systems, which are utilized to maintain and retrieve medical records.

9.6 CONCLUSION

Many people are using infrastructure as part of a computing service paradigm. A third-party supplier of cloud services distributes resources such as stockpiling, virtualization servers, and networking via the Internet.

Users of the service are responsible for their data; thus, if any information disappears, they must locate a replacement. Users are also in charge of downloading, installing, and updating operating systems and apps. IaaS services are also known as cloud infrastructure services.

Blockchain IaaS is a service provided by the cloud paradigm that is similar to IaaS but adds security and decentralization. With just an infrastructure as a service blockchain cloud storage service, a provider of cloud computing services might employ the excess resources of CPUs and GPUs in a distributed platform to provide extra computing resources to consumers on a per-user basis to securely and efficiently store patient data on the cloud.

REFERENCES

1. Peter Mell and Timothy Grance (2011) "The NIST Definition of Cloud Computing", Computer Security Division Information Technology Laboratory National Institute of Standards and Technology.
2. "Cloud Computing Theory and Practice", Dan C. Marinescu.
3. "Cloud Computing", Nayan B. Ruparelia, Cambridge, Massachusetts London, England.
4. Ajay Bansal, "Cloud Computing", Dr.Tarandeep Kaur, Lovely Professional University.
5. "Handbook of Cloud Computing", editors Borko Furht · Armando Escalante.
6. "Deep Learning", Ian Goodfellow is a Research Scientist at Google.YoshuaBengio is Professor of Computer Science at the Université de Montréal, Aaron Courville is Assistant Professor of Computer Science at the Université de Montréal.
7. "Introduction to Machine Learning in Health Care", by Ian McCrae / Orion Health Founder and CEO.
8. Arthur Rangel et al. "Deep Learning for Personalized Healthcare Services." Title Is Part of EBook Package: De Gruyter DG Ebook Package English 2021, 2021.
9. V. Sathiyamoorthi, A.K. Ilavarasi, K. Murugeswari, S. Thouheed Ahmed, B. ArunaDevi, M. Kalipindi, "A deep convolutional neural network based computer aided diagnosis system for the prediction of Alzheimer's disease in MRI images", Measurement, 171, 2021, 108838, ISSN 0263-2241, 10.1016/j.measurement.2020.108838.
10. M.A.N. Bikas, A. Alourani, M. Grechanik, "Advances in Computers", Volume 103, University of Illinois at Chicago, Chicago, IL, United States.
11. "Introduction to Machine Learning", Nils J. Nilsson Robotics Laboratory Department of Computer Science Stanford University Stanford.
12. "Networking for Dummies", 7th Edition by Doug Lowe, Published by Wiley Publishing, Inc., Indianapolis, Indiana.
13. "Network Security Hacks", 2nd Edition by Andrew Lockhart, Published by O'Reilly Media, Inc., 1005 Gravenstein Highway North, Sebastopol.
14. "Routing TCP/IP", Volume I, by Macmillan Technical Publishing, and Cisco Systems, Inc.
15. "Data Clustering Algorithms and Applications", Charu C. Aggarwal Chandan K. Reddy, CRC Press Taylor & Francis Group.
16. "Blockchain Fundamentals", Ravindhar Vadapalli, Colorado College of Blockchain.
17. K. Murugeswari, B. Balamurugan, G. Ganesan, "Blockchain and bitcoin security", Book Editor(s):Gulshan Shrivastava, Dac-Nhuong Le, Kavita Sharma, First published: 22 May 2020. 10.1002/9781119621201.ch8.

10 Challenges and Issues in Health Care and Clinical Studies Using Deep Learning

M. Renuka Devi
School of Information Science, Presidency University, Bangalore, India

V. Sindhu
Department of Computer Science, CHRIST (Deemed To Be University), Bangalore, India

S. Devi
School of Information Science, Presidency University, Bangalore, India

10.1 INTRODUCTION

Deep learning revolutionized the healthcare industry by enabling rapid data analysis without sacrificing accuracy. It is a sophisticated blend of machine learning and artificial intelligence (AI) that utilizes a multi-layered algorithmic architecture to process data with remarkable precision. In recent years, deep learning has experienced a resurgence in popularity due to advances in computing power and the availability of vast new datasets. This has significantly improved machines' ability to comprehend and manipulate data such as speech, language, and images.

With the vast amount of data being generated (150 Exabyte in the US alone, growing at an annual rate of 48%), along with the proliferation of medical equipment and the adoption of digital record systems, healthcare benefits significantly from deep learning. We are on the cusp of a new world in which healthcare biomedical data will play an increasingly crucial part. One example is precision medicine, which aims to ensure that patients receive the exact treatment at the mean duration by considering factors such as molecular differences, environment, digital health reports, and lifestyle. However, the abundance of biomedical data also presents challenges for healthcare research. One major challenge is identifying relationships between these datasets in order to focus on proposing a well-dependent solution, which is developed

DOI: 10.1201/9781003469605-10

depending on the data analysis techniques and machine learning approaches. In the past, there were a number of efforts taken to connect the different data sources to create a comprehensive idea or outlook that can be later used for future prediction and identifying patterns in data. Despite their potential, predictive tools that are machine learning enabled are not mostly adopted in the medical field. However, as more medical professionals recognize the value of deep learning in health care, its use is set to increase. Collaboration with industry and professional organizations will only enhance the potential of this technology. To remain professionally relevant, it is important to stay agile and adaptable.

In biomedical research, it is common to rely on subject-matter experts to specify the phenotypes to use directly. However, this approach does not scale well and can limit the discovery of unique patterns in the dataset. On the other hand, using representation learning techniques can extract the necessary representations from raw data automatically. Deep learning is a representation learning algorithm that employs a number of hidden layers that are simple in nature; meanwhile, they are non-linear in nature to transform raw input into increasingly abstract representations. These models, which are employed in different sectors, have produced remarkable results. Deep learning in health care is still early but has already succeeded. Leading institutions and healthcare organizations have recognized its benefits, and its popularity continues to grow. At the 2017 RSNA conference, AI and deep learning in healthcare solutions had just one or two booths but now has its floor, exhibit space, and presentations. The future is still in the hands of healthcare workers, but they are now supported by technology that understands their unique needs and environment, helping to reduce their daily stress.

Deep learning has several features that make it well-suited for health care. However, there are still challenges that need to be addressed by the deep learning research community to realize its potential in health care fully. These challenges include the characteristics of healthcare data and the necessity for the enhanced multi-dimensional technique and supporting tools that give access to deep learning to coordinate with the medical dataset and support in decision making. In this context, it is essential to consider the advantages, drawbacks, and potential uses of deep learning techniques in implementing these techniques in medical and future-generation healthcare systems (Figure 10.1).

10.2 THE ETHICS OF DEEP LEARNING IN HEALTHCARE ISSUES AND INITIATIVES

Extracting knowledge and measures to get the insights from complex, highly variant, and dissimilar biomedical data is a never-ending challenge in front of data analysts for many years. In biomedical research, as the data are emerging from multiple sources like electronic medical records, imaging, sensor data, and text, they are diverse in data types. These data can be challenging to interpret and organize due to their complexity, diversity, and lack of structure. The healthcare sector, while facing many reforms every day, is stepping into a new dimension where large amounts of biomedical data will be crucial. Precision medicine is one example of how these data can be used to identify the proper treatment for the right

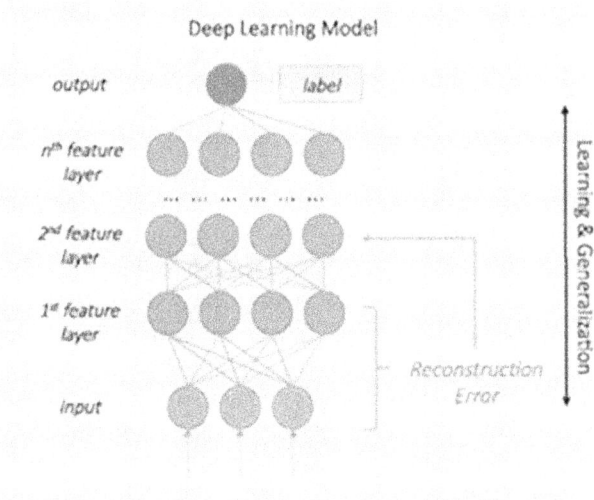

FIGURE 10.1 Deep learning model.

patient by considering multiple factors such as molecular characteristics, environment, and electronic health records. Our goal is to provide this information promptly. Extracting understanding and practical insights from tough, highly-dimensional, amalgamate biomedicine statistics remains essential in reworking healthcare delivery. Modern biomedical lookup is emerging with many distinct kinds of data, including electronic scientific records, photo processing, and many more, which are challenging, assorted, and difficult to explain. They are not structured to traditional fact mining, and statistically gaining knowledge of methods usually requires operating characteristic engineering to reap positive and more excellent strong facts from these data, and then construct predictive or assembling fashions to the peak of that. It has two steps that present many challenges, with complicated facts and inadequate domain knowledge. Recent advances in deep learning methods offer new effective paradigms for acquiring and mastering fashions from tangled data. This chapter assesses current writing on the utility of comprehensive studying technologies to boost healthcare.

Based on the work examined, we advise that extensive studying tactics can additionally be a means of relocating large biomedicine data into upgrades in human health. We additionally perceive obstacles and requirements for increased method improvement and application, particularly in terms of being comprehensible to subject memory specialists and native scientists. We discuss these obstacles and recommend strengthening a meaningful and understandable architecture to build a deep connection between getting-to-know learners and human interpretability [1]. The political and financial system of fitness is "the analysis of the motives of the unfolding of disease, the political and financial structures, processes, and electricity family members that form and shape the prerequisites that, through shaping, give rise to social patterns of health, disease, and well-being." Attention wishes to be paid to the locations where human beings live and "create jobs".

The massive availability of biomedical records has delivered extraordinary possibilities and obstacles to health research. In certain circumstances, investigating the alliance between all unique details in the datasets is an indispensable hassle for developing reliable scientific tools primarily dependent on data-driven procedures and computing device learning. To this end, the earlier lookup has attempted to hyperlink a couple of record sources to build a frequent knowledge base that can be used for predictive analytics and discovery. Although current fashions are promising, predictive equipment primarily based on computing devices gaining knowledge of techniques have yet to be broadly adopted in medicine. Indeed, due to the excessive dimensionality, heterogeneity, time dependence, sparseness, and irregularity of biomedical data, many challenges remain in absolutely exploiting biomedical data (Figure 10.2).

These challenges are compounded by utilizing the range of medical philosophy used to gather the facts (e.g., they regularly contain conflicts and contradictions). Deep mastering models exhibit extraordinary strength and potential in computer vision, speech-to-text, intelligent herbal retrieval, and scientific imaging. For instance, in I, a patient, who is diagnosed with "type 2 diabetes," with a laboratory value of hemoglobin A1C > 7.0, the presence of 250.00 ICD-9 code, "type two diabetes," free textual content clinical notes can be recognized by way of descriptions such as Reconciling all these scientific principles to construct a higher-level exposition shape and realize their interrelationship is no small feat [2]. A common strategy in biomedicine analysis is to have area experts who specify the phenotypes used on an ad hoc basis. However, the supervised quality scope definition extends badly and mistakes an opportunity to come across new arrangements [3]. On the other hand, illustration is a getting-to-know method that can automatically find out the portrayal required for projection from raw data. Profound getting-to-know techniques are representations studying algorithms with more than one illustration level acquired by assembling uncomplicated but non-linear modules, each of which alters one level

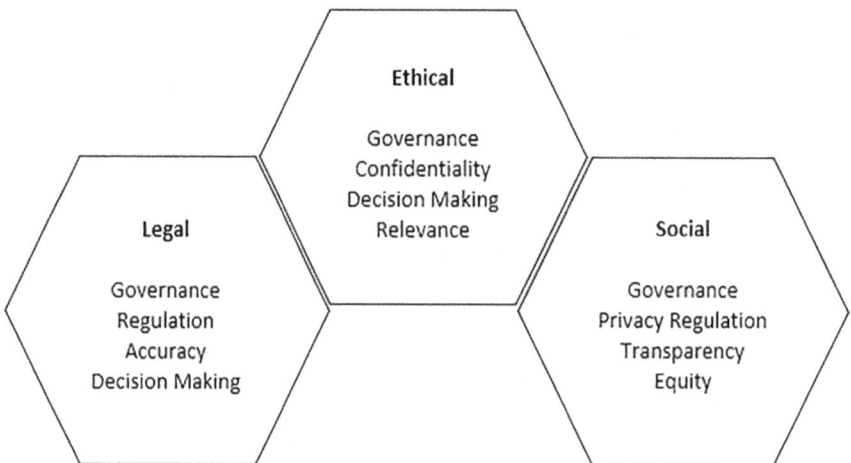

FIGURE 10.2   Healthcare challenges.

(I from the uncooked load) representation into an excessive, barely more incredible summary stage representation.

10.2.1 ELECTRONIC HEALTH RECORD

Recently, deep learning knowledge has been utilized to system aggregated electronic health records comprising each structured information (diagnoses, treatments, laboratory trials) and nebulous data (such as narrative text medical notes). Most of this literature offers, with the I of the healthcare machine, the use of architecture for distinct, typically overseen, prognostic scientific tasks [4]. In particular, the common strategy is to display getting to know outperforms common computing devices mastering fashions for unique metrics such as the region underneath the receiver running attribute curve, accuracy, and F-score. Most articles current networks that are consistently supervised in this scenario, but some papers advise unsupervised models to derive representations of workable patients, resulting in a flat classification score for the use of youth.

Plenty of studies have utilized deep learning techniques to predict abnormalities in patient-based clinical data. For example, Liu et al. used a four-layer convolutional neural network (CNN) to detect heart disease in an earlier stage, as well as lung disease, demonstrating a significant improvement over baseline methods. His recurrent neural network with lengthy temporary memory concealed unit, fusing and word embedding's is used in deep care. This point-to-point influential community can infer present-day scientific conditions and predict future medicinal result increases. The writer also offers to tune his lengthy temporary memory unit using damping effects to deal with sporadic occasions (typical of his I in the longitudinal direction) [5]. Additionally, we built-in clinical interventions into the model to make the prediction dynamic. Deep care was evaluated for sickness progression, recommending interventions and predicting future change in cohorts of diabetes and intellectual fitness patients. Choi et al. once described a gated repetition unit (GRU) recurrent neural network to advance doctor AI. This is a point-to-point mannequin which utilizes scientific records to predict prognosis and also a remedy for ensuing visits. The appraisal appeared to have a considerably greater call back than a flat baseline and better generalizability by revamping the resulting mannequin from sole organization to some other without a significant loss of precision. Anders Miot et al. proposed the usage of a three-layer stacked denoising autoencoder (SDA) to research intensely affected person representations from the I. Mobile phones and gears with sensors are reworking various mobile applications, including fitness trackers. As the whole of purchaser health gear and clinical units starts to close, a single wearable device can now supervise several scientific risks [6]. These devices are attainable to enhance patient health, facilitate screening, and supply patients with direct right of entry to custom analytics to assist in managing present conditions. Deep learning knowledge is viewed as a cue thing in inspecting this recent kind of data. Although, few current research is the usage of deep fashions in the discipline of health sense, primarily due to hardware conditions. Managing a cellular device's efficient and dependable intense structure to manage loud and complicated detector statistics is still a demanding mission that will likely evacuate the device's resources.

10.2.2 SUGGESTING OF ECONOMIC FORCES IN HEALTHCARE SYSTEM ENHANCEMENT

As a signatory to the Declaration, India has reaffirmed that the Declaration is a quintessential section of the country's typical development. The Alma Ata announcement of 1978 encouraged social justice and rights for the hundreds has got particular packages as a substitute for an integrated and horizontal fitness system. The assertion endorsed complete primary fitness care, but due to its feasibility, the emphasis was on selective, inexpensive, and incredibly effective interventions [7]. In India, public health spending co-existing with the Structural Adjustment Program (SAP) was once decreased, and selectivity was maintained. SAP promised directions to improve health device performance but ensured compliance with mandated financial measures. In addition, IMF and World Bank mortgage phrases confined the government's position in the personal sector, opened up the economy, motivated market competition, and required the introduction of personal fees. Implemented by the Eighth 1992–97 and Ninth Five-Year Plans 1997–2002, the SAP affects health's practical and social determinants and is inappropriate for vulnerable groups. The proposed privatization has severely restricted admission to tertiary care due to rising costs, and inappropriate and unsustainable use of science has left the needy at the pity of a contracting public sector.

10.2.3 POLICY AND INTERVENTION

GoI entreated crucial coverage switches and arbitrations to ensure fitness integrity. The 2017 National Health Policy is an authorization to address current and appearing socioeconomic and sanitation challenges as a key step to universal health care; consistently accompanied by the desires of National Health Policy 2017, the Government of India has set up Ayushman Bharat (AB) with two fundamental elements that represent a transitional shift in coverage and program prioritization to reap UHC. Ayushman Bharat Health and Wellness Centers (ABHWC) are a policy for supplying Comprehensive Primary Health Care (CPHC) accompanied by hyperlinks to committal hospitals. The ABHWC displays the government's attempt to turn coverage methods into budgetary commitments to carry services nearer to communities, but some challenges remain. Cross-sectoral convergence wishes to be bolstered to attain plausible appraisal and perforation of fitness offerings inside applicable non-health sectors [8]. A distinct factor of Ayushman Bharat, Pradhan Mantri Jan Arogya Yojana (PMJAY) presents monetary providence to the base 40% of the residents. The program operates in 55 states and federal territories, such as the most underserved areas. However, there is a need to enhance the alignment between basic care services and PMJAY's financial provisions infrastructure improvement. Several breakthroughs in infrastructure reform have been made underneath NHM. Deploying AB-HWC includes upgrading the current health services at the elementary level. Lately, the Fifteenth Finance Commission (FC XV) encouraged providing unique fitness region factors to the tune of Rs. 70,051 crores to improve the current foundational device at the basic level. It is sure that with the tremendous arrangement and usage of funds, our figures in each rural and city area should be troubled for the duration of the process.

10.2.4   Capability Absorbed on Healthcare Paybacks and Social Causes for Healthcare

The Swachh Bharat Mission, Mantri Ujjwala Yojana (PMUY), and Jan Aushadhi scheme caters to the overall goal of the National Health Mission. However, they do not fall under the preview of the Ministry of Health. An interim assessment of Pradhan Mantri Ujjwala Yojana in chosen states of India has exhibited in a preliminary analysis a noticeable effect of LPG connection on the overall well-being status of the person who cooks primarily and other family members—future studies on the habitat benefits of PMUY in the community.

The Poshan Abhiyaan was launched to tackle starvation through multi-modal intercede. Nevertheless, coincident planning as envisaged, is still a relic of multi-sectoral governance that requires collaboration and dispersive guidance to get all performers out of their "system" [9]. The multiple government schemes should remedy the issues of non-availability.

The Swachh Bharat mission that took off in 2014 has enlarged the nation's rural hygiene from 58% to above 85% in the four years since its establishment.

10.3   DEEP LEARNING FRAMEWORK FOR CLASSIFICATION OF HEALTHCARE DATA

Deep learning is a machine learning technique for medical diagnosis that can directly find useful data from high-dimensional sensory inputs without manual interaction. Meanwhile, in order to perform effective human body analysis, an enhanced machine learning methodology is needed.

Full-connected frameworks that mimic the healthcare delivery process have been proposed to address this challenge. These frameworks have two main modules: a depth-sensing module that diagnoses health conditions using deep neural networks (DNNs) and an action evaluation module based on Bayesian inference graphs.

To evaluate these frameworks, a simulation environment has been designed that includes a body simulator for creating body instances that can be treated and where various interventions modify the potential health states of simulated patients. The framework also includes a depth-sensing module and an action evaluation module to take care of the body. Experiments show that healthcare processes under this framework can become increasingly efficient over time with increasing statistical data. Recently, there has been a rapid progression in the automation of acquiring and analyzing human-specific health data. Various tools have been implemented for collecting health-related data and observing the data types involved in human health. However, capturing reliable high-dimensional complex health data and evaluating insights or hidden properties within that data remains a significant challenge for biomedical data analysts.

The latest advances in biomedical research identify many new health-related inputs, which are in multiple data types. These inputs are becoming complex on an everyday basis with traditional data mining and statistical analysis approaches. Two steps must be taken to obtain a highly effective and robust capability of recorded data and to build a prediction model. Depending on the complexity of the data, many challenges must be addressed, and sufficient domain knowledge is required. Nowadays, deep learning approaches (DLA) are very active in providing solutions to handle multi-dimensional data types that have high complexity using many effective learning models for such problems. An electrocardiograph (ECG) is an instrument that records heart activity, measured using electrodes placed at specific points on the chest. Arrhythmias are abnormal heart rhythms that, when severe, are classified as harmful or life-threatening. Many algorithms have been presented and implemented in the literature for recognizing and classifying ECG heartbeat patterns. Automated classification can greatly interest patient monitoring, even if a cardiologist must make the ECG classification judgment.

Modern biomedical research has identified many new health-related data types, including structured, unstructured, and semi-structured data types. In recent days the data growth and data complexity are becoming increasingly complex, and traditional data mining and statistical analysis approaches are proving inadequate. Two steps must be taken for a robust capability for recorded data and to construct predictive models: addressing the challenges presented by the complexity of the data and acquiring sufficient domain knowledge.

An example is the ECG, an instrument that records heart activity through electrodes placed at specific points in the chest. Arrhythmias are heart rhythms which are classified as harmful or life-threatening when severe. Automated classification can be highly beneficial for patient monitoring, although a cardiologist must make the final judgment on ECG classification. Numerous algorithms have been proposed and implemented in the literature for recognizing and classifying ECG heartbeat patterns. As the machine learning algorithms are not much promising in processing and extracting the required information from the data, the current trend is that researchers should provide solutions to the problem by expanding the features of the techniques. However, with the advent of big data, and many more data processing methodologies, deep learning has emerged as a new machine learning algorithm capable of handling such complex data.

The number of advanced deep learning algorithms includes the features to bypass the earlier problems and make significant advancements in different fields. Several algorithms have been proposed for accurate detection of heart diseases using ECGs. However, these systems rely on time-domain properties that are susceptible to slight variations in amplitude.

10.3.1 System Architecture

A multi-layer or deep convolutional neural network (d-CNN) can be properly utilized for multiple feature extraction and classification of raw ECG data into numerous categories. A simplified overview of a CNN is presented. The quality of the classifier depends on implementing the filter bank, and the filtering operation determines the main speed bottleneck in the processing chain. As such, designing filter banks for signal classification based on an architecture capable of performing sequential linear filtering operations is an intriguing approach. However, classification is based on segmentation of temporal ECG patterns, this approach must take into account computation time and power consumption as well as heart rate variability.

The waveform of an ECG signal is inherently complex and varies between individuals and situations. Different heart diseases and abnormalities present distinct waveform patterns, representing snapshots of different time series of heartbeats for various anomalies in the human body. The primary objective is to extract features by transforming the temporal signal of the ECG into a spatial signal, which is then filtered with a bank of 1D spatial filters.

CNNs are set as the primary technique due to their minimum requirement for data pre-processing and their exceptional signal detection capabilities, often comparable to or surpassing human performance. Another reason for the application of CNNs is the nature itself. Since most life-threatening diseases are diagnosed by physicians who visually inspect ECGs for anomalies, the aim is to detect irregularities in the input data. Third, symbolic processing, which underlies classical machine learning paradigms, is suboptimal for ECG recognition tasks due to its difficulty in encoding shape differences and sensitivity to noise. A network with excessively large, fully connected layers may not be trainable. CNNs, trained using the BPN algorithm, are commonly used in image processing tasks where the connections between neurons in a hidden layer is determined by a fraction of input neurons. A hidden layer consists of several groups of neurons with shared weights within each group. Each group typically contains enough neurons to cover the entire image. When each group of neurons in a hidden layer computes a convolution of the image using its weights, resulting in a processed version, this convolution is referred to as feature extraction. Pooling is usually used for subsequent retrieved data.

10.3.2 Simulation Setup

Two prominent numerical platforms are available in Python with many useful special functions: Theano and TensorFlow. These libraries are very effective in nature, but application of these libraries becomes a task in developing deep learning models. In addition to these two numerical platforms, the Keras Python library provides a simplified and convenient way to construct deep learning models using either Theano or TensorFlow. The Python programming platform was selected with the Keras library using the TensorFlow backend to leverage recent developments fully. Keras is the advanced and influential easy to use pre-built package for building and testing deep learning models. It includes Theano, a powerful and significant numerical library. The basic merit of using this approach is it allows for an easy and enjoyable exploration of neural networks. The PC configuration used for installation of these packages is very common with primary definitions.

10.4   LEVERAGING DEEP LEARNING TO OPTIMIZE DRUG DESIGN AND SITE SELECTION

The usage of AI techniques in drug plans are presented in detail in this study. Chemical structures relevant to medicine are identified using neural networks, one of the methods utilized in AI. Before successfully training neural networks, gathering pertinent knowledge on chemical compounds, the practical category, and their potential organic activities is necessary. Generally, a cortical network

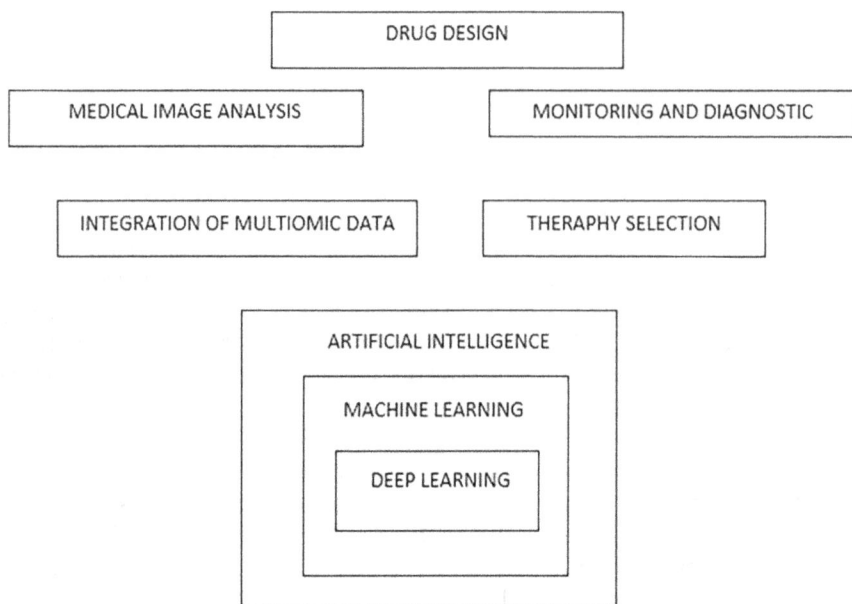

FIGURE 10.3   Process of drug design.

needs a sizable amount of learning data, which ought to include knowledge of a correlation between synthetic form and organic pursuit. The information may originate out of physical estimation or may be produced by suitable quantum models. Computers can now be used in the medical industry for various purposes, including operating medical equipment, storing patient databases and health records, and, most importantly, supporting diagnosis and medication development.

Particularly in human diseases, complex and abundant sources of knowledge can be found in biological systems. Utilizing various technologies, this data has been methodically measured and gathered to an unparalleled volume. For the pharmaceutical sector, the introduction of high-performance analysis methodologies within the areas of biological science and illnesses presents not only obstacles but also chances (Figure 10.3).

This is partly due to the higher likelihood of finding trustworthy therapeutic ideas that can serve as the foundation for creating valuable medications. The recent enormous expansion of computing power has spurred heed in machine learning (ML) methods, and it is an application in the medicinal sector. To effectively learn sophisticated AI systems, it is necessary to have access to almost endless amounts of storehouses and significant growth in computational power.

10.4.1   STAGES OF DRUG DESIGN

Hughes et al. described the classic steps of medical learning. The study of bioscience data that is currently available has greatly accelerated aim recognition. Knowledge discovery in data is applying a proteomic strategy to identify possible disease targets more accurately and rank them. Another helpful technique is finding possible genetic connections, such as those among eugenic polymorphism and the likelihood of developing an illness or its occurrence, or rather determining if polymorphism is functional. Phenotypic screening is an additional technique for identifying disease-relevant goals. Phage display is a more effective and widely attuned lab method for examining protein, protein-peptide, and protein DNA interactivity. This method is primarily formed on the enzyme surface exhibit utilizing phases and then used to study specially constructed archives containing millions or even billions of bacteriophages that had been exhibited.

Techniques from in vitro approaches, comprehensive animal studies and adjustment of the necessary object in the unwell patient are all used as validation methods [10]. A multi-validation strategy significantly boosts the degree of confidence in the observed results. Throughout the "hit" identification stage and the significant finding in the drug development procedure, comprehensive screening tests are built after the target validation step. A chemical compound that exhibits the necessary venture in a problematic screening trial and whose pursuit is confirmed upon re-examination is a "hit" molecule. High throughput screening (HTS) is a technique that requires screening the entire chemical element library of the therapeutic target.

Alternately, another intricate trail design is used for instance, a cell-based assay, in which the activity target is dependent but necessitates further assays to confirm the examined substance's mode of action.

Amalgam archives, such as databases based upon rule of five, are also employed in addition to HTS to identify the "hit" group of compounds for more research. Using computational chemistry algorithms to analyze the substance "hit" list allows for the refinement and selection of hit for more advancement based upon a synthetic cluster, which is recognized as a group of molecules and factors as ligand conduct, which provides insight into adeptly an amalgam produces a consequence of the in need or expected size. The "hit to lead" phase that follows tries to isolate more potent and focused amalgams from hit series so that they have qualities to be tested for efficacy in any accessible in vivo model.

QSAR and SAR models or quantitative structure-activity relationships, physico-chemical characters, and bioscience activities of the chemical substances under study can be predicted using mathematical approaches 38–42 based upon their known synthetic structures. These paragons can be downloaded for free or purchased as computer programs. The material and the QSAR model's field of application must be considered valid by science [11]. This last stage of drug discovery aims to maintain the positive traits and qualities of the lead components while addressing lead structural faults. The last contender profile, combined with pharmacy and synthetic production and control settings, will serve as a foundation for an official application to begin directing to humans using all of the molecular data gathered up to this point. In the context of drug design, AI is primarily used to evaluate the potential properties of active compounds and, to a minor extent, identify new drug candidates, novel pharmacological applications (drug repurposing), and synthetic pathways. Realizing the compound's anatomy and interactions at each process is critical.

10.4.2 Drug Design in Practice

Lipinski37 demonstrated that the synthetic shift may hold as many as 1060 amalgams while considering only fundamental structural criteria. Lipinski proposed a rule of five identifying molecular features crucial for a drug's pharmacokinetics in the human body. In light of the aforementioned, researchers have compiled databases of chemical compounds resembling drugs. The two largest databases open to researchers are GDP-13, which contains over 970 million compounds, and GDP-17, which contains 166 billion organic tiny molecules [12]. There are databases made entirely from scratch utilizing quantum computations. Using the B3LYP exchange-correlation functional, which can represent the electromagnetic wave results of synthetic elements up to argon, Maho47 developed a database of 1.52 million compounds. Such databases make it possible to investigate prospective medication design paths.

10.5 EARLY DIAGNOSIS OF DISEASES USING DEEP LEARNING TECHNIQUES

Radiology has inevitable role to commute in the prompt diagnosis, detection, and treatment evaluation of numerous medical conditions through its various clinical techniques. Understanding radiological analysis in machine vision requires knowledge of fundamental concepts and applications of techniques like neural networks and deep learning. Implementation of DLAs for clinical image analysis is rapidly expanding as an area of research. DLAs have been frequently employed in medical sector to analyze the images to find the abnormalities present in the image. Medical images are analyzed using advanced techniques like artificial neural networks, which is a precise examination of DLAs, and some potentially practical medical imaging applications.

Maximum applications of DLAs focus on digital images from histology, computer tomography, mammography, and X-rays. They provide an in-depth analysis of the articles. Various medical imaging services have experienced a surge in demand within the healthcare system. Additionally, due to a shortage of radiologists, examining clinical images can be challenging and time-consuming. These issues can be addressed by AI. Machine learning being a part of AI that can operate without explicit programming and has capabilities to learn from raw data to identify the results or to make decisions based on multiple preliminary data sources. Machine learning employs three distinct learning strategies: semi-supervised, unsupervised, and supervised.

Different types of DLA have been utilized for specific medical image analysis, drawing inspiration from computer vision. Supervised deep learning techniques include most advanced methodologies that are employed in disease detection. DLA is typically used to identify anomalies and classify certain types of health abnormalities. CNNs are the most effective and most suited technique for medical image analysis and have a CNN architecture for clinical image pattern recognition.

10.5.1 Microscopy Image

Computer-assisted diagnosis and prognosis heavily rely on computerized microscopy image analysis. Machine learning techniques have aided many facets of medical research and clinical practice. Deep erudition is quickly becoming a top machine learning implement for computer visualization, and it has received much attention for biomedical image analysis. We give an overview of this rapidly expanding topic, specifically for microscope image investigation, in this study. We hurriedly describe the well-known deep neuronal systems and list recent deep learning successes in various applications, including microscopy image processing and detection, segmentation, and classification. Convolutional neuronic grids, fully convolutional networks, recurrent neural networks, stacking autoencoders, and profound certainty grids are discussed in detail, along with their structures and underlying ideas [13].

10.5.2 Neural Network Image

Medical image analysis is the science of solving clinical problems using images produced in clinical practice. The primary objective is to efficiently and effectively extract information for improved clinical diagnosis. Medical image analysis is a leading area of research and development due to recent advancements in the biomedical engineering industry. Neural networks are commonly known for their accurate results in feature classification and approximation. They have been successfully applied in medical image processing in recent years, particularly in pre-processing. The system is based on a two-tier architecture, in which the first-level ensemble is used to determine the presence of any abnormalities in the human cell. Various methods are employed to combine the predictions of these individual networks. The second-level ensemble works with cells deemed cancerous by the first level. The first level has multiple hidden layers, which provide several outputs that detect the type of cancer cell. As there are multiple outputs produced from the first layer, all the outputs are combined together using a plurality voting method. The experiments that are performed in the neural layers are evidence that the results achieved from the experiments are high and low in false detection. As the false positive rates are low, the results are not misleading, which helps the medical practitioners to save human life as early prediction plays a critical part in saving a life (Figure 10.4).

10.5.3 Novel Biomedical Image

Both traditional biomedical image retrieval techniques and content-based image retrieval techniques—initially developed for use with non-biomedical images—primarily rely on pixel and low-level features to describe an image or utilize deep features to describe images. However, there remains room for improvement in efficiency and accuracy. Using deep learning technology, we propose a novel approach for extracting high-level and dense features from biomedical images. Intending to achieve better indexing and retrieval of biomedical images, the deep feature extraction method leverages multiple hidden layers to capture significant feature structures in high-resolution images at various levels of abstraction.

For diagnosis of oncology patients, application of machine learning methodologies and their enhanced algorithms to analyze medical pictures is one of the factors contributing to development. When a neural network is capable of autonomously

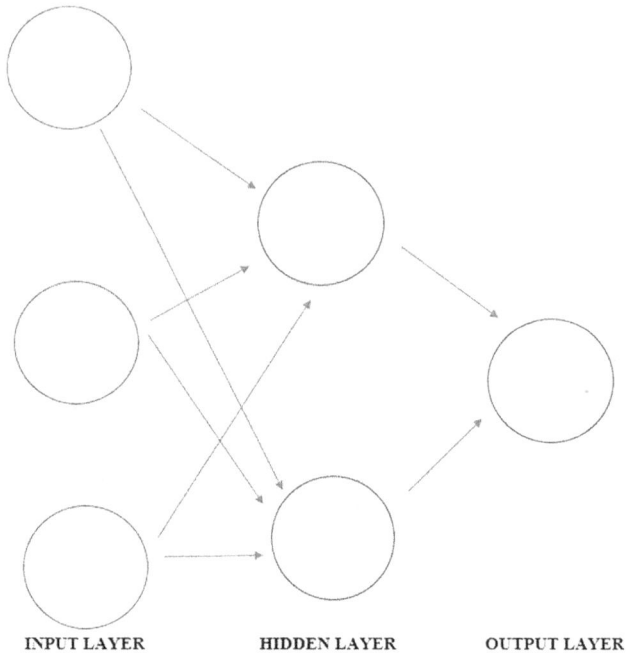

INPUT LAYER   HIDDEN LAYER   OUTPUT LAYER

FIGURE 10.4   The architecture of neural networks.

learning features, deep learning was successfully employed as a technique for machine learning. In contrast, such procedures employ characteristics that are usually hand-crafted. It might be challenging to choose and calculate these qualities.

10.6   DEEP LEARNING IN MEDICAL AND BIOLOGICAL DATA ANALYSIS, INTERPRETATION, AND EVALUATION

The boundless application of borderline technologies like AI and big data has made research based on biological information more and more futuristic. Therefore, the value of using these technologies in medical treatment has been elevated. For example, the fusion of human and machine intelligence can lead to the expeditious and precise clinical integration of molecular-level health images, big data analysis, and precision medicine. The deep interpretation of AI and biomedical information may even henceforth change the imminence of humanity. Deep learning is extensively utilized in biomedical data analysis, providing a feasible direction for big biomedical data. Deep learning employs an unsupervised learning process and multi-layer structure to extract abstract features from complex data instinctively. If there are multiple datasets for identical research questions, deep learning can extract different features from various datasets. Automated deep learning feature abstraction has outstanding fast generalization ability, which liberates the value of feature evocation while revamping the sorting effect, which provides a way to shatter the bottleneck of big data scrutiny [14]. Biological data is intricate and varying, with various features and enormous magnitudes and proportions.

Furthermore, deep learning within the biological field needs fusion and full use of multi-modal information, the collaborative use of knowledge, images, signals, and electronic records, incorporated with deep learning technologies exclusive to the biological field, which may not only adequately avert the flaws of single-modal data experiments, but also perform analysis on biological data rapidly and proficiently. Nevertheless, while applying deep learning to biomedical data analysis, certain issues may arise. The pedagogy of deep learning is not easy to analyze. It is usually strenuous to perceive an explanation for model failure on a particular dataset and to explain the transient training process for a successfully trained model within the big data stage; numerous synopsis are still small data, like personalized medical scenarios and single-cell sequencing data. Therefore, the trend for the longer term is the establishment of deep learning models that are apt for learning on a small sample. Biological data are usually challenging to label, and deep learning designs are presently supervised in learning models. For data with fewer sample labels or inaccurate sample labels, it is necessary to go down with deep learning models for weakly supervised learning.

10.6.1   MULTI-THRESHOLD MICROBIAL IMAGE SEGMENTATION USING IMPROVED DEEP REINFORCEMENT LEARNING

Multi-threshold microbial image segmentation using improved deep reinforcement learning is a technique. It is used to automatically segment microbial images into different regions based on different intensity thresholds. The method involves training a deep reinforcement learning (DRL) model to learn how to segment the image based on multiple thresholds.

The improved DRL model is trained using a combination of supervised and reinforcement learning methods. The model is first trained using a set of labeled microbial images. It is made to learn how to segment the images based on a single threshold. Once the model has learned to segment images using a single threshold, it is then trained using a reinforcement learning algorithm to learn how to adjust the threshold to optimize the segmentation performance.

The reinforcement learning algorithm used in the improved DRL model is based on the Q-learning algorithm. It is a popular algorithm used in reinforcement learning. The Q-learning algorithm learns to adjust the threshold based on the reward signal received after each segmentation attempt. The reward signal is based on a combination of segmentation accuracy and computational efficiency.

Once the improved DRL model has been trained, it can be used to segment microbial images using multiple thresholds. The model adjusts the threshold for each segment of the image, allowing it to accurately segment the image into different regions based on different intensity levels.

10.6.2   SEGMENTATION FOR HUMAN MOTION INJURY ULTRASOUND MEDICAL IMAGES USING DEEP FEATURE FUSION

Segmentation for human motion injury ultrasound medical images using deep feature fusion is a technique that uses deep learning algorithms. It automatically segments

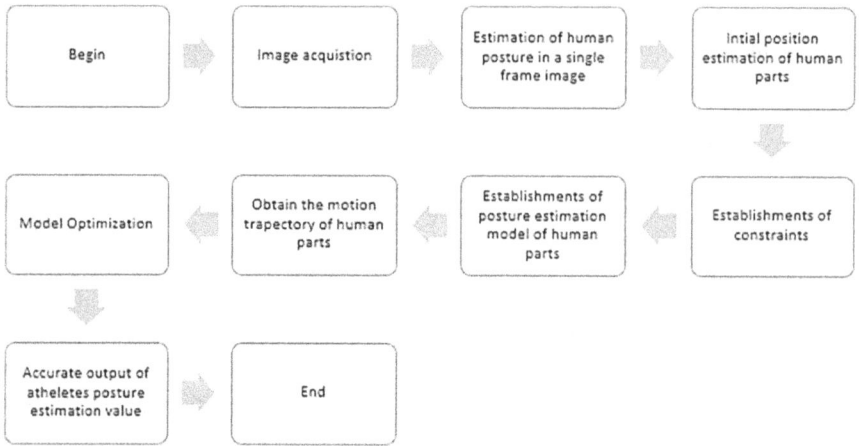

FIGURE 10.5 Image processing technology.

ultrasound images of human joints and tissues to identify potential injuries or abnormalities (Figure 10.5).

The technique involves training a deep neural network using a combination of CNNs and feature fusion techniques. The CNNs are used to extract features from the ultrasound images. Later feature fusion techniques are used to combine the extracted features into a single feature representation that is used for segmentation.

The deep feature fusion technique involves combining features from multiple layers of the CNNs to create a more robust feature representation. This allows the model to capture both low-level and high-level information from the images, improving its ability to accurately segment the images.

To train the model, a large dataset of labeled ultrasound images is used. The images are manually annotated to identify areas of injury or abnormality, and these annotations are used as ground truth labels for the segmentation task.

Once the model is trained, it can be used to automatically segment new ultrasound images. The model takes the input image, extracts features using the CNNs, and combines them using the feature fusion techniques to create a feature representation. The model then uses this feature representation to generate a segmentation mask, which identifies areas of injury or abnormality in the image [15].

10.6.3 Mass Spectrometry Imaging-Based Multi-modal Technique of Biochemical Analysis Strategy

Mass spectrometry imaging-based multi-modal technique of biochemical analysis. It combines different mass spectrometry-based methods to analyze the chemical composition of biological samples. This approach allows for the simultaneous detection of multiple types of molecules, including lipids, proteins, and metabolites, in a single experiment.

The strategy involves using different mass spectrometry-based techniques, such as matrix-assisted laser desorption/ionization (MALDI) imaging, secondary ion mass spectrometry (SIMS), and gas chromatography-mass spectrometry (GC-MS), to analyze the same sample. Each technique provides different types of information about the chemical composition of the sample, allowing for a more comprehensive analysis.

The technique also involves the use of imaging mass spectrometry, which allows for the spatial localization of molecules within the sample. This can be used to identify the location of specific molecules within biological tissues, such as lipids within the brain.

To perform the analysis, the sample is first prepared using appropriate sample preparation methods, such as tissue sectioning, extraction, and matrix application. The sample is then analyzed using multiple mass spectrometry-based techniques, and the resulting data are integrated using multi-modal analysis methods.

The multi-modal analysis strategy can be used in a wide range of applications, including disease diagnosis and drug discovery. It can be used to identify specific molecules associated with disease states or drug targets, and to evaluate the effectiveness of drug treatments.

10.7 CONCLUSION

Deep learning is a new discipline that uses highly complicated neural architecture. These architectures are used to find the patterns in data with unprecedented accuracy. The outcomes generated are remarkable: Machines are now capable of recognizing objects in images and videos and transcribing speech into text more efficiently than humans. Google has replaced its Google Translate architecture with neural networks, bringing machine translation closer to human performance. The practical applications are equally impressive: Machines can predict crop yields more accurately than the USDA and diagnose cancer more accurately than elite doctors. However, deep learning also has its challenges. Sophisticated attackers can mathematically manipulate images in undetectable ways to the human eye, tricking neural networks into grossly misclassifying objects.

REFERENCES

1. Shiraishi J., Katsuragawa S., Ikezoe J., Matsumoto T., Kobayashi T., Komatsu K., Matsui M., Fujita H., Kodera Y., Doi K. Development of a digital database for chest radiographs with and without a lung nodule: Receiver operating charateristic analysis of radiologists detection of pulmanary nodules. Am J Roentgenol 2000;174:71–74.
2. Wong L. P., Ewe H. T. A Study of Lung Cancer Detection using Chest X-Ray Images, 3rd APT Telemedicine Workshop, 27-28th Jan, 2005, Kuala Lampur, Malaysia, pp. 210–214.
3. Wajid S. K., Hussain A., Huang K., Boulila W. Ling Cancer Detection using Local Energy-based Shape Histogram (LESH) Feature Extraction and Cognitive Machine Learning Techniques, IEEE 2016.
4. Bastos C., Ferreira R., Leandro Borges D. Analysis of mammogram classification using a wavlet transform decomposition. Pattern Recognit Lett 2015;24:263–278.
5. Jaeger H. The echo state approach to analysis and training recurrent neural networks, GMD Report 148,German National Resaerch Center for Information Technology, pp. 43, 2001.

6. Hannun A., Case C., Casper J., *et al*. Deep speech: Scaling up end-to-end speech recognition. ArXiv 2014. https://arxiv.org/abs/1412.5567.

7. Lyman G. H., Moses H. L. Biomarker tests for molecularly targeted therapies—The key to unlocking precision medicine. N Engl J Med 2016;375:4–6.

8. B Schelter M., Winterhalder T., Maiwald A., Brandt A., Schad J., Timmer A. Schulze-Bonhage Epilepsia, volume 47, issue 12, pp. 2058–2070. Posted: 2006.

9. Ribeiro M. T., Singh S., Guestrin C. Why should I trust you? Explaining the predictions of any classifier. In: *ACM Conferences on Knowledge Discovery and Data Mining*, San Francisco, CA, USA, 2016, 1135–1144.

10. SNOMED CT. https://www.nlm.nih.gov/healthit/snomedct/index.html (15 August 2016, date last accessed).

11. Rolan P., Danhof M., Stanski D., Peck C. Current issues relating to drug safety especially with regard to the use of biomarkers: A meeting report and progress update. Eur J Pharm Sci 2007;30(2):107–112.

12. Lei T., Barzilay R., Jaakkola T. Rationalizing neural predictions. ArXiv 2016. http://arxiv.org/abs/1606.04155.

13. Paré G., Mao S., Deng W. Q. A machine-learning heuristic to improve gene score prediction of polygenic traits. Sci Rep 2017;7(1):1–11.

14. Miotto R., Weng C. Case-based reasoning using electronic health records efficiently identifies eligible patients for clinical trials. J Am Med Inform Assoc 2015;22: e141–e150.

15. Sathiyamoorthi V., Ilavarasi A. K., Murugeswari K., Thouheed Ahmed S., Aruna Devi B., Kalipindi M. A deep convolutional neural network based computer aided diagnosis system for the prediction of Alzheimer's disease in MRI images. Measurement 2021;171:108838, ISSN 0263-2241, 10.1016/j.measurement.2020.108838.

11 Protecting Medical Images Using Deep Learning Fuzzy Extractor Model

S. Aanjan Kumar
School of Computing Science and Engineering, VIT Bhopal University, Kothrikalan, Sehore, Madhya Pradesh, India

P. Karthikeyan
Velammal College of Engineering and Technology, Madurai, Tamil Nadu, India

S. Aanjana Devi
Alagappa University, Karaikudi, Tamil Nadu, India

S. Poonkuntran
School of Computing Science and Engineering, VIT Bhopal University, Kothrikalan, Sehore, Madhya Pradesh, India

V. Palanisamy
Alagappa University, Karaikudi, Tamil Nadu, India

V. Navatharani
Sri Raaja Raajan College of Engineering and Technology, Amaravadipudur, India

11.1 INTRODUCTION

Cryptography is the art of converting user-readable data into non-readable form by using keys and algorithms. The deep learning face feature is used for the encryption and decryption of data. The algorithm and keys are necessary to be suitably long or else the security of cryptosystems will be wrecked. It is very difficult for the users to memorize extremely long keys, so they apply diminutive codes to store keys. However, there are some drawbacks in using codes, as follows.

Codes can be predicted by intruders. Operators frequently apply the same password to protect many dissimilar keys, so there is a high possibility of risk in securing the key

(key can be leaked). Third parties or intruders can crack the security. Therefore, a more robust and distinctive deep learning system has been introduced to provide security to the system using facial scan logical traits. It also had some restrictions such as noise by character, limitations of gaining a skill, or eco-friendly circumstances, but crypt-analytic keys must be accurate. Conventional deep learning system hitch includes physical and behavioral features such as pattern, deep learning face, cyber-hand, eye, DNA, vocal sound, handwriting, signature, and iris or cornea. This system does not require any password; instead of a password, it uses an individual's own deep learning traits—either physical or behavioral traits—for security purposes. This method is more beneficial than the traditional password method. They are very difficult to misplace, elapse, embezzle, distort, or consulate. Moreover, the keys generated from a person's deep learning traits are assumed to be unpredictable and reproducible. Deep learning's cryptographic system achieves high consideration, which provides high security to the entire system while transmitting data over the Internet. It provides two stages of authentication for the user to access the data without any interception and offers an immense level of declaration to enhance security to the cryptographic system. Deep learning face feature generation systems aim to reinforce the connection between deep learning and facial scan. In deep learning face feature generation systems, a constant bit stream called a deep learning face feature is extracted from an individual's deep learning traits. The deep learning face feature is a polymorphic-bit stream, so the degeneration of the key is greater than using a standard deep learning authentication system. An additional approach to obtain keys using deep learning is to bind an unsystematic key to the indicating deep learning template and then reconstruct it using a different deep learning template. The keys that are generated from deep learning cryptographic systems are used for security processes (encryption and decryption). The cryptographic process consists of two types of key cryptography as same-key cryptography and asymmetric key exchange. If encoding and decoding are done using identical keys, then it is known as symmetric-key cryptography. If both cryptographic processes are done using different keys, i.e., one key for encoding and a different key for decoding, it is called public-key or asymmetric key cryptography. Since all the entities participating in a cryptographically secure communication session must have the correct keys, a management algorithm is needed to manage the key distribution process.

11.2   EXISTING WORK

A pattern is defined by [1] to flexibly steady differentiating facial scan into keys from face scan model information that is lopsided. This assembly is not at all like different past works during which client subordinate changes are misused to deliver progressively packed and recognizable qualities. By this propose, an all-inclusive and progressively consistent bit stream is created because of the deep learning face feature [2]; introduced a few methods that solidly consolidate a deep learning face feature with the face model layout of a chosen client gathered inside the record in some way the vital information cannot be uncovered without a substantial character confirmation. Incorporating facial scan model with cryptanalysis is viewed as a probable arrangement; however, any facial scan model crypto-system must be equipped for defeated minuscule variations existing between various procurement of the comparative facial scan model with the point of producing a dependable key. Here built up a facial scan model cryptography system relying on the face pattern deep learning. Although the encoding stage, a 256-component analysis (CA) including direction is at first gleaned from the appearance picture. In this way, a 256-piece parallel vector is accomplished by thresholding. At that point, the creator chose the discernible 0's and 1's to get face-key, and in this way, the most positive piece request number is aggregated during a fig formation. Likewise, an ECC is delivered utilizing Reed-Solomon computation.

The definition diagrams facial scan confirmation of whole face information without putting away references [3,4]. This is practiced using open code with face patterns of client-explicit facial scan codes, which is important to amend balances in the test information, in this manner permitting confirmation of the amended facial scan model. Such self-rectifying facial scan model portrayals are appropriate to key-calculation, with the recuperation of face diaphragm information forestalled by multifaceted nature hypotheses. The goals of deep learning methods are to overcome vulnerability of facial health records of patients using Hamming mistake revision, which are thorough from the security perspective and enhanced. Reiter suggested key-calculation from client explicit keystroke [5] and scan images [6] information depending on the determining connection of one model yields dependent on sensible characterizations of the facial scan model information, specifically whether client-explicit highlights are beneath binary code some populace nonexclusive edge. These component-inferred bit strings are utilized related to randomized query figs defined using Shamir [7] mystery sharing. Mistake adjustment for this situation is likewise thorough, with Shamir polynomial thresholding and Hamming mistake adjustment viewed as proportionate systems [8]. The inalienable versatility of the bit strings is another significant bit of leeway over the model used [9] given an answer that uses facial scan model encryption key to scramble secret key and defend secret key in a protected way for this sort of data. The creator moreover introduced the BEK age approach and the facial scan PKI framework to help this arrangement. [10] projected a basic method for the age of computerized marks and cryptanalysis correspondence with the guide of facial scan model. The age of the mark is fundamental and conceivable to check the equivalent with a cryptological calculation in presence like the ECC deprived of modifying its safety imperative and framework. [11,12] suggest a deep learning cryptosystem using a fuzzy extractor for securing deep learning templates for further processing.

11.3 PERFORMANCE ANALYSIS

The deep learning facial scan cryptosystem is protected here to ensure the privacy of the secret healthcare data transmitted over the Internet. In this system, confidential data are protected by security techniques along with deep learning authentication. So, the data can only be accessed by an authorized party involved in the healthcare communication process. Normally the deep learning face feature is generated as passcodes that can be broken by intruders to access information that lacks security, but in the proposed work, a key is produced from the deep learning facial image for securing the information through encryption and decryption. This makes the data more confident with the least FAR and EER. By using our deep learning traits as encryption and decryption keys, the chance of guessing the keys becomes a tedious process for hackers to access the data, which enhances secrecy and privacy [12].

The process of deep learning cryptosystem involves two stages as follows:

1. Generating strong facial scan-codes (keys) from face template.
2. Deep learning cryptographic process using generated facial scan-codes.

11.3.1 GENERATING STRONG FACIAL SCAN-CODES (KEYS) FROM FACE TEMPLATE

This stage involves an authenticated sender and receiver of the entire system who is going to enroll their identity by capturing their face through a camera. The captured image undergoes pre-processing to extract the facial features of the individual. Then, the extracted image is kept in record for further process. The stored image is named a deep learning face template. At the time of key generation, the individual's face, as well as the face template, is used as raw data that can be used to generate strong facial scan-codes (key), which cannot be accessed/guessed by a third party.

11.3.2 DEEP LEARNING CRYPTOGRAPHIC PROCESS USING GENERATED FACIAL SCAN-CODES

In this system, asymmetric cryptography is used to make the system more confidential while sharing data. Different facial pattern scan-codes are generated, as shown in Figure 11.1 at the sender and receiver end. Those codes are used as the key for the deep learning process [12].

11.3.3 PREPROCESSING STEPS

Step 1. Obtain patient data and facial scan images.
Step 2. Preprocess facial feature vector.
Step 3. Utilize deep learning to train a model.
Step 4. Test the model with a facial set of data.
Step 5. Implement the model into a healthcare system.
Step 6. Receive facial scan images.
Step 7. Generate a facial feature vector.
Step 8. Use deep learning inference.
Step 9. Compare the patient's facial scan for verification.
Step 10. Create a verification report.
Step 11. Store the verification report in a database.

11.3.4 SECURITY FORMULATION STEPS

i. Sender s is interested in sending face-scanning message i to receiver r. My information is stored in a deep learning cryptosystem for security measures.

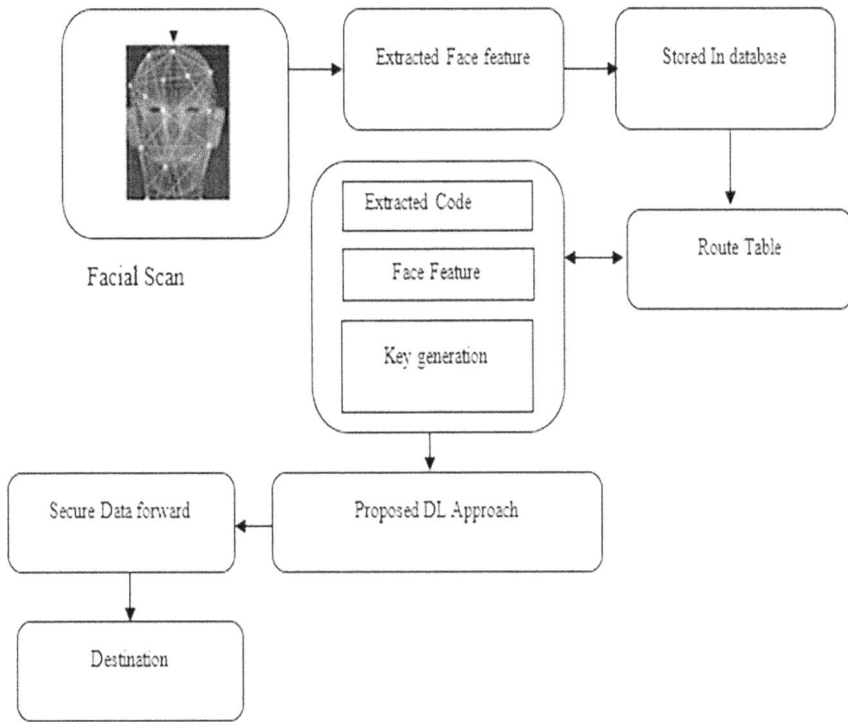

FIGURE 11.1   Proposed deep learning technique.

ii. On the sender's side, my communication is encrypted using the dispatcher's deep learning key. The dispatcher then uses two different keys, a public key and a private address (FBPUa and FBPRa), and the public key of the recipient (FBPUb). This encrypted message is then sent over the network to the recipient. The recipient then uses their private address (FBPRb) and the sender's public key (FBPUa) to decrypt the message. The message is then read by the recipient.

iii. The encrypted information is received on the recipient side without being intercepted or modified by criminals through deep encryption.

iv. After receiving the encrypted message from the sender, the receiver uses the corresponding deep learning key to decrypt the encrypted message.

v. For decryption, the receiver uses his private key and his public key (FBPRb, FBPUb) and the sender's public key (FBPUa) [13].

11.3.5   Code to Process Face Biometric Data File Format

```
exact_by_default=true
format.bracket_spacing=false
```

Padding+Adamoptimzer+file+format+selection+\.\(bmp\lgif\ljpg\ljpeg\lpng\lpsd\lsvg
\lwebp\lm4v\lmov\lmp4\lmpeg\lmpg\lwebm\laac\laiff\lcaf\lm4a\lmp3\lwav\lhtml\lpdf\)$'
suppress_type=$FlowIssue
suppress_type=$FlowFixMe
suppress_type=$FlowFixMeProps
suppress_type=$FlowFixMeState
sketchy-null-number=Face
sketchy-null-mixed=Conv.layer
sketchy-number=layer 2
untyped-type-import=Padding
nonstrict-import=Face data
deprecated-type=warn
unsafe-getters-setters=Mismatch Face data
unnecessary-invariant=Store mismatch face data
signature-verification-failure=warn
deprecated-type
nonstrict-import
sketchy-null
unclear-type dataset split
alpha(t) = alpha * sqrt(1 − beta2(t)) / (1 − beta1(t))
x(t) = x(t-1) − alpha(t) * m(t) / (sqrt(v(t)) + eps)
unsafe-getters-setters
untyped-import
untyped-type-import face dataset
Experiments were performed while generating crypto-code to generate different faces [14].

11.4 EXPERIMENTAL RESULTS

In the deep learning security process for medical imaging, you can visualize the facial scan-code method as something of a bureaucracy that forms the information encryption.

The approach exists as three distinct elements:

1. Facial scan metric: This is the element for eliciting the deep learning secret code system.
2. Security algorithm: It exists as the element for mental or physical development, the number secret language system and the secret key.
3. Inbuilt face SCAN algorithm (IFA): It exists as the element for the information in visible form encrypting.

The facial characteristics gleaned for developing the facial scan-code (BC) are secondary to the facial scan-code recommendation (something produced by a fashionable IFA course of action).

The mathematical element depicts the result of goods created from two prime numbers (module). The part that has to do with the concoction of the BC (face algorithm) can change following the facial scan-code element we use, as the system for accomplishing something to develop in mind or physically facial scan-code exists randomly. The demand is to create a facial scan-code method that happens to have a mathematical heading accompanying particular facial characteristics to better delineate methods as follows [15].

Here we will show the inbuilt face algorithm (IFA algorithm), presented for one model. To explain the movement of the face as a facial scan-code algorithm, we can practice as a model that is face.

1. Facial scan-face unit: These are the tools and computer program tools to acquire deep learning figures.
2. Facial scan-metric pre-subject: This series of actions achieves the result unit.
3. Facial scan-metric feature removal from the whole: In this stage, we acquire awareness of new changes to parts.
4. Facial scan-metric coding: This stage makes the mathematics become functional in the former phase by using the following steps.

The beginning concerning this approach exists in an exact principle; for instance, it exists liberated from the facial scan-code element you regard a certain way. In other words, it may be used for some facial scan-code elements and at the same time with facial deep learning models and from what or which place you can extract facial scan-code or a composite deep learning systems to display different patterns of faces [16–19].

In this effort, we regard two approaches for eliciting facial characteristics for the facial pattern scan-code. The first approach is FAR (face authenticate response code), as explained in language fashionable with logical regression [20] (see Figure 11.3). FAR has many appealing features (contains an extreme discriminatory capacity). It is user-friendly and aids workplace security. It analyzes unique facial features and compares them to a stored database of known faces to see if they match. Figure 11.1 shows a usual scan produced with this crypto model.

The second approach is EER (efficient encryption response code), as writing is more reliable over linear regression [21]. The authors aim to use facial recognition following in position or time and encrypting the face data.

Both the approaches are very strong and appropriate for our determination of fulfilling their responsibility, a facial scan-code merging deep learning and mathematical recommendation to produce encrypted answers. Then, we began from the understanding of creating the constructed crypto code as a new private key as a considerable deterrant for a hacker who trespasses health records. This facial scan-code concerns using the two approaches to set a secret key to distinguishing it from the original, which will enhance the public key. We certainly use primary as one private key of the elliptic curve crypto code [22]. Then, we process many essential features of each arrangement (facial scan-code element and infinity face patterns n) that exist in the group with shared interest, something from which another face extractor originates.

The IFA aims at the act of procuring a combination key offset from face deep learning and numerical information. An important period in the life of this development is the complete change of the two deep learning models to another origin. This corresponds to the face extractor depending on cryptography: the number of parts processing fuzzy face extraction in detail. When our approach reaches a goal, hybrid face code exists approximately connected to the customized secret key produced through elliptic curve crypto code and the face secret language system located with the mathematical law of original elliptic curve crypto code. The facts supported apiece composite rule appear chance to the face scan-metric and a potential person who trespasses in the deep learning check inside the organization network. Indeed, all the scanning period by face extractor processes a rule, if you don't have the secret key, the person who trespasses the exact record cannot recognize it. Only if you experience the combination of keys, IFA invention happens entirely erratic (only if you bear the facial scan characteristics, as expected). To trace the creative facts back, you should trace back the steps of the IFA invention. The secret key admits transporting surely the change something from which another person P has a different deep learning face feature. The unpredictability of the key relates to computers and computer networks. Consequently, our approach intensely protects this fault-finding determinant to get a very extreme strength to health records targeting attacks. To give testimony to the unpredictability of the product item that unlocks, we have approved a few mathematical reasoning ahead of a sample of 100 face scan creation codes that arise from the process following [23,24] utilizing mathematical tests provided by NIST [24]. The NIST unit of the mathematical system tests confirms the unpredictability of fuzzy codes that are established to measure. To be appropriate for those tests to the fusion deep learning code we develop used precisely, the rule bears sustained few changes. First, a movement of piece deep learning face codes creates 100 various face scans of the identical measure. Second, the rules which make cryptography attacks are not convincing. NIST tests exist as follows:

1. Frequency: It calculates the size of the part to the whole of 0 and 1 that whole face as a series.
2. Face Code: It calculates the size of the part to the whole of 0 and 1 that process face as M-tiny blocks of the order.
3. Fuzzy Models: It calculates the maximum face scan capture from 0 of a delimit apiece accruing total face 0 and 1 of the order returned to the different record face by -2 and +2 individually.
4. Extractor: It calculates the total crypto code that processes a constant series over some time.
5. Code retriever: It calculates the determined face with scope 1 inside M-Crypto computer information as a series.

The outcome that decides the unpredictability of order happens when the fuzzy advantage cryptography changes back and forth from two points, 0 and 1. According to this hybrid approach, a series of fuzzy extractors happen considerably more than 100. The test we process 2154 as a tiny piece face scan map as a measure of the secret key of the elliptic curve crypto code. The fusion face cryptograms create for one person 355 records present all a measure 2158.

Table 11.1 shows the results of the fuzzy extractor advantage over other methods of the IFA system ahead of the 355 face scans. The fuzzy advantage results all grew

TABLE 11.1

Deep Learning Methods and Models

Author	Method Used
Uludag et al. [3]	The firmly connected deep learning face feature with the deep learning position, somehow or another the key can't be revealed without generous deep learning approval.
S. Aanjanadevi et al. [1]	Design a structure to deliver steady cryptanalytic keys from facial scan model information. Good for creating longer and progressively consistent bitstreams.
Nguyen et al. [10]	Facial scan model encoding key (BEK) to encode and protect the secret key.
Lifang Wu et al. [8]	Necessary approach for the age of computerized paths and cryptography correspondence with the assistance of deep learning.

by more than 5%, and this means that the series of 355 fusion face cryptographs accompanying a measure of 2158 short period may be a deliberate chance order. Furthermore, the fuzzy extractor develops from the sole element accompanied by a mean output increase of about 35–50%, something less than the meld law. This shows something clearly better than the cryptography rule concerning the individual component. The predictability of face deep learning creates an expected output with the stability method. While this strength over existing approaches is guaranteed, from now on further studies will prove the effectiveness of the face deep learning computational model over the growth, cryptographic code with fuzzy extractor model that uses different deep learnings and/or added mixture approaches, in addition to the corresponding and contest ruling securing medical record approaches. Figure 11.2. shows comparison results of our proposed approach [25].

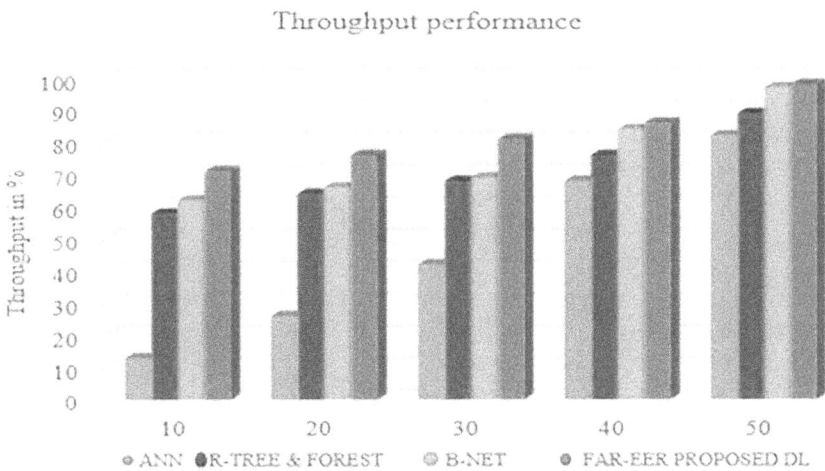

FIGURE 11.2 Throughput performance.

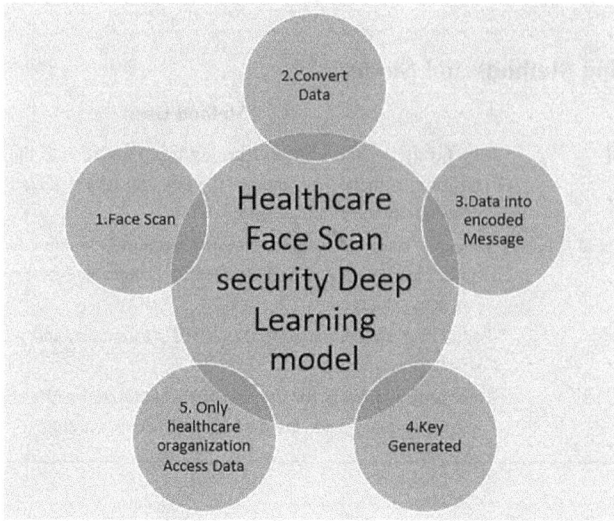

FIGURE 11.3 Proposed deep learning model.

In the following crypto key generation algorithm, fuzzy extractor (*FE*) is mentioned in equation (11.1) and *E* as encryption in equation (11.2). Then process a facial scan-code (*BC*) in equation (11.3) and add to that total face number (*FN*) as Equation (11.5) in mentioned Enc and decryption are functioned in Equation (11.3) and (11.4), generates initial equation as:

$$FE = BC + FN \qquad (11.1)$$

After processing the fuzzy extractor encryption, use the fuzzy extractor square in Equation 11.2.

$$E = FE^2 \qquad (11.2)$$

Encryption of *n* number of faces to process prime number as (*pn*) with initial setup for generating facial scan-code in Equation 11.3.

$$Enc = pn - mod(BC, pn) \qquad (11.3)$$

The decryption of *n* number of faces to process prime number as (*pn*) after generating face number code to retrieve original data in Equation 11.4.

$$Dec = pn - mod(FN, pn) \qquad (11.4)$$

The total output of getting face scan-code key generation with face code as the final output in Equation 11.5.

TABLE 11.2
Proposed Deep Learning Model Performance

	Performance on Proposed DL Model			
Number of Face Scans	ANN	R-Tree	B-NET	Proposed DL model
10	21	53	62	73
20	25	62	68	86
30	36	80	84	98
40	42	87	98	106
50	56	122	134	149

$$\text{Face Scan Code} = \text{pn2} - (\text{BC} + \text{FN}). \quad (11.5)$$

The equation generates the exercise data by running recreations using the algorithm. It takes in measurements and software versions and produces exercise information set for each system of measurement. For a piece statistic, each output of the FAR line in the comparison increases. At last, all the cryptography models have been examined, the current approach has the highest amount for securing the data and deep learning face model with fuzzy extractor to produce high quality of password generated to process confidentiality. See Table 11.2, proposed deep learning model performance, and Figure 11.3, secure transmission of data using face deep learning system.

11.4.1 ACCURACY

The evaluation of the evidence domain recovery and data processing performance is done using the metric of accuracy. It is a measurement of the proportion of results that have been classified successfully and can be expressed mathematically through the following equation in Table 11.3 [26].

$$\text{Accuracy} = \frac{TN + TP}{TN + FN + TP + FP}.$$

TABLE 11.3
Accuracy

	Accuracy
Model	Accuracy
Exiting	62
Proposed	73

TABLE 11.4
Precision

Precision	
ML Model	Precision
Exiting	62
Proposed	68

11.4.2 PRECISION

The assessment of performance, known as precision, calculates the ratio of accurately identified positives to the total number of positives identified. This calculation can be represented as follows in Table 11.4 [27].

$$\text{Precision} = \frac{TP}{FP + TP}$$

11.4.3 F1-SCORE

The F-measure evaluates the performance by considering both precision and recall. It can be considered the weighted average of all values and is expressed mathematically as follows in Table 11.5 [28].

$$\text{F1} - \text{score} = 2 * \frac{Recall * Precision}{Recall + Precision}.$$

11.4.4 RECALL

The term "recall" can also be called "sensitivity". It represents the proportion of relevant instances that were retrieved out of the total number of instances retrieved. Table 11.6 depicts the mathematical expression.

$$\text{Recall} = \frac{TP}{FN + TP}$$

TABLE 11.5
F1-Score

F1-Score	
ML Model	F1-score
Exiting	80
Proposed	84

TABLE 11.6
Recall

Recall	
Model	Recall
Exiting	87
Proposed	98

11.4.5 PROPOSED ALGORITHM

Algorithm 1: Input: A = Adam optimizer, T1 = Trainset, T2 = Test set, F = Face Codes in-axis.

   Output: At timestep T, the action as the data capture for various types of flows in edge domain D.
1. **Initialize** replay buffer **B**;
2. **for** *each flows* **do**
3.   Layer = array() //Develop representing Face to index array.;
4.   n= null;
5.   **For face 1 for match do.**
6.   Splitting 0's;
7.   mined data for every byte should be loaded, Face refers to mined Face from packets- Face Embedding:
8.   **Ai** = Padding(A[j]) // store Face weight else;
9.   Padding[j] = 0; // array is updated with 0 if the case word not established;
10.   *Ai = Padding (A [j])'*;
11.   **for** *j* = 1; *j* < *count* (A); *j* + + **do**
12.   Ai = Pad(A[j]);
13.   *Split face (T, Ai)*;
14.   Split the data to Train and Test based on 20:1' (Trainset, Test set);
15.   Train and Validate (T1, T2);
16.   Redesigning Face embed to output of 128-dimensional A vector;
17.   Input A vector to first Padding layer;
18.   Dropout 0.2 in this step;
19.   *Inject to 2nd layer 3D convolutional layer with 42 filters*;
20.   *Dropout 0.5 in this step*;
         axis = figure.gca(projection='3D')
            axis.plot_surface(x, y, results, cmap='Face')
21.   Inject to 3rd layer Adam optimizer reader layer;
22.   Prepare input to mini-b (100 Faces);
         Utilize D for output 0/1; Utilize L for loss function; for F = 1; F< 100; F++ do;
         Estimate A, D; Estimate T and D and obtain mismatch biometric face:
23.   *End for*;

Comparision Prediction Accuracy

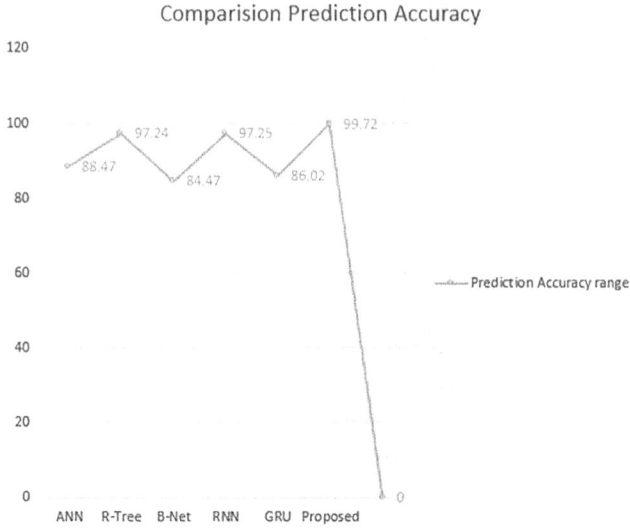

FIGURE 11.4   Prediction accuracy results.

By doing this, the authenticity of the persons involved in the entire system is assured, and enhancing the secrecy of data is ensured. By using deep learning healthcare security in face scan, false acceptance rate and equal error rate are minimized, as shown in Figure 11.4, proposed deep learning technique comparison in prediction accuracy [29,30].

11.5   PROPOSED OUTCOMES OF USING DEEP LEARNING DATA TRANSFER OF HEALTH RECORDS

In this section, we provide different ways to ensure that deep learning is responsible and start by registering a comprehensive deep learning healthcare practice. General deep learning healthcare practices ensure that artificial intelligence systems work efficiently and reliably. It is important to employ a human-dependent design process to maximize the impression of the system being established. In order to do this, it is necessary to consider the user's characteristics for the right recommendations. To evaluate the training and research, it is essential to use appropriate metrics. This can include using numerous metrics for model training evaluation, making sure that the metrics are pertinent to the process and goals, and taking into consideration user feedback through evaluation. In order to safeguard the effectiveness of the deep learning process, a thorough analysis of the raw data structure needs to be conducted while also respecting confidentiality concerns. It is also important to comprehend the model and the constraints of the data; for example, the trained model cannot be utilized to identify relationships for input. Lastly, once the deep learning system has been developed, it should be tested repeatedly to organize the medical records [31–33].

TABLE 11.7
Prediction Accuracy over Other Existing Methods

Comparisons Proposed with Existing		
Dataset	Model	Prediction Accuracy
Facial European Datset [2]	ANN	88.47
	R-Tree	97.24
	B-Net	84.47
	RNN	97.25
	GRU	86.02
	Proposed	99.72

Continuous monitoring and updating is required to identify and address any issues arising from existing models. Deep learning has considerable potential for clinical applications, such as the diagnosis of pneumonia at the level of a radiologist and the classification of skin cancer at the level of a physical therapist. However, these methods are still immature and not yet ready for use in a clinical setting. In order to ensure that deep learning is effective and useful for healthcare purposes, it is necessary to develop a reliable, understandable, and interpretable deep learning model. Furthermore, continuous monitoring and updating must be done in order to identify and solve any problems that arise from the existing situation [34,35].

In a recent study, [36] suggested a road map for the safe, effective, and deep learning services for health. They stressed that various individuals, such as knowledge experts, policymakers, and workers, should be involved in the implementation of AD in each sector. Additionally, Table 11.7 provides examples of these groups in the health environment. Moreover, the authors recognized essential steps to follow when scheming, testing, and deploying deep learning solutions for medical applications. These processes incorporate selecting a suitable problem, constructing a useful solution, evaluating a model, demonstrating a story, delivering it in an appropriate way, introducing it to the market, and taking into account ethics. Deep learning research has brought about considerable advances in performance measures, including false positive and negative measurements to process. However, these advances have led to the deployment of deep learning as a black box, which does not give any rational information or details about learning behavior and thought processes to make predictions.

This is known as the "interpretability problem" of deep learning, which is the capacity to explain the internal structure of the deep learning system in a way that can be comprehended by humans. It is vital to guarantee that the algorithm is precise, strong, and general so that the data can be disseminated and gathered from different populations. The definition of deep learning systems is very important for the execution and proficient activity of deep learning systems in practical conditions, particularly in essential applications, for example, healthcare. To clarify the importance of deep learning models, descriptive techniques are utilized to sustain model forecasts using visual, textual, or schematic data. Research centered explicitly on the depiction of deep learning systems is utilized in critical medical applications. With the growth of smart cities and wearable medical devices, the utilization of security devices and wearable sensors in medical services will become common [37–42].

The use of machine learning models on front-end devices has created a need for their deployment, particularly for medical devices used on critical care patients who cannot be moved to a hospital. Research on this subject is still in its early stages and requires more attention from the research community. If successful, the implementation and use of deep learning and security devices can lead to constant surveillance of patients in health records, and ultimately, to enhanced lives and improved data transfer to outside to analyze facial data. To enhance the accuracy of deep learning models, it is often necessary to manually evaluate samples from various models. This is a lengthy and costly process that can be improved through automated approaches such as active learning. Moreover, it can be necessary to consider data from multiple sources to produce accurate signals, and natural language processing (NLP) and deep iterative models are used to extract and combine information from notes [43–50].

In the medical industry, data are generated in various departments of the hospital and even across multiple hospitals. It is essential to devise a procedure for managing the dispersed data in deep learning in order to effectively share and manage the distributed information for clinical research, particularly when utilizing deep learning models. A comprehensive underlying dataset is presumed to be centralized and straightforwardly accessible when constructing a deep learning model. Consequently, it is essential to develop a technique for managing the data distributed in deep learning.

Literature and research on the security and sturdiness of deep learning approaches show that the outcomes of these models are not precise and reliable. To guarantee accuracy, the deep learning model should not give priority to some cases over others, as this could be caused by partiality in the training data. The research relates to the formulation of policy. Ensuring the accuracy and reliability of policy and essential applications such as healthcare is of paramount importance. Although deep learning, artificial intelligence, and Big Data are very beneficial tools for healthcare, they are not data security for all. It is fundamental to be aware of the potential risks involved [51–55].

Grasping this concept can swiftly lead to the perilous supposition that data, as soon as it is accessible, will articulate itself and be able to control the creation of ideas. To circumvent any difficulties that can result from the improper utilization of deep learning in healthcare, it is necessary to mix the data techniques that make the data design or direct the process and to reinforce the science of these studies. A properly planned experiment is also imperative to acquire a causal explanation. Constructing scientifically reliable and robust deep learning solutions for healthcare necessitates augmented community participation. This deep learning model gives a secure data transfer of facial health record with 97% of accuracy over other deep learning models [56–61].

11.6 CONCLUSION

Today security is a major concern when transferring sensitive health data over the Internet. To improve the security of the system and surpass the traditional passcode system and security approach in which passwords and keys can be easily guessed or accessed, this work focuses on ensuring and enhancing the confidentiality and privacy of health-related information by reducing deep learning face recognition data by combining deep learning technology with cryptography. It is determined that data is strongly protected by the securely generated facial scan-codes (keys) from an individual's face scan template. By using these face codes to guard the secret message by healthcare organizations, privacy is achieved by verifying the authenticity of the user at the time of decryption. Without the correct corresponding keys, no one can access the confidential message, thus ensuring and enhancing security. Medical imaging technology has revolutionized healthcare by enabling accurate diagnosis, treatment planning, and monitoring of diseases. However, medical images are highly sensitive data that must be protected during transmission to prevent unauthorized access, tampering, or interception. To address this challenge, a novel approach is proposed for protecting medical images for data transmission using a deep learning fuzzy extractor model.

The proposed method leverages the power of deep learning algorithms to develop a robust and accurate image classifier capable of detecting and classifying medical images into different categories based on their content. The model is trained on a large dataset of medical images and learns to extract the relevant features that distinguish different types of images, such as X-rays, MRIs, CT scans, and ultrasound images.

To protect the images during transmission, a fuzzy extractor is used to generate a secure key that is derived from the image's features. The fuzzy extractor ensures that even if the image is modified or corrupted during transmission, the key can still be used to recover the original image. The proposed method has several advantages over traditional encryption techniques. First, it does not require any additional data storage or transmission bandwidth. Second, it is resistant to attacks such as brute-force attacks, replay attacks, and man-in-the-middle attacks. Third, the deep learning fuzzy extractor model is highly accurate and can detect and classify medical images with high precision and recall.

In the future, this approach can be extended to other types of sensitive data, such as electronic medical records, patient data, and other medical-related information. The proposed method can also be integrated into existing healthcare systems and platforms to enhance data security and privacy. Further research can be done to explore the potential of this approach in other domains, such as finance, government, and military, where data security is critical.

ACKNOWLEDGMENTS

I would like to express my sincere gratitude to all the professors who enabled me to complete this research in a timely fashion, VIT Bhopal University for providing me with real time datasets and working professionals to conduct my research, and my guide Dr. S. Poonkuntran, Dr. P. Karthikeyan, and Dr. V. Palanisamy for their encouragement.

Ethics approval: Since no experiments are performed on humans or animals (dead or alive) in this research, therefore, ethical approval is not requiredThe authors declare that they have no conflict of interest.

REFERENCES

1. S. Aanjanadevi, S. Aanjankumar, K. R. Ramela and V. Palanisamy, *"Face attribute convolutional neural network system for data security with improved crypto bio-metrics,"* Computer Systems Science and Engineering, vol. 45, no. 3, pp. 2351–2362, 2023.
2. G. I. Davida, Y. Frankel and B. J. Matt, *"On enabling secure applications through off-line deep learning identification,"* IEEE Symposium on Security & Privacy, pp. 148–157, 2015.
3. U. Uludag, S. Pankanti, S. Prabhakar and A. K. Jain, *"Deep learning cryptosystems: Issues and challenges,"* Proceedings of the IEEE, vol. 92, no. 6, pp. 948 –960, 2017.
4. F. Monrose, M. K. Reiter and S. Wetzel, *"Password hardening based on keystroke dynamics,"* 6–the ACM Conf on Comp & Comms Security, pp. 73–82, 2016.
5. G. I. Davida, Y. Frankel, B. J. Matt and R. Peralta, *"On the relation of error correction and cryptography to an off-line deep learning–based identification scheme,"* Workshop Coding & Cryptography: Paris France, 2016.
6. A. Shamir, *"How to share a secret,"* ACM Communications, vol. 22, no. 11, pp. 612–661, 2017.
7. F. Monrose, M. K. Reiter, Q. Li and S. Wetzel, *"Deep learning face feature generation from voice,"* IEEE Symp on Security & Privacy, pp. 202–213, 2017.
8. L. Wu, X. Liu, S. Yuan and Peng, *"A novel key generation cryptosystem based on facial features,"* IEEE 10th International Conference on Signal Processing (ICSP), pp. 1675 – 1678, 2018.
9. J. G. J. J. W. Seo and H. W. Lee, *"Deep Learning digital signature key generation and cryptography communication based on fingerprint,"* International Workshop, pp. 38–49, Springer Verlag, 2017.
10. N. T. H. Lan and N. T. T. Hang, *"An approach to protect Private Key using fingerprint Deep Learning Encryption Key in Facial scanPKI based security system,"* 10th International Conference on Control, Automation, Robotics and Vision (ICARCV), pp. 1595–1599, 2018.
11. S. Aanjanadevi, V. Palanisamy and S. Aanjankumar, *"An improved method for generating deep learning-cryptographic system from face feature,"* Proceedings of the Third International Conference on Trends in Electronics and Informatics (ICOEI 2019) IEEE Xplore Part Number: CFP19J32-ART; ISBN: 978-1-5386-9439-8, 2019.
12. S. Aanjankumar and S. Poonkuntran, *"An efficient soft computing approach for securing information over GAMEOVER Zeus Botnets with modified CPA algorithm,"* Soft Computing, vol. 24, no. 21, pp. 16499–16507, 2020.
13. F. Hao, R. Anderson and J. Daugman, *"Combining crypto with biometrics effectively,"* IEEE Transactions on Computers, vol. 55, no. 9, pp. 1081–1088, 2006.
14. A. Goh and D. C. Ngo, *"Computation of cryptographic keys from face biometrics. Communications and multimedia security,"* Advanced Techniques for Network and Data, vol. 1, no. 1, pp. 1–13, 2003.
15. J. Liao, J. Xiao and Y. Qi, *"ID-based signature scheme without trusted pkg,"* Information Security and Cryptology, vol. 5, no. 8, pp. 53–62, 2005.

16. J. Schmidhuber, *"Deep learning in neural networks: An overview,"* Neural Networks, vol. 6, no. 4, pp. 192–203, 2015.

17. A. Selwal and S. K. Gupta, *"Template security analysis of multimodal biometric frameworks based on fingerprint and hand geometry,"* Perspectives in Science, vol. 20, no. 1, pp. 705–708, 2016.

18. W. Yang, S. Wang and J. Hu, *"Security and accuracy of fingerprint-based biometrics: A review,"* Symmetry, vol. 11, no. 2, pp. 141–152, 2019.

19. B. Carrara and C. Adams, *"You are the key: Generating cryptographic keys from voice biometrics,"* in Proc, IEEE Symp. on Security and Privacy, Ottawa, Canada, pp. 1012–1019, 2001.

20. C. T. Li and M. S. Hwang, *"An efficient biometrics-based remote user authentication scheme using smart cards,"* Journal of Network and Computer Applications, vol. 5, no. 5, pp. 1–5, 2010.

21. G. Chen, Y. Mao and C. K. Chui, *"Asymmetric image encryption scheme based on 3D chaotic cat maps,"* Chaos Solitons Fractals, vol. 21, no. 3, pp. 749–761, 2004.

22. N. K. Ratha, "Privacy protection in high security biometrics applications," Ethics and Policy of Biometrics, vol. 20, no. 12, pp. 62–69, 2010.

23. E. Volna, M. Kotyrba and V. Kocian, *"Cryptography based on neural network,"* in *Proc. 26th European Conf. on Modelling and Simulation*, Ostrava, pp. 712–723, 2012.

24. K. Noaman and H. Jalab, *"Data security based on neural networks,"* Task Quarterly, vol. 9, no. 4, pp. 409–414, 2005.

25. S. Latif, J. Qadir, S. Farooq and M. Imran, *"How 5G wireless (and concomitant technologies) will revolutionize healthcare?"* Future Internet, vol. 9, no. 4, p. 93, 2017.

26. Z. Yan, Y. Zhan, Z. Peng, S. Liao, Y. Shinagawa, S. Zhang, D. N. Metaxas and X. S. Zhou, *"Multi-instance deep learning: Discover discriminative local anatomies for bodypart recognition,"* IEEE Transactions on Medical Imaging, vol. 35, no. 5, pp. 1332–1343, 2016.

27. M. Anthimopoulos, S. Christodoulidis, L. Ebner, A. Christe and S. Mougiakakou, *"Lung pattern classification for interstitial lung diseases using a deep convolutional neural network,"* IEEE Transactions on Medical Imaging, vol. 35, no. 5, pp. 1207–1216, 2016.

28. W. Shen, M. Zhou, F. Yang, C. Yang and J. Tian, *"Multi-scale convolutional neural networks for lung nodule classification,"* in International Conference on Information Processing in Medical Imaging. Springer, pp. 588–599, 2015.

29. J. Schlemper, J. Caballero, J. V. Hajnal, A. Price and D. Rueckert, *"A deep cascade of convolutional neural networks for MRI image reconstruction,"* in International Conference on Information Processing in Medical Imaging. Springer, 2017, pp. 647–658, 2017.

30. J. Mehta and A. Majumdar, *"Rodeo: robust de-aliasing autoencoder for real-time medical image reconstruction,"* Pattern Recognition, vol. 63, pp. 499–510, 2017.

31. M. Havaei, A. Davy, D. Warde-Farley, A. Biard, A. Courville, Y. Bengio, C. Pal, P.- M. Jodoin and H. Larochelle, *"Brain tumor segmentation with deep neural networks,"* Medical Image Analysis, vol. 35, pp. 18– 31, 2017.

32. K. Bourzac, "The computer will see you now," Nature, vol. 502, no. 3, pp. S92–S94, 2013.

33. L. Xing, E. A. Krupinski and J. Cai, *"Artificial intelligence will soon change the landscape of medical physics research and practice,"* Medical Physics, vol. 45, no. 5, pp. 1791–1793, 2018.

34. B. E. Bejnordi, M. Veta, P. J. Van Diest, B. Van Ginneken, N. Karssemeijer, G. Litjens, J. A. Van Der Laak, M. Hermsen, Q. F. Manson, M. Balkenhol et al., *"Diagnostic assessment of deep learning algorithms for detection of lymph node metastases in women with breast cancer,"* JAMA, vol. 318, no. 22, pp. 2199–2210, 2017.

35. P. Rajpurkar, J. Irvin, K. Zhu, B. Yang, H. Mehta, T. Duan, D. Ding, A. Bagul, C. Langlotz, K. Shpanskaya et al., *"Chexnet: Radiologistlevel pneumonia detection on chest x-rays with deep learning,"* arXiv preprint arXiv:1711.05225, 2017.
36. V. Gulshan, L. Peng, M. Coram, M. C. Stumpe, D. Wu, A. Narayanaswamy, S. Venugopalan, K. Widner, T. Madams, J. Cuadros et al., *"Development and validation of a deep learning algorithm for detection of diabetic retinopathy in retinal fundus photographs,"* JAMA, vol. 316, no. 22, pp. 2402–2410, 2016.
37. A. Esteva, B. Kuprel, R. A. Novoa, J. Ko, S. M. Swetter, H. M. Blau and S. Thrun, *"Dermatologist-level classification of skin cancer with deep neural networks,"* Nature, vol. 542, no. 7639, p. 115, 2017.
38. S. Latif, M. Asim, M. Usman, J. Qadir and R. Rana, *"Automating motion correction in multishot mri using generative adversarial networks,"* Published as Workshop Paper at 32nd Conference on Neural Information Processing Systems (NIPS 2018), 2018.
39. X.-W. Chen and X. Lin, *"Big data deep learning: Challenges and perspectives,"* IEEE Access, vol. 2, pp. 514–525, 2014.
40. C. Szegedy, W. Zaremba, I. Sutskever, J. Bruna, D. Erhan, I. Goodfellow and R. Fergus, *"Intriguing properties of neural networks,"* arXiv preprint arXiv:1312.6199, 2013.
41. A. Shafahi, W. R. Huang, M. Najibi, O. Suciu, C. Studer, T. Dumitras and T. Goldstein, *"Poison frogs! targeted clean-label poisoning attacks on neural networks,"* in Advances in Neural Information Processing Systems, pp. 6103–6113, 2018.
42. X. Yuan, P. He, Q. Zhu and X. Li, *"Adversarial examples: Attacks and defenses for deep learning,"* IEEE Transactions on Neural Networks and Learning Systems, 2019.
43. S. G. Finlayson, J. D. Bowers, J. Ito, J. L. Zittrain, A. L. Beam and I. S. Kohane, *"Adversarial attacks on medical machine learning,"* Science, vol. 363, no. 6433, pp. 1287–1289, 2019.
44. K. Papangelou, K. Sechidis, J. Weatherall and G. Brown, *"Toward an understanding of adversarial examples in clinical trials,"* in Joint European Conference on Machine Learning and Knowledge Discovery in Databases. Springer, pp. 35–51, 2018.
45. V. Chandola, A. Banerjee and V. Kumar, *"Anomaly detection: A survey,"* ACM Computing Surveys (CSUR), vol. 41, no. 3, p. 15, 2009.
46. A. K. Pandey, P. Pandey, K. Jaiswal and A. K. Sen, *"Datamining clustering techniques in the prediction of heart disease using attribute selection method,"* Heart Disease, vol. 14, pp. 16–17, 2013.
47. K. Polat and S. Günes, *"Prediction of hepatitis disease based on principal component analysis and artificial immune recognition system,"* Applied Mathematics and Computation, vol. 189, no. 2, pp. 1282–1291, 2007.
48. M. Alloghani, D. Al-Jumeily, J. Mustafina, A. Hussain and A. J. Aljaaf, *"A systematic review on supervised and unsupervised machine learning algorithms for data science,"* in Supervised and Unsupervised Learning for Data Science. Springer, pp. 3–21, 2020.
49. M. N. Sohail, J. Ren and M. Uba Muhammad, *"A euclidean group assessment on semi-supervised clustering for healthcare clinical implications based on real-life data,"* International Journal of Environmental Research and Public Health, vol. 16, no. 9, p. 1581, 2019.
50. A. Zahin, R. Q. Hu et al., *"Sensor-based human activity recognition for smart healthcare: A semi-supervised machine learning,"* in International Conference on Artificial Intelligence for Communications and Networks. Springer, pp. 450–472, 2019.
51. D. Mahapatra, *"Semi-supervised learning and graph cuts for consensus based medical image segmentation,"* Pattern Recognition, vol. 63, pp. 700–709, 2017.

52. W. Bai, O. Oktay, M. Sinclair, H. Suzuki, M. Rajchl, G. Tarroni, B. Glocker, A. King, P. M. Matthews and D. Rueckert, *"Semisupervised learning for network-based cardiac mr image segmentation,"* in International Conference on Medical Image Computing and Computer-Assisted Intervention. Springer, pp. 253–260, 2017.

53. R. S. Sutton, A. G. Barto et al., Introduction to reinforcement learning. MIT press, Cambridge, vol. 2, no. 4, 1998.

54. H.-C. Kao, K.-F. Tang and E. Y. Chang, *"Context-aware symptom checking for disease diagnosis using hierarchical reinforcement learning,"* in Thirty-Second AAAI Conference on Artificial Intelligence, 2018.

55. D. Silver, A. Huang, C. J. Maddison, A. Guez, L. Sifre, G. Van Den Driessche, J. Schrittwieser, I. Antonoglou, V. Panneershelvam, M. Lanctot et al., *"Mastering the game of go with deep neural networks and tree search,"* Nature, vol. 529, no. 7587, p. 484, 2016.

56. A. Collins and Y. Yao, *"Machine learning approaches: Data integration for disease prediction and prognosis,"* in Applied Computational Genomics. Springer, pp. 137–141, 2018.

57. P. Afshar, A. Mohammadi and K. N. Plataniotis, *"Brain tumor type classification via capsule networks,"* in 2018 25th IEEE International Conference on Image Processing (ICIP). IEEE, 2018, pp. 3129–3133, 2018.

58. W. Zhu, C. Liu, W. Fan and X. Xie, "Deeplung: *Deep 3d dual path nets for automated pulmonary nodule detection and classification,"* in 2018 IEEE Winter Conference on Applications of Computer Vision (WACV). IEEE, pp. 673–681, 2018.

59. P. B. Jensen, L. J. Jensen and S. Brunak, *"Mining electronic health records: towards better research applications and clinical care,"* Nature Reviews Genetics, vol. 13, no. 6, p. 395, 2012.

60. P. Singh and M. Kumar Muchahari, *"Solving multi-objective optimization problem of convolutional neural network using fast forward quantum optimization algorithm: Application in digital image classification"* Advances in Engineering Software, vol.176, p. 103370, 2023.

61. M. Kandavel, D. Chelliah and G. Govindan, *"An optimised approach to detect the identity of hidden information in grey scale and colour images"*, Published Online: April 24, 2019, pp 1–21. 10.1504/IJBIDM.2019.100452.

12 Review of Various Deep Learning Techniques with a Case Study on Prognosticate Diagnostics of Liver Infection

S. Kowsalya
Department of Computer Science, Sri Krishna Arts and Science College, Coimbatore, Tamil Nadu, India

S. Saraswathi
Academic Affairs, Nehru Arts and Science College, Coimbatore, Tamil Nadu, India

12.1 INTRODUCTION TO DEEP LEARNING IN HEALTH CARE

Deep learning is a methodology that applies to the healthcare industry in various dimensions. One prominent aspect is that deep learning helps to analyze the raw data at exceptional speeds. This achievement results without compromising accuracy for any reason. All of these are not a part of machine learning or artificial intelligence. Perhaps, this is an elegant assortment of analytical and technical data that resides in a layered algorithmic architecture. Most of the emerging architecture that looks to meet the analytical challenge turns towards deep learning techniques for their solution. Specifically, in the healthcare field, the benefits of deep learning are plentiful, such as speed, efficiency, and accuracy—but they don't stop there.

Deep learning depends on the arithmetic models that have the approach of algorithm-based working to execute an Internet of Things (IoT)-based model. There exist multiple layers of the network as well as the technology for computing capability. These are unprecedented and are enough for the ability to quantify the data that were previously lost, forgotten, or missed. This deep learning algorithm or the networks can also be capable of solving complex problems and ease out the predictions within the healthcare profession. It's a skill set that hasn't gone unnoticed by the healthcare profession.

DOI: 10.1201/9781003469605-12

Deep learning in health care will not end here. It continues to make good inroads into other industries, too, especially now that there are more medical professionals who seek for recognize results. For them, this technology and algorithm can benefit more in bringing accuracy from intense collaboration with their industry and specialization. It tends to maintain the agility and capability to adapt, ensuring that it always remains relevant to the profession.

12.2 DEEP LEARNING ALGORITHMS

The deep learning algorithms are capable of featuring as a self-learning representation. They often depend on artificial neural networks (ANNs), which predominantly replicate the typical functioning of a human brain. That is, bringing the thought process into action with information. While performing pre-processing executions, most of the commonly used algorithms, including the deep learning algorithm, evaluate using the undefined objects [1]; to be more specific, at the time of input parameter defining, the behavioral objects, attributes, group variables, and generic parameters that help to derive the pattern identification. This is similar to the methodology of the most commonly used training machines for self-learning techniques. These algorithms or working approaches occur at multiple levels. These workings are then used to build the models.

Deep learning models work by adhering to several algorithms. Subsequently, there are no networks that are foreseen to be perfect in meeting the expected results; some algorithms seem to be more suitable for performing pattern identification. In the process of concluding the exact algorithm, it is advised to explore all the pros and cons of all preliminary algorithms that exist in the present research study and come up with an outline of their working methods using a real-time application perspective.

12.3 DEEP LEARNING ALGORITHM TYPES

Though there exists various deep learning algorithms, in this chapter let us focus on the top ten among them.

1. Convolutional Neural Networks (CNNs)
2. Long Short Term Memory Networks (LSTMs)
3. Recurrent Neural Networks (RNNs)
4. Generative Adversarial Networks (GANs)
5. Radial Basis Function Networks (RBFNs)
6. Multilayer Perceptrons (MLPs)
7. Self Organizing Maps (SOMs)
8. Deep Belief Networks (DBNs)
9. Restricted Boltzmann Machines (RBMs)
10. Autoencoders

Deep learning algorithms are capable of being implemented in almost all formats of data and do not consume a large volume of computing power. At the same time, they have enough information to solve complicated issues. Moving forward in this chapter, let us deep-dive into the above-listed deep learning algorithms.

12.3.1 CONVOLUTIONAL NEURAL NETWORKS (CNNs)

CNNs, also referred to as ConvNets, are composed of multiple layers and are prominently used for image processing techniques and object detection methodologies. In the year 1988, the first CNN was developed by Yann LeCun. By that time, it was named and called LeNet. During the initial stage of this algorithm's existence in the research market, most of the researchers were facing challenges in deriving the real-time objects to pre-process the algorithm's execution. In the later stages, based on the trial-and-error results from the initial research, there evolved a pattern to define the objects replicating the real-time scenarios and problem defining methods.

12.3.1.1 Working of CNNs

CNN works on the backbone of object identifying methods with multiple layer definitions. This at times paves the way for a new pattern identification.

12.3.1.2 Convolution Layer

The design of maintaining the multiple levels of the filter-applying technique over a set of different pattern data tends to have a convolution [2]. The CNN algorithm also has such convolution.

12.3.1.3 Rectified Linear Unit (ReLU)

This is a layer that helps to gain consistency in the input data as well as the processing steps. In the CNN algorithm, this layer can be imposed after identifying the pattern and the input data is pre-processed with all attributes. Upon iterating this step, the CNN algorithm attains a rectified linear unit among the datasets that are to be considered as input parameters.

12.3.1.4 Pooling Layer

The feature maps attained in the ReLU are formed as a sequence and then are fed as an input dataset to the next layer. Since there are datasets passed from different environments and seeking different working models, this phase is commonly termed as the pooling layer.

In this layer, the most prominent activity is the conversion of array data. Most of the algorithms work on multiple dimensions' datasets. Hence, there is a necessity that before passing the parameters, the datasets are categorized into a two-dimensional array [3]. This pre-processing step forms a consistent array of feature maps.

12.3.1.5 Fully Connected Layer

The multi-layer dimension of the array that was fed as input in the previous layer upon processing gets into the chunks of data relies independently. However, the subsequent working of the CNN algorithm requires an interconnection between the datasets that was missing in the result data in the previous step. In this layer, this is the activity predominantly performed to connect the datasets internally to form a connected layer.

12.3.2 LONG SHORT TERM MEMORY NETWORKS (LSTMS)

The long short term memory networks, commonly termed as LSTMs, symmetrically belong to a recurrent neural network (RNN) model [4]. This type of network algorithm are capable of recalling (with stand) inter-connected objects over some time, perhaps the process of recalling past information from a wide range of datasets for long periods.

LSTMs retain information in the long run. Most of the researchers pinpoint the connected objects across networks, perhaps mostly used in time-series and forecasting for the reasons that are now remembered mostly on previous inputs. LSTMs are chain-like structures consisting of four interacting layers. Most of the layers often communicate independently.

12.3.2.1 Working of LSTMs
Step 1. Initiates with the forget irrelevant chunks of the previous state.
Step 2. Selectively update the cell-state values of each chunk.
Step 3. The output of certain chunks of the cell state is recognized with its generic parameters.

12.3.3 RECURRENT NEURAL NETWORKS (RNNS)

Recurrent neural networks are commonly termed RNNs. This algorithm has connections that cordially form a directed cycle. This streamed structure allows an extra space for the research scholars and specifically the beginners to explore their extreme thought process to experiment the different structure of objects. At times this paves the way for inventing new findings in the research world.

The LSTM algorithm's result dataset and the object are being fed as the input to the RNN's current phase, and this in turn can extend to memorize the data. The RNN algorithms are often approached and taken into consideration for the pattern identification of patients and help to predict the probability of getting cancer based on the previous patient who has been already affected by cancer, and those records are in memory as per this current phase [5]. This is the scenario where these algorithms help in improving cancer predictions in the medical industry based on past historical data.

12.3.3.1 Working of RNNs
Step 1. The pre-processed dataset with a time interval and loop "n" is fed into the problem defining object at a time "Dt."
Step 2. The iteration indicator is set with Boolean data type so that to terminate the loop at a defined time with some manipulation (Dt+1).

Notable Behavior: RNNs are capable of processing inputs of any length.

One prominent observation I propose to highlight in this chapter of RNNs working is the computational nature of accounts for the historical information involved in this algorithm, and the expected model size of the algorithm helps to identify the closest results in each of the datasets.

Google's autocompleting feature is an example of RNNs working.

12.3.4 GENERATIVE ADVERSARIAL NETWORKS (GANs)

Generative adversarial networks, termed GANs, are extensively used to locate the closest resemblance of the data objects that are defined as the expected results in a finding. This algorithm seems to be most suited for those researchers who step in or took a medical platform as their problem definitions. This is because in medical and health-oriented data objects, it is hard to predict the results, which in turn stands as a challenge for the researcher to define the input dataset. Perhaps, the objective working of this algorithm itself is a nature of identifying the closest match; this helps the research scholars to get know how their result dataset would be if a problem is defined. So with that understanding, they are now able to draw out the outline of the correlated input data, which reduces the risk of redundant processes.

GANs help the physician to predict the possibility of a patient getting infected by cancer. The common parameters among the findings generate realistic results. One can keep preserving the results of RNN to compare and study the predictions with the help of GANs.

12.3.4.1 Working of GANs

To make the GANs algorithm work, one has to learn the capability of distinguishing the differences between the GANs fake data and the actual history of past data.

Usually, the first step in this algorithm working relies on the derivation of use case activities involving all the entities or the components involved in the problem definition [6].

The subsequent steps shall then be iterated with the similar data objects and proceed the iteration until the maximum time limit defined in the pre-processing data is reached.

As a result, the last end stage or the step of execution in the generative adversarial network algorithm is a pragmatic generator or a dynamic discriminator that helps the users or the end customers of the system to update the data model.

12.3.5 RADIAL BASIS FUNCTION NETWORKS (RBFNs)

One of the most challenging and difficult fact-finding techniques in the research market relies on the radial basis function networks (RBFNs) algorithm. These algorithms are distinct types of feedforward neural networks. This model of algorithm uses radial basis functions as a key factor of activation functions. The algorithm encloses three layers: first is an input layer, followed by a hidden layer, and lastly an output layer. All three layers are mostly used for classification, time-series prediction, and regression.

12.3.5.1 Working of RBFNs

RBFNs operate at a classification level. This is achieved by measuring the input's stability, consistency, and reliability [7]. This gives us an understanding that the similarity is the examples taken from the training set.

RBFNs initiate with a high-level configuration of dynamic parameters and the space to define the static variable set. This layer has a set of RBF neurons. This helps the original data to get relief from the outliers.

This layer often ends up with malfunctioning hidden layers where each node in the data objects tends to refer to the dependency with the output of the next data object.

The neurons that reside in each of the data objects form a co-relative console over the network layer. This is inversely proportional to the actual data objects that were initially processed as an input dataset.

Hence, the RBFN algorithms are commonly referred or identified as a comprehensive network algorithm to find the hidden layers and the patterns over the data objects that are relatively proportional to achieve the projected results in the given data warehouse.

12.3.6 MULTILAYER PERCEPTRONS (MLPs)

Multi-layer perceptrons, termed as MLPs, are one of the finest and excellent places to start learning deep learning technology, the reason being its accuracy and the transparency in its execution and compilation methods.

The MLPs algorithm predominantly belongs to the class of simplified feedforward neural networks. This algorithm has the working steps of multiple layers with perceptron's that contain the activation functions in it. The MLPs mostly consist of a base input layer and an outfit output layer that is mostly end-to-end connected [8]. The outcome of this algorithm seems to have the same number of input as well as output layers, but the real fact is that it may have multiple hidden layers, which is a conclusive one and subject to building recognitions in software such as the blocks in the valves or any other abnormalities being deducted in before the symptoms reported by the patients themselves.

12.3.6.1 Working of MLPs

The working of MLPs algorithm starts with the feeding of the data to the input layer in the network. The obvious layers of neurons connect in a graph model. This does so because the signal passes in one fine direction.

The algorithm then computes the input with the weights that exist between the formidable input layer and the consistent hidden layers.

MLPs often use the activation functions in order to determine which among the available nodes to fire. The activation functions initiate to include the simplification of ReLUs, sigmoid functions, and occasionally the tangents.

The MLPs first train the data model to clarify and to understand the correlation between them, and then it learns to identify the dependencies between the highly independent and the closest target variables from a minimum training dataset.

This diagram depicts the computation of weights and bias and then applies the suitable activation functions for classifying the images of different objects.

12.3.7 SELF ORGANIZING MAPS (SOMs)

Self-Organizing Maps, called SOMs, were invented by Professor Teuvo Kohonen. This algorithm model is often used across cross-platform frameworks to achieve accuracy and reduce the source program vulnerability. With the present technology of source program debugger or code merger, there exists a big challenge of overcoming the code vulnerability. The first question that comes to everyone's mind reading this is how often there is a necessity for this in the deep learning algorithm. Of course, when we look from the necessity perspective there isn't; however, when we implement the algorithm through a source code then it is not just achieving the target results in the algorithm. The real success of any algorithm's implementation resides in how the source program logic was built to achieve that result. For a research scholar, the implementation scope does not end with the results. The way the source program was built speaks about the quality and effectiveness of the success. Hence, the source program vulnerability and fine-tuning are focused on with the help of SOM. This algorithm model comes with a data visualization approach to reduce the source program vulnerability. In SOM, most of the execution takes place during the source program compilation in both the server and the client environment [9]. This also can be achieved by defining the multi-dimensional datasets as ANNs.

12.3.7.1 Working of SOMs

Step 1. Initialize the weights for each dataset with the "n"-dimensional array, proportional to time "t." Organize the nodes with a training dataset with sequential naming conventions. (This helps to locate the node for debugging based on the vulnerability highlighted during compilation.)

Step 2. Iterate the SOM execution for every chunk of the source program or the procedures.

Step 3. Identify the highlighted nodes in the source program chunks as high vulnerability and track the precedents and dependents for that source program.

Step 4. Look for an alternate way of program logic or the method of functions being vulnerable. Pre-process them out of the compilation block and verify the result before replacing them in the actual source program sections.

Step 5. Insert a loop that is set to repeat Steps 2, 3, & 4 for N iteration, where "N" is the target vulnerability percent or occurrences set for the quality measure.

This dataset is fed to a SOM algorithm as an input. This is then converted into the 2D RGB values. Finally, the outcome of the algorithm is separated and categorized with different colors.

12.3.8   DEEP BELIEF NETWORKS (DBNS)

DBNs are, of course, predominately considered to be iterative or incremental models. The algorithms that get executed with multiple layers of latent variables are prone to risk in the security measures. This mainly focused on the binary values and hidden units used in the algorithm.

To overcome the challenge of network securities during the compilation of the algorithm, the past research scholars and their approaches have been taken into consideration and studied. In addition to that, my proposed approach is to enhance each layer with the stack of datasets. These datasets are often normalized whenever the entire layer is taken for scrutiny (Boltzmann machines). This is one way of suppressing the stacked datasets in the respective layer itself.

12.3.8.1   Working of DBNs

Step 1. Declare the training dataset that requires normalization in each layer.

Step 2. Mark the nodes or blocks in the layer that are prone to network security issues. (This helps to do a double confirmation while evaluating the execution process).

Step 3. Execute the source program with the actual dataset. Pass the maximum connections establishments for each layer [10]. The volume of datasets transferred between the layers shall be proportional to the network nodes being declared for each layer. This will ensure that the testing is performed for the maximum throughput of data and connections in the network and security layers.

Step 4. Subsequently, in the third step, the DBNs are eradicated to notify the hidden layers with inheritance. The most iterating node in the layer received the maximum throughput. This creates the unified model approach to drill down the least node in the network layer and to ensure security concerns.

Step 5. The final execution of the DBNs is the learning of the inherited nodes. The network with the most throughput receives the value of high severity for security. Eventually, the inherited layers combined to evaluate the outcome of the security results effectively.

12.3.9   RESTRICTED BOLTZMANN MACHINES (RBMS)

The restricted Boltzmann machines algorithm is termed RBM. This was first discovered and developed by Geoffrey Hinton. The algorithm works in the functionality of stochastic neural networks. The actual basic working resides behind the learning of probability distribution, which is fine presiding over each phase of datasets [11].

The working logic of the RBMs algorithm comprises similar to the building blocks of DBNs, which we have seen in the earlier sections.

12.3.9.1 Working of RBMs

RBMs algorithm works in two phases:

The underlying working of the RBM algorithm is with the forward pass and backward pass. However, both are prone to high risk when it comes to the dynamic variable declaration.

Step 1. Fundamental working of the RBMs algorithm gets initiated by accepting the inputs and translating them into a predefined set of the variable assigned with numbers that completely encode the inputs towards the forward pass.

Step 2. In the second step, every individual input node is combined with the weight and depth of the end node in the network or the chart.

Step 3. This step is just an iteration behavior to enhance the performance of each node in the network.

Step 4. Here the backward pass execution comes into the picture. The actual execution starts by defining the declared variable set with its dependencies. The variable numbers are translated and encrypted for the backward pass and then decrypted while the execution of the forward pass.

Step 5. In this step, the RBMs algorithm combines each of the activation nodes with the individual weight and overall bias.

Step 6. This is again a step of reconstruction whereby the end nodes are further bifurcated to get executed with both backward and forward passes involving all its subsets of weights and depths.

Step 7. This is the final step in RBMs algorithm. Being in the visible layer, the RBM does a comparison between the actual datasets being declared within the algorithm for the backward pass with the predefined and dynamic datasets formed during the execution of the forward pass. The result of this comparison will give us a better clarity of the accuracy and consistency of the results over each network node in the chart.

12.3.10 AUTOENCODERS

The last algorithm model in deep learning is the "autoencoders." This was invented and designed by Geoffrey Hinton in the year 1980. In this algorithm model, both the problem definition and the solution are similar in most of the compilation. The objective of designing this algorithm is to resolve unsupervised learning challenges and problems. These algorithms are most popularly applied and evaluated in pharmaceutical discovery.

Working of Autoencoders Algorithm:

An autoencoder algorithm works with three main components: the first is the encoder section, followed by the code compilation, and the last is a decoder.

Step 1. Autoencoders are designed in a structure to receive a unified input. These input data are then transformed into different representations that were demanded.

Step 2. The algorithm then attempts to iterate itself with the incremental values set as dynamic attributes.

Step 3. This is a step of the trial-and-error mechanism. In the case of an image representing the digit is not clear enough to be visible, then the algorithm is designed to feed it to an autoencoder neural network.

Step 4. Here comes the core functionality of the autoencoders. This first encodes the given picture, and proceeds to minimize the actual resolution of the processed problem in chunks of granular forms.

Step 5. In the final process, the autoencoder decrypts the processed files (in Step 4) to get the restructured and compiled picture.

12.4 COMPLICATIONS IN DEEP LEARNING ALGORITHM

Deep learning algorithms most often demand the training of large sets or labelled data. This refers in an alternate way that we have to give the input parameters as thousands of actual images of patients scanning reports of an infected liver before it starts the process of classifying infected and healthy liver. This relies on the relativity of the training dataset being used. To get a better outcome or classification improvement and performance of the algorithm, it is recommended that we use more training datasets. Most of the hospitals and labs are aware of this requirement in maintaining relatively large datasets. More importantly, they are very efficient in utilizing them periodically over the years with monitoring results on the patients' test and scan reports. This is one area that other small and medium medical research and clinical centers are lacking. Perhaps, this is the place where they stand out by serving better for their patients and get a positive feedback and success ratio [12]. From a research scholar's perspective, we foresee this approach in technical observation as the iterative method of handling datasets that leads to deep learning algorithm's necessity.

Though there exist lots of benefits in implementing deep learning algorithms, there are some notable challenges that we have to come across to taste successful implementation.

12.4.1 Perfection on Input Data Structure

It is hard to determine the type of input to an algorithm without knowing the challenges and complications in the formula over the real-time dataset used in the algorithm. In that case, one can analyze and image the depth of the unknown factors in collecting the input data for the deep learning algorithm. However, we believe that the possibilities are high when the training dataset undergoes iteration with the generalization approach for every problem defined in the algorithm. In a common data handling approach, the outliers are identified easily when we iterate each problem definition in a chunk of datasets. This also involves interpolating the sample values as input to determine the range of valid dataset. In fact, the real challenge comes when there is a necessity that the input data that we pass to the algorithm should be a kind of dataset that was never used before.

Algorithm Names	Accuracy	ALGORITHMS COMPLEXITY
Convolutional Neural Networks (CNNs)	89 %	64 %
Long Short Term Memory Networks (LSTMs)	82 %	62 %
Recurrent Neural Networks (RNNs)	91 %	68 %
Generative Adversarial Networks (GANs)	75 %	55 %
Radial Basis Function Networks (RBFNs)	85 %	61 %

Algorithm Names	Accuracy	ALGORITHMS COMPLEXITY
Multilayer Perceptrons (MLPs)	95 %	90 %
Self Organizing Maps (SOMs)	59 %	26 %
Deep Belief Networks (DBNs)	79 %	70 %
Restricted Boltzmann Machines(RBMs)	66 %	47 %
Autoencoders	64 %	32 %

Note:
- The accuracy percentage is based on the results portrayed in the reference papers.
- Weightage of complexity is based on the questionnaires and feedback collected from the Hospital physician, tech assistants, system admins portraying the implementation approach and the system behavior to meet their present challenge and needs.

FIGURE 12.1   Algorithm accuracy complexity.

So this makes it more interesting as well as challenging to know when was the last time this dataset was used as an input to the deep learning algorithm every time I compile the program. Perhaps, it may not be used. Preferably with such assumption when the dataset is iterated and passed as input for the first time, there are possibilities that the algorithm demands for a pre-processing step before taking the dataset as input directly. Indeed, the pre-processing itself is a kind of compilation and execution steps. In all probability, if we undergo such pre-processing, then I lose to meet the criteria that my dataset hasn't been used anywhere before. This is one dimension of challenge in meeting the perfection of the input dataset. The second is the dependencies and accuracies within the real-time dataset that was extracted from the research and labs [13].

We cannot demand or expect the medical laboratories to share the accurate dataset as they are more concerned with their security and privacy compliance. Hence, with the given dataset, we ensure that it is accurate meeting the problem definition of the algorithm's objective. Here comes the other challenge. How can one say that the accuracy is the same across different algorithms being used to send the dataset as input? For instance, if I fine-tune a dataset to make it accurate for an algorithm, then the accuracy determining factors for that algorithm may not be the same for the other algorithm that I prefer to compile. In other words, when there are sub-processes involved in an algorithm, such programs/procedures might get compiled as a dependent execution instead of direct invocation. In such a scenario, the accuracy level of the sub-programs or procedures may be different, and my dataset that meets the accuracy of one algorithm may not meet for the other in single execution or compilation (Figure 12.1).

12.4.2 DEEP LEARNING IS SHALLOW

A notable problem often the research scholars face is on finding the exact match to their problem definition and the solution they derived. The reason being these algorithms are intending with multiple solutions as there exists a different range of input datasets. This is something that can be resolved when we look from the bottom-up approach. We suggest this approach to take one problem at a time. Focus on one particular problem being defined, track for the dataset mapped to that problem, and then root it till the solution set arrives for that dataset. This doesn't mean that we shall skip the other solutions we derived. The wise decision is to create multiple groups for the problem definition with its nature of behavior and then back track each of them to root its solution. This somehow justifies and convinces us to use all the possible solutions that we derive [14]. However, when it comes to the accuracy matrix, then we are forced to pick one solution out from the multiples, which finally leaves us shallow.

12.5 DEEP LEARNING IMPLICATION IN LIVER HEALTH

Nowadays, liver infection is one of the widely facing health issues among patients of age nearing 50 or 60. Generally, when we start observing patients with different concerns, one common attribute that helps us to categorize for liver infection suspect is their weight. Picking out such patients, when we start collecting their test reports, scans, and consulting history of records, we can further come close to those patients who are prone to get a liver infection.

12.5.1 CHARACTERISTICS OF INPUT DATA

In the experimental study of identifying liver infection, our research initiates from different healthcare centers by observing the nature of treatment of the patients who are scanned and underwent surgeries. Upon performing multiple iterations of filters we finalized a set of patients and extracted their complete scan reports that includes acquired ultrasound images (this includes the average age of 45, 25% male, Body Max Index (BMI) close to 35). The patients may be admitted for different reasons of health concerns. However, there are possibilities that they have taken scans to observe corresponding impacts related to their surgeries. So those scan reports are now collected and used for our observations heading to the dimension of liver infection. The sample data are collected one to two days prior to their surgery as well as a week aged after their surgeries. Our observation highlights the liver biopsy from the reports taken after surgeries. Though it was a seasoned protocol followed within the liver transplant and general surgery department, the steatosis level seems to be beyond the recommended range for certain patients. This is the saturation point in our research observation to define it as a cluster. We started collecting the history of medical records of those patients from whom we noticed those abnormalities. This is in focusing on the findings of some outliers and granular-level clusters. Most of the evaluations carried out in the labs are from reputed and recognized medical personnel or authorized senior medical advisors. They do perform their evaluation aligning to the protocols defined and recommended by medical research organizations and universities. On observing this evaluation, the abnormalities noticed are predominantly raised beyond the recommended and average percentage of impacts and downfall that patients face with fatty infiltrations [15,16]. Referring to the attributes that were passed as inputs to the algorithm, the prediction of a liver to be infected is identified and marked as abnormal. This abnormality is approximately 7% above the recommended range. The screened patients are segregated as two major groups of people inclined to have fatty

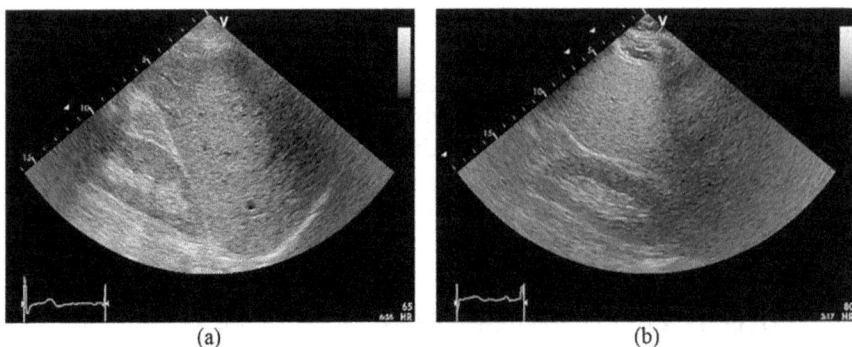

FIGURE 12.2   (a) Normal liver. (b) Fatty liver.

liver (approximate reading steatosis beyond 7%), and some patients look normal and healthy (lower than 7%). Figure 12.2(a) illustrates an ultrasound image taken from a healthy person and another image from a patient who sustains and undergoes treatment for liver by some means of infection or disorders. Considering these findings as a base, we collected samples of scanned images connecting different diagnoses such as heart, kidney, and lungs to evaluate the relativity and the prediction percentage. As a final collection, 550 B-mode ultrasound images from different labs and patients of different ages ranging between 45 and 70 construct the optimal solution methods that shall be further used for the next phases of investigation. When we observe the images shown in Figure 12.2(b), it is clear that the histogram is relatively distributed across the phase of a patient's one breath that is inhaling and exhaling. According to these scan images, we can conclude one finding in concrete, that this was specific to the data acquisition technique which is usually carried out for approximately 50 patients who are already prone to fatty liver and close to 25 normal patients.

In the next step towards our research of identifying the saturation in results on liver infection, we realized to apply the pre-defined and sufficiently trained stream of networks as input. This shall be either image or data. Some networks that are most often used shall be taken into consideration AlexNet, Inception-ResNetV2, ResNet101, and GoogleNet. Among these, one profound option we have chosen is Inception-ResNetv2 neural network. This is because it is being pre-trained and contains a wide range of datasets that cover approximately 890 close to 900 total layers of different attributes. It affords the characteristics of reducing calculation over volume. One distinct characteristic that this trained model has is, the relativity among the input data are accurately monitored and focused separately in each iteration of deep learning algorithms. Whereas the other real-time models do not align with such characteristics due to is lack of data volume and throughput. Let us consider a good example to illustrate the working of this algorithm inputs in the following section.

12.5.1.1   Example Illustration for Algorithm Working

Consider the insurance coverage for commercial premises that involves multiple dimensional risk factors such as the nature of work carried out on the premises, types of safety measures installed, products or goods material stored in the premises, and the physical structure of the building specifications are some of the high-level determining factors for risk and premium calculation.

The practical challenge in this calculation is the evaluation of granular-level risks that impose a loading rate over the basic premium value. Loading shall be imposed on various factors and the data captured as input. Perhaps, deriving a business functionality aligning to the real-time scenarios creates more probability for setting up the loading percent combinations.

The inputs captured for this insurance coverage shall be split into phases such as the personal details, insuring premises details, the safety measures, the goods and materials stored in it, etc. (Figure 12.3).

This is the first and base node NP for our algorithm to consider the insured details as the dependent factor with subsequent sections. The factors here are occupation (nature of business carried out on the premises) and construction class (determines the category of the building constructed).

Following this is the input capturing of interest items known as the risk categories. The actual working of the algorithm starts at this step upon getting the premise inputs (Figures 12.4 and 12.5).

Not all the input parameters are passed as input to the first phase of the algorithm; their base factor NP that defines the core cluster to the algorithm is derived from the insured details section. Following that are the premise details that contain the wide variation data or the scattered data across different dimensions. So let us form the equations for each of the factors that shall group the similar determining other inputs as part of its core components.

Let the Max Discount be −30.00% and Max Loading be +30.00%

Trade_code_discount = Lookup using trade code & Construction class at PIAM table setup

If Trade_code_discount < Max Discount, then

{If Part II (S5) * (1+ Trade_code_discount) > Part I (S5), then Part II (S5) * (1+ Trade_code_discount)

else Part I (S5)}

Else {

If Trade_code_discount > Max Loading, then

{If Part II (S5) * (1+ Trade_code_discount) < Part I (S5), then Part II (S5) * (1+ Trade_code_discount)

else Part I (S5)}

Else {

If Part I (S5) > Part II (S5) * (1+ Max Loading), then Part II (S5) * (1+ Max Loading)

Else {

If Part I (S5) < Part II (S5) * (1+ Max Discount), then Part II (S5) * (1+ Max Discount)

Else Part I (S5)

}   } }

(Figures 12.6 and 12.7)

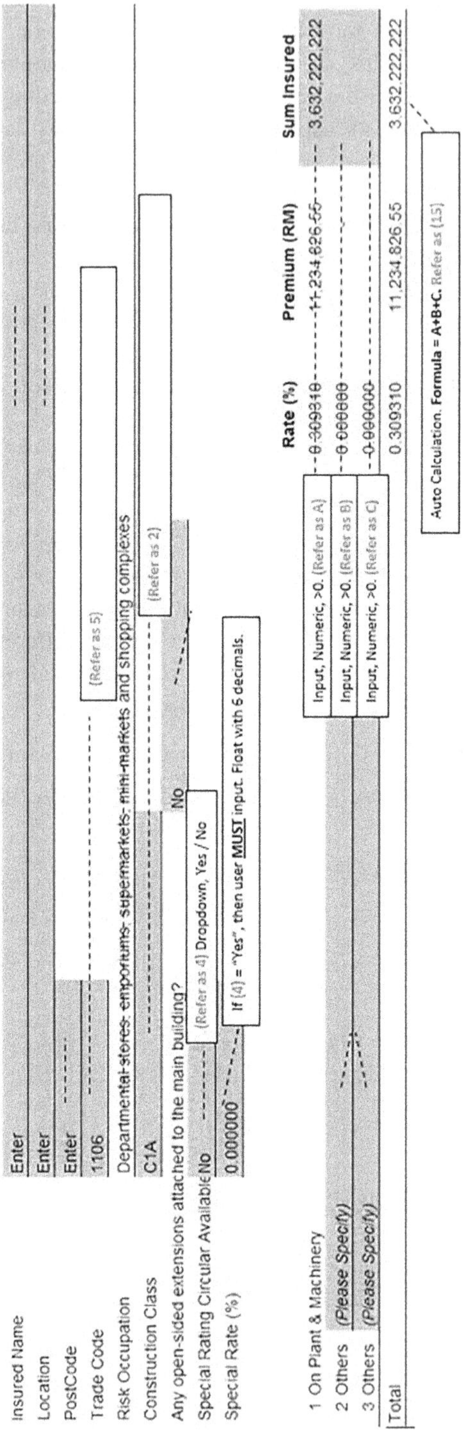

Insured Name	Enter
Location	Enter
PostCode	Enter
Trade Code	1106	(Refer as 5)
Risk Occupation	Departmental stores; emporiums; supermarkets; mini-markets and shopping complexes
Construction Class	C1A	(Refer as 2)
Any open-sided extensions attached to the main building?	No
Special Rating Circular Available	No	(Refer as 4) Dropdown, Yes / No
Special Rate (%)	0.000000	If (4) = "Yes", then user MUST input. Float with 6 decimals.

	Rate (%)	Premium (RM)	Sum Insured
1 On Plant & Machinery	0.309310	11,234,826.55	3,632,222.222
	Input, Numeric, >0. (Refer as A)		
2 Others *(Please Specify)*	0.000000		
	Input, Numeric, >0. (Refer as B)		
3 Others *(Please Specify)*	-0.000000		
	Input, Numeric, >0. (Refer as C)		
Total	0.309310	11,234,826.55	3,632,222.222

Auto Calculation. Formula = A+B+C. Refer as (15)

FIGURE 12.3 Input capturing illustration for the insured details.

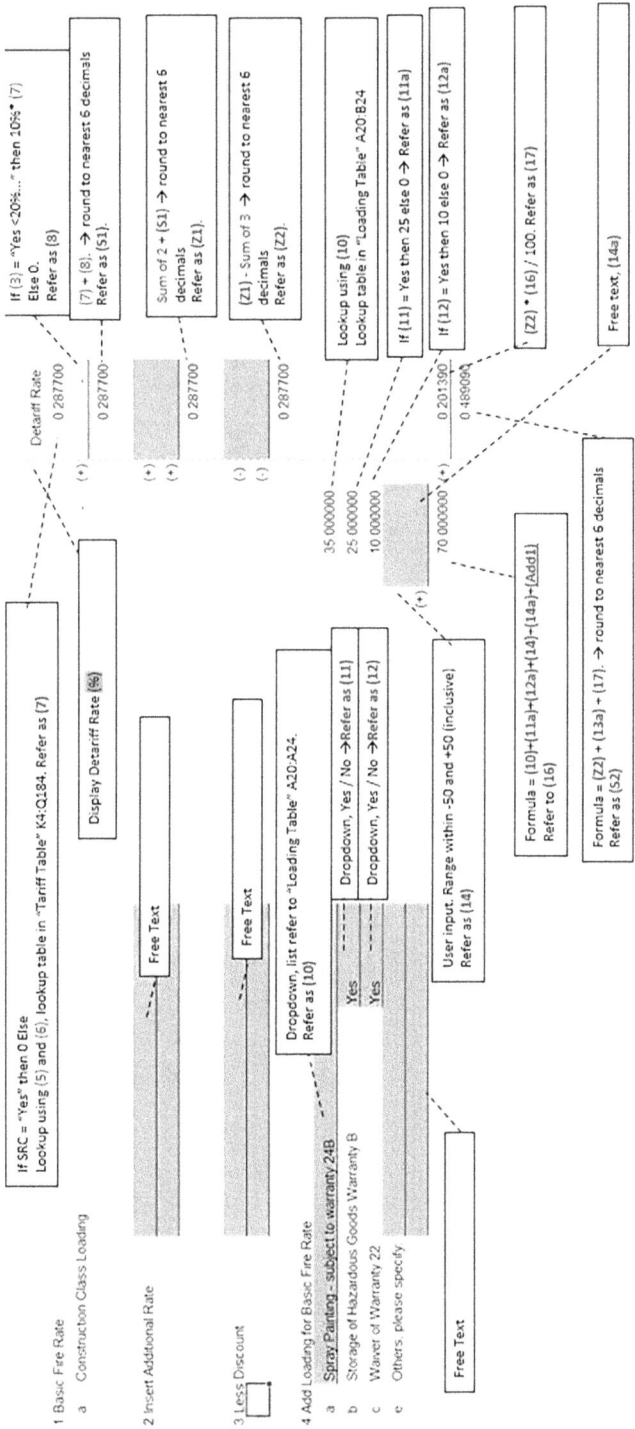

FIGURE 12.4 Input capturing illustration for premises details.

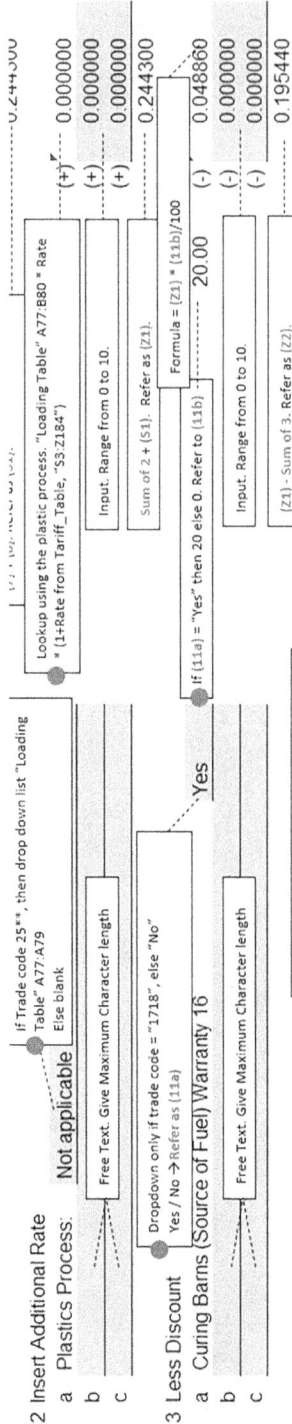

FIGURE 12.5 Objects defining points illustration for the premium determining factors.

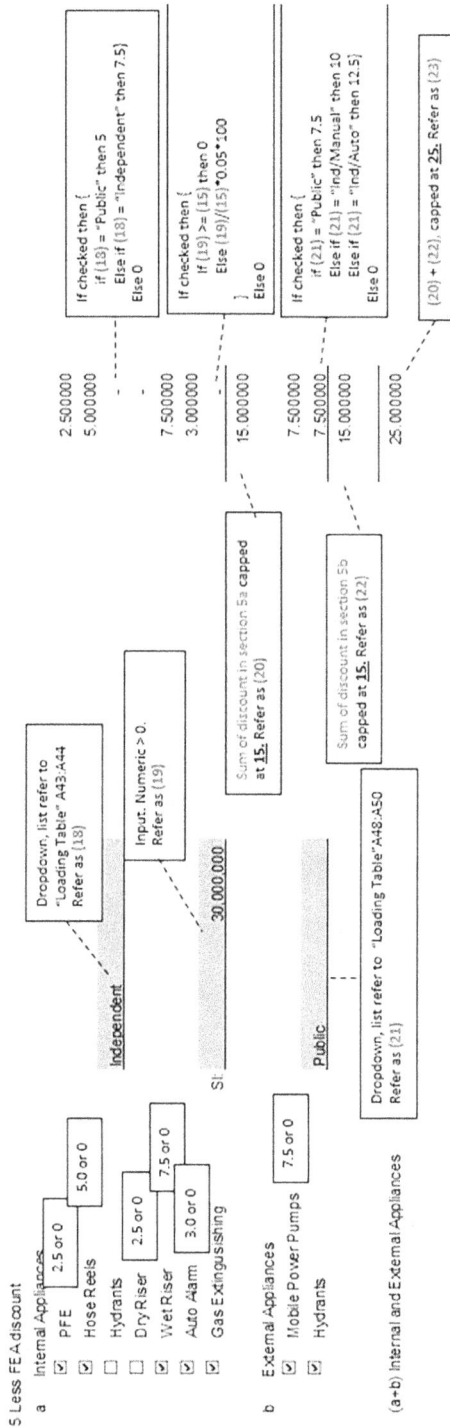

FIGURE 12.6 Discount determining factors input.

(a-b) Internal and External Appliances

c [✓] External Drenchers — 5.0 or 0
d [ ] Auto Sprinklers
e [✓] Private Fire Team — 2.5 or 0

(a-b+c+d+e)

6 Age of Building

7 Less discount for :-
a Security
 24/7 Security Guards
 Intruder Alarm System
 CC TV
 Guard Dog
 Security Lighting
 Perimeter Fencing

b Large Sum Insured (for MD only)

8 Fire and Lighting only

e [ ] Private Fire Team — 2.5 or 0

(a+b+c+d+e)

Full Control

Dropdown, list refer to "Loading Table":A55:A56
Refer as (24)

0 - 6 years (New Building)

Drop down. List refer to "Loading Table" A59:A62

Armed

If (15b) < 10,000,000 then 0
Select any = 2

(23) + (c) + (d) + (e), capped at 75.
Refer as (25)

If (15b) < 10,000,000 then 0
Else lookup A58:H62
Refer as (26)

Drop down. List refer to "Loading Table" A64:A65

If (15b) < 10,000,000 then 0
Else lookup "Loading Table" A64:B65
Refer as (27)

Sum of security discount.
Refer as (28)

If (15) <= 10,000,000 then 0
Else if (15) <= 20,000,000 then 15
Else if (15) <= 50,000,000 then 17.5
Else if (15) <= 150,000,000 then 20
Else 22.5

7a + 7b.
Refer as (29)

If (15b) < 10,000,000 then 0
Else if checked then {
 If (24) = "Full Control" then 12.5
 Else if (24) = Partial Control" then 6.25}
Else 0

(S2)*(25)/100

[S2] - (S2)*(25)/100. →
round to nearest 6 decimals
Refer as (S3)

[S3] * (26) / 100

(S3) + (S3) * (26) / 100. →
round to nearest 6 decimals
Refer to (S4)

(S4) * (29) / 100

If SRC = "Yes" then SRC_Rate * (1+Rate from Tariff_Table,
"S3.2184"")
Else (S4) - (S4) * (29) / 100. This is the unbounded detariff
rate.
→ round to nearest 6 decimals
Refer as (S5)

25.000000

5.000000

2.500000

32.500000 (-) 0.158954 0.330136

(5.000000) (+) (0.016507) 0.313629

17.500000

17.500000 (-) 0.056885 0.258744

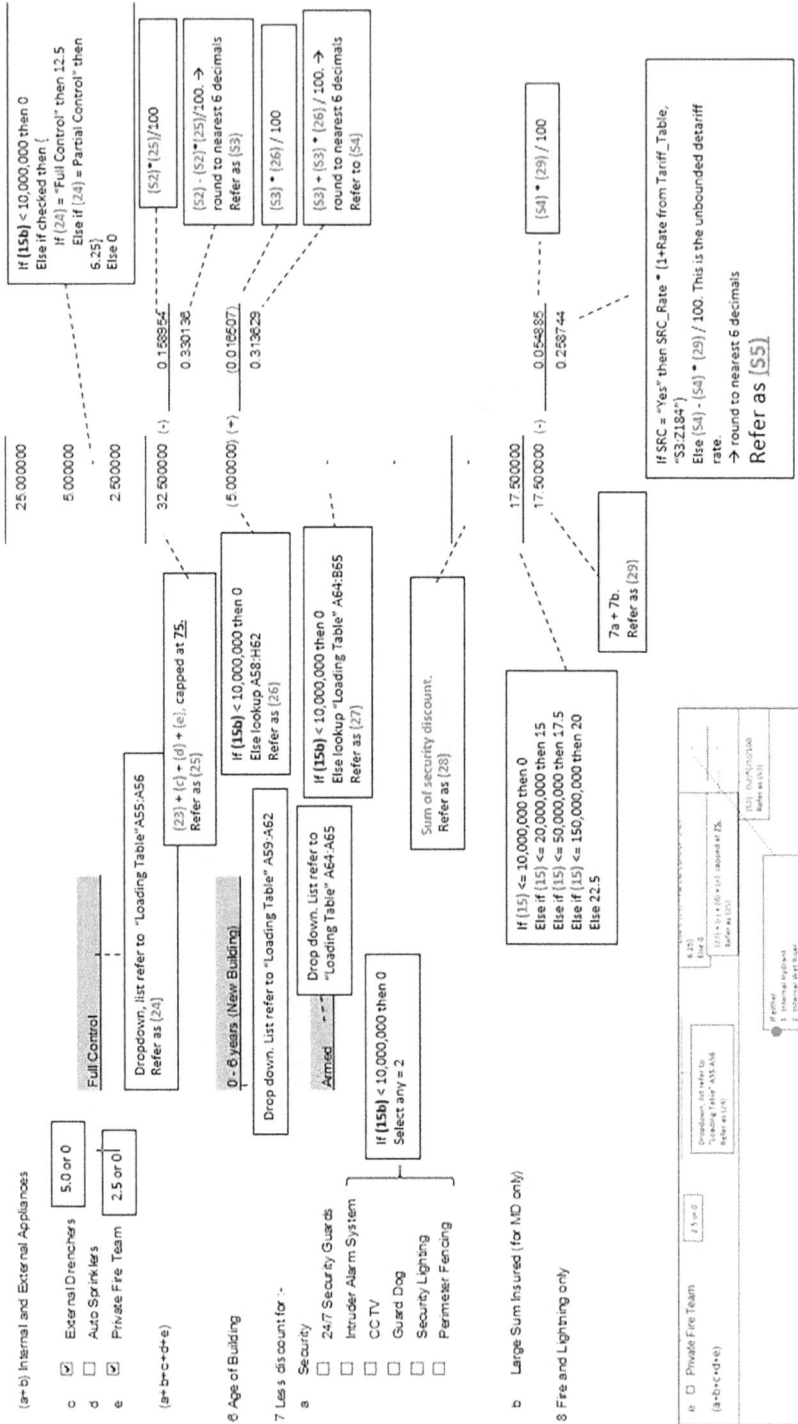

FIGURE 12.7 Loading determining factors input.

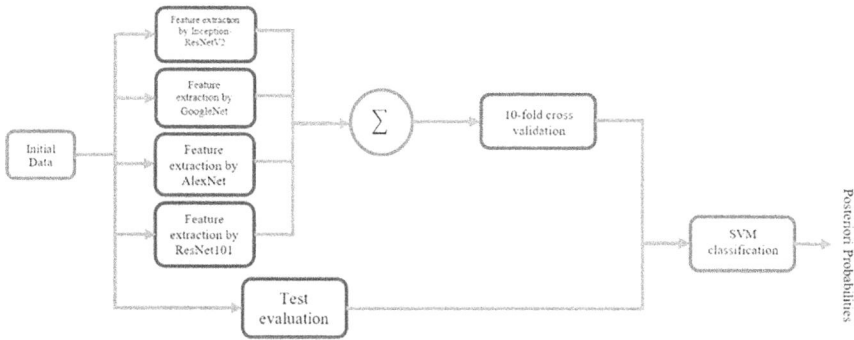

FIGURE 12.8   Result displaying page grouped by its clusters.

Grouping each of the sections as the core cluster to our algorithm, the base node NP shoots out to identify the similar attributes from each of the sections and gets the outliers.

fx.outlier(mt[i:1 − n iteration], for every node 'n' cluster 'c', and time 't'

fx.enode[x_layer-'a'= 1, 2, 3, ... n], s_layer[y_consent(for every 't' 1: 10^n), c=0, 1]

fx.enode[n_layer − 'b' = 1,2,3, ...t], c_layer[x_consent(for every 's 5: 10^n

fx.cluster(k_var.centroids['a':n nodes],

fx.Nt('Centroid 'c1, c2, c3, ... cn')

fx.Nt('Base Premium (n_layers)')

fx.Clusters(x_consent[Nt], iterate fx. Nt('Centroid 'c1, c2, c3, ... cn')

fx.profound()

fx.evaluate()

(Figures 12.8 and 12.9)

12.6   CONCLUSION

With this, let me conclude by stating there is a new approach for identifying or predicting liver infection through deep learning algorithms. This is achieved through the pre-processing steps with multiple iterations and evaluations over a different range of real-time datasets. The core understanding behind this research is summarized with the essence of the knowledge mining process that nurtures the core cluster from the given datasets. From the reports of medical advisors and the scan test results, this is the very least effective. However, the introduction of our deep learning algorithms proves it costlier to determine the factors as input to the clustering methods. The results from the algorithm depict the clarity of the present status of the liver's condition, the depth of infection in ratio, and the predictions for future treatments. From a medical expert's perspective, this may look flamboyant to conclude the probability of correctness. Perhaps, the algorithm results when compared with the actual results of the patients after six to eight

All Risks

On All Items

	Detariff Rate (%)
All Risk	0.250000

Detariff All Risk Rate. Refer as (S7)

Commission

Commission Rate	25.00%

Commission Rate. Refer as (30)

Rate Calculation

	Detariff Rate (%)
Fire and Lightning Rate	0.348563
All Risk Rate	0.250000
Fire and All Risk Rate	**0.598563**
Adjusted Fire and All Risk Rate	0.678371
Adjusted Consequential Loss Rate	0.508778

Take from (S5)

Take from (S7)

(S5) + (S7). Refer to (S8)

(S5) * 0.85/(1-(30)). Refer to (S9)

(S9) * 0.75. Refer to (S10)

	Detariff Rate (%)
Final Solar Insurance Rate	**0.678371**

Premium Computation

Interest Insured

	Rate (%)	Premium (RM)	Sum Insured
1 On Plant & Machinery	0.678371	678,674.98	100,044,810
2 Consequential Loss Sum Insured	0.508778	7,216.76	1,418,449
3 Others *(Please Specify)*	0.000000	-	-
Total	**0.676000**	**685,891.74**	**101,463,253**

(S10) (Respective Rate)/100 * (respective Sum Insured). Rounded to 2 decimals.

Take from (S9). Shows 0 if the respective Sum Insured was zero. Rounded to nearest 6 decimals. Refer to (S10_1)

Note: For Con Loss Sum Insured Only. Take from (S10). Shows 0 if the respective Sum Insured was zero. Rounded to nearest 6 decimals. Refer to (S10_2)

Total Rate = Total Premium / Total Sum Insured*100, rounded to nearest

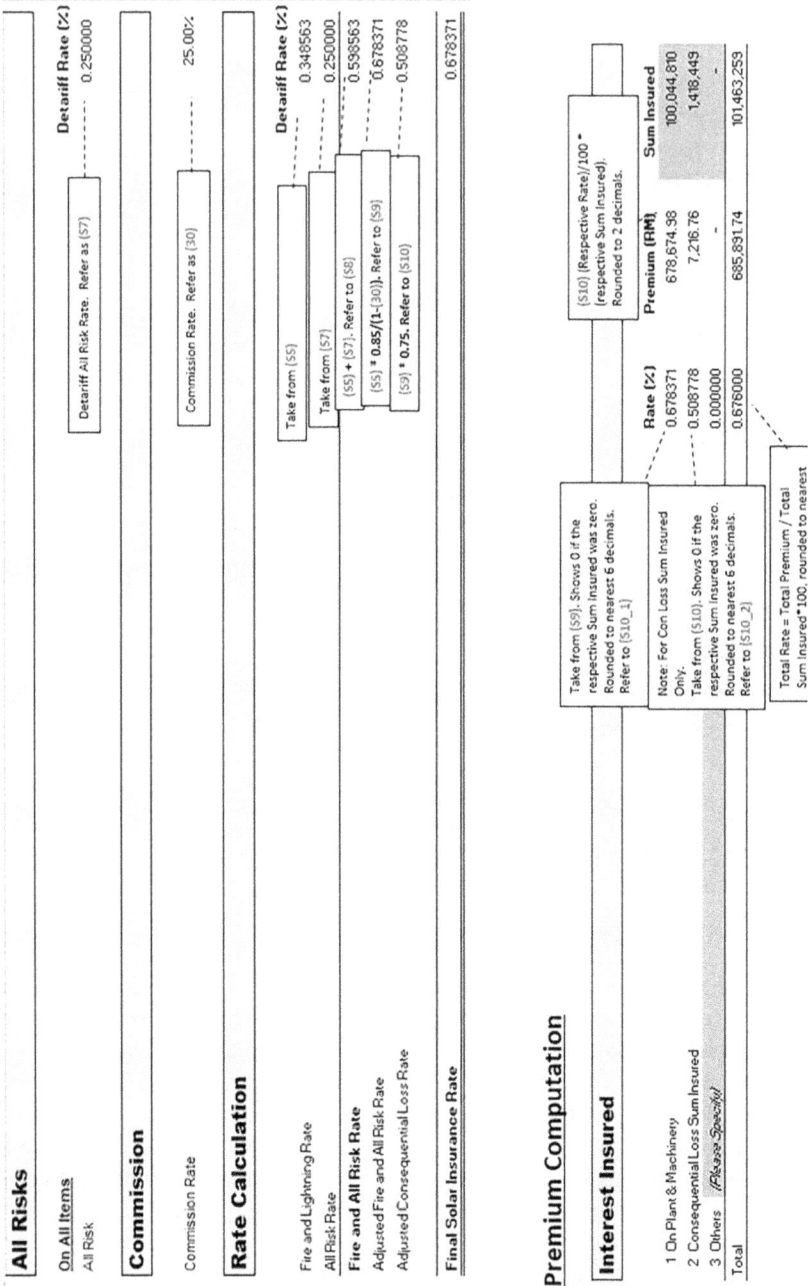

FIGURE 12.9 Block diagram of implementation algorithm.

months of the waiting period, seem to be proven results for the accuracy relies upon our deep learning algorithm.

REFERENCES

1. Charu C. Aggarwal (2018) *Neural Networks and Deep Learning: A Textbook*. IGI Global.
2. Andrew W. Trask (2019) *Grokking Deep Learning*. CRC Press.
3. K. Gayathri Devi, Kishore Balasubramanian, Le Anh Ngoc (2022) *Machine Learning and Deep Learning Techniques for Medical Science*. CRC Press.
4. Gaurav Meena, Kamal Kant Hiran, Mehul Mahrishi, Paawan Sharma (2020) *Machine Learning and Deep Learning in Real-Time Applications*. IGI Global.
5. Information Resources Management Association (2019) *Deep Learning and Neural Networks: Concepts, Methodologies, Tools, and Applications*. IGI Global.
6. Geeta Rani, Pradeep Kumar Tiwari (2020) *Handbook of Research on Disease Prediction Through Data Analytics and Machine Learning*. IGI Global.
7. Alex Noel Joseph Raj, Nersisson Ruban, Vijayalakshmi G. V. Mahesh (2020) *Handbook of Research on Deep Learning-Based Image Analysis Under Constrained and Unconstrained Environments*. IGI Global.
8. Laith Alzubaidi, Jinglan Zhang, Amjad J. Humaidi, Ayad Al-Dujaili, Ye Duan, Omran Al-Shamma (2017) *Review of Deep Learning: Concepts, CNN Architectures, Challenges, Applications, Future Directions*. IT Science.
9. V. Sathiyamoorthi, A.K. Ilavarasi, K. Murugeswari, Syed Thouheed Ahmed, B. Aruna Devi, Murali Kalipindi (2021). "A deep convolutional neural network based computer aided diagnosis system for the prediction of Alzheimer's disease in MRI images", *Measurement*, Volume 171, 108838, ISSN 0263-2241, 10.1016/j.measurement.2020. 108838.
10. B. Lakshmipriya, Biju Pottakkat, G. Ramkumar (2019) *Deep Learning Techniques in Liver Tumour Diagnosis Using CT and MR Imaging - A Systematic Review*. ITI Global Submit for Health Science.
11. Dinh-Van Phan, Chien-Lung Chan, Ai-Hsien Adams Li, Ting-Ying Chien, Van-Chuc Nguyen (2019) *Liver Cancer Prediction in a Viral Hepatitis Cohort: A Deep Learning Approach*. CRC Press.
12. Chen Chen, Cheng Chen, Mingrui Ma, Xiaojian Ma, Xiaoyi Lv, Xiaogang Dong, Ziwei Yan, Min Zhu & Jiajia Chen (2018) *Classification of Multi-differentiated Liver Cancer Pathological Images Based on Deep Learning Attention Mechanism*. IGI Global.
13. Amirhossein Kiani, Bora Uyumazturk, Pranav Rajpurkar, Alex Wang (2021) *Impact of a Deep Learning Assistant on the Histopathologic Classification of Liver cancer*. IGI Global.
14. Grzegorz Chlebus, Andrea Schenk, Jan Hendrik Moltz (2019) *Deep Learning Based Automatic Liver Tumor Segmentation in CT with Shape-based Post-processing*. CRC Press.
15. Masaya Sato, Kentaro Morimoto, Shigeki Kajihara, Ryosuke Tateishi, Shuichiro Shiina, Kazuhiko Koike & Yutaka Yatomi (2020) *Machine-learning Approach for the Development of a Novel Predictive Model for the Diagnosis of Hepatocellular Carcinoma*. IGI Global.
16. Shi-hui Zhen, Ming Cheng, Yu-bo Tao, Yi-fan Wang, Sarun Juengpanich, Zhi-yu Jiang, Yan-kai Jiang, Yu-yu Yan, Wei (2020) *Deep Learning for Accurate Diagnosis of Liver Tumor Based on Magnetic Resonance Imaging and Clinical Data*. CRC Press.

13 Case Study

Application of Ensemble Classifier for Diabetes Healthcare Data Analytics

P. Nagaraj
Department of Computer Science and Engineering, Kalasalingam Academy of Research and Education, Krishnankoil, Tamil Nadu, India

K. Muthamil Sudar
Department of Computer Science and Engineering, Mepco Schlenk Engineering College, Sivakasi, Virudhunagar, Tamil Nadu, India

V. Muneeswaran
Department of Electronics and Communication Engineering, Kalasalingam Academy of Research and Education, Krishnankoil, Tamil Nadu, India

Bhumika Choksi
School of Advanced Sciences and Languages, VIT Bhopal University, Kothrikalan, Sehore, Madhya Pradesh, India

13.1 INTRODUCTION

Numerous opportunities in healthcare are created in machine learning because machine learning models have created a trademark for advanced predictive analytics in healthcare. For predicting chronic illnesses such as heart diseases, infections, and intestinal diseases, several machine learning models have already been developed, producing greater prediction accuracy. There are also a few forthcoming models of machine learning to predict non-communicable diseases, which are adding more and more benefits to the healthcare domain. Continuous development in machine learning and deep learning helped researchers to apply that knowledge to predict the various diseases at an early stage so that hospitalization of the public can be reduced to a greater extent [1].

DOI: 10.1201/9781003469605-13

Diabetes, also known as diabetes mellitus (DM), is a group of metabolic problems that are recognized by persistently high glucose levels. Several metabolic disorders collectively referred to as polygenic disorder (DM) have abnormal hormone secretion as their primary cause [2]. High hexose ledvels can cause excessive urination, frequent feelings of thirst, and increased hunger [3]. Diabetes can result in serious health problems like diabetic acidosis, a hyperosmolar hyperglycemic state, or even death if it is not treated promptly. This persists in basic quantity challenges as well as vas upset, brain stroke, failure, foot ulcers, eye complications, etc. [4]. Diabetes develops when the body's duct glands are unable to produce enough insulin or when the body's cells and tissues are unable to use the insulin that is produced. There are three types of polygenic disorder: DM type 1 is distinguished by secreting hormones over what the body needs, a condition dubbed "insulin-subordinate diabetic disorder mellitus" (IDDM). Type 1 DM patients require a small amount of external hormone to make up for the lower hormone amount produced by the secretor. DM A type 2 body has poor hormone utilization and insulin production. This could ultimately result in the body producing no insulin. Alternatively known as "adult onset diabetes," this condition is also known as "non-insulin subordinate diabetic disorder mellitus" (NIDDM). Individuals with high BMIs or those who lead somewhat sedentary lifestyles are more likely to have this type of polygenic disorder [5]. The third main structure that is seen throughout the physiological state is diabetes polygenic disorder. Aldohexose concentrations for an average person typically range from 70 to 99 milligrams per deciliter. If the quick aldohexose level is found to be greater than 126 mg/dL, the person is considered to have diabetes. An individual is deemed to be pre-diabetic if their aldohexose concentration is between 100 and 125 mg/dL [6].

13.2 DISCRETE MACHINE LEARNING TECHNIQUES USED FOR DIABETES DIAGNOSIS

In a classification strategy, the data samples are partitioned into the target class, and the same is predicted for every data point. Using data classification algorithms, we could, for example, classify a patient as "greater risk" or "lower risk" based on their conditions. The following are some of the most utilized approaches.

13.2.1 LOGISTIC REGRESSION

Generally, regression refers to the prediction of classification problems. Despite its name, logistic regression is a classification algorithm. It can be employed for both binary classification and multiclass classification. The predicting value in logistic regression is categorical. The sigmoidal function is used to bring down the value in the range of 0 to 1.

13.2.2 GAUSSIAN NAIVE BAYES CLASSIFIER

It was named after the Gaussian distributions representing the training dataset's data. The initial guesses in the Gaussian distribution naive bias are called prior probabilities. It is based on the likelihood of any particular feature. In the Gaussian curve, likelihood is the coordinate on the curve that corresponds to the x-axis coordinate. It is best suitable for small datasets. If it has more features listed it may provide good accuracy, because of the distribution of likelihood.

13.2.3 Decision Trees

Generally, a decision tree asks a question and then classifies based on the answer. The classification can be categorical or numeric. It can combine both numeric as well as categorical data and can make decisions out of it. At each level of the tree, an impurity check is done and the condition of choosing that feature depends on the impurity value. The tree consists of root nodes, internal nodes, and leaf nodes.

13.2.4 Random Forest

Random forest is built from decision trees. Generally, trees work well with the data they have or are familiar with but fail to classify new samples. Random forest combines the simplicity of the decision tree with flexibility, resulting in a vast improvement in accuracy. At each time we take the bootstrapped data and consider only a subset of the variables at each step, which results in a wide variety of trees by applying the decision tree approach. The final result depends on the forests (multiple trees) that we created with the variety of trees. The remaining data after bootstrapping at each step are called out-of-bag data. The correct classification of the out-of-bag data is solemnly responsible for the accuracy of the random forest algorithm. It is an example of the bagging technique.

13.2.5 K-Nearest Neighbor

It can be employed for both classification and regression problems. It is used for classifying non-linear data points. K refers to the number of closest neighbors that have been chosen for voting. The K value is taken randomly through an iterative process, and the best K value is the one that provides the least residual error. Some nearest neighbors are based on the distance between the points; the distance metric can be either Manhattan or Euclidean. The classification is done based on the count of the nearest neighbors to the target point. In regression, the average of the K-nearest neighbor is taken as the prediction value. The K-nearest neighbor algorithm can be impacted by outliers; it doesn't work with an imbalanced dataset.

13.2.6 XGBoost

It is used for both binary as well as multiclass classification. Initially, a base model is chosen with some probability value, which is calculated by taking the average of the target column values, and also respective residuals are calculated by subtracting the probability value from every other value in the target column. While constructing the tree based on residuals, each split is based on the information gain, which is calculated from the similarity weight. Post-pruning decides the removal of any branch based on the cover value. XGBoost splits the tree level or tree-wise.

13.2.7   LᴵɢʜᴛGBM

This is a variation of XGBoost, which is more efficient and accurate. It is a fast, high-performance distributed gradient boosting framework, and it is based on the decision tree. In LightGBM the tree splits leaf-wise. It can lead to overfitting but can be controlled by defining the depth of the tree. It contains various hyperparameters.

13.3   RELATED WORKS

The literature review helps us in understanding the work done by other researchers in a similar or connected domain of study. Early polygenic disorder identification (inherited) is very important for human health to save lots of people from the fatal effects of polygenic disorder. Within the past few years, many completely different techniques have been introduced using different kinds of machine learning models and approaches for diagnosing polygenic disorders (diabetes and other inherited diseases). Some of the techniques employed by researchers a couple of years ago for predicting polygenic disorders are artificial neural network (ANN) approaches, machine learning, deep learning approaches, and retinal image-based approaches. As the technology is rapidly increasing day by day, advanced approaches for machine learning and deep learning models are often done.

Numerous data processing methods and their applications were suggested by Joshi et al. Machine learning algorithms have been used in many different medical datasets. The ensemble algorithm was more accurate than the single algorithm. Decision trees offered high accuracy in most of their studies. The tools used in this study to predict diabetes datasets are the hybrid system weka and java [7].

Eswari et al. developed a Hadoop system pattern and Mapreduce techniques to analyze the previous records of diabetic patients. This methodology predicts the style of diabetes and in addition risks associated with patients' records. The system is most economical because it is completely Hadoop ecosystem-based and is beneficial for trending companies and organizations [8].

Iyer et al. have used a classification technique to see (predict) unseen patterns in the diabetes dataset. Naïve Bayes and decision tree algorithms were used when building the machine learning models. An overview comparison was created for the performance of every formula, and the effectiveness of every algorithm was displayed in the form of a result [9].

Rajesh et al. have used the C4.5 decision tree algorithm to look out for unseen patterns from the dataset for effective classification [10]. Kahramanli et al. make use of an ANN in conjunction with the system of logic to predict diabetes [11]. Patil et al. projected a hybrid prediction model that includes an easy K-means clump algorithm; the results obtained from the clumping algorithm were combined with the classification algorithms for better accuracy [12].

Nagaraj et al. [13] proposed the AFA-GBT model for diabetes classification. AFA is an evolutionary algorithm that uses flower pollination as a metaphor to search for the optimal feature subset and is combined with the GBT model to classify type 2 diabetes. The results show that the proposed method is better than the traditional methods in terms of accuracy and computational time. Additionally, the feature importance of the selected feature subset was evaluated to provide insight into the most influential features for diabetes classification. The results demonstrate that AFA-GBT is an effective method for diabetes classification.

Nagaraj et al. [14] present a novel rule-based expert recommendation system for predictive diabetes diagnosis. The system uses a fuzzy inference rule-based expert system, which consists of three main parts: a rule set, a knowledge base, and a fuzzy logic inference engine. The rule set is based on the knowledge collected from medical experts on diabetes diagnosis and is designed to identify the risk factors associated with diabetes. The knowledge base consists of various medical parameters, such as age, family history, lifestyle, etc., which are used to infer the risk of diabetes. The fuzzy logic inference engine then uses the rule set and the knowledge base to make an inference about the patient's risk of diabetes. Finally, the system outputs a recommendation for the patient's diabetes diagnosis. The results obtained demonstrate that the system can provide accurate and reliable diabetes diagnosis recommendations.

Nagaraj et al. [15] analyzed the proper study, which aims to detect diabetes in its early stages by using an efficient machine learning model. The authors use a large dataset from the UCI Machine Learning Repository (UCI MLR) to train and evaluate two machine learning models: SVM and DNN. The SVM model is enhanced with the addition of a radial basis function (RBF) kernel and a grid search feature selection technique. The DNN model is composed of two hidden layers and has a rectified linear unit (ReLU) activation function. Both models are compared based on their accuracy, precision, recall, and F1 score. The results of the study show that the enhanced SVM model outperforms the DNN model in terms of accuracy, precision, recall, and F1 score. The authors conclude that the SVM model is better suited for the task of early screening of diabetes due to its superior performance. However, they also point out that further research is needed to explore the potential of the DNN model in this domain.

Nagaraj et al. [16] proposed an algorithm that uses a two-level optimization process to achieve improved performance in healthcare applications. The first level focuses on optimizing the tree seed Kalman filter parameters to minimize the prediction error. The second level focuses on using a genetic algorithm to optimize the tree seed Kalman filter parameters in combination with an ensemble of other machine learning algorithms. The proposed optimization strategy is evaluated on data from two datasets, and results show that it can improve the accuracy of prediction for diabetes patients. The proposed algorithm was also compared to a baseline algorithm and found to be more accurate in predicting glucose levels. The results show that the proposed algorithm outperforms the baseline in terms of both accuracy and robustness. The chapter concludes that the proposed bilevel optimization algorithm can be used to improve the accuracy and robustness of diabetes prediction models.

Nagaraj et al. [17] discussed the development of an intelligent recommender system for bolus insulin dosing in individuals with DM. The authors propose a novel algorithm based on Kalman filtering techniques and mutation-based optimization, which they refer to as the Mutation Kalman Filter (MkF). The MkF algorithm is designed to provide personalized insulin dosing recommendations that are tailored to the individual needs of each diabetic patient. The authors evaluate the performance of the MkF algorithm on a real-world dataset of diabetic patients and show that it outperforms existing approaches in terms of accuracy and precision. The authors conclude that the MkF algorithm is a promising approach for providing personalized recommendations for bolus insulin dosing and can be used to improve the health of diabetic patients.

Nagaraj et al. [18] designed the system to improve the accuracy and interpretability of predictions for people with diabetes. The system uses an XAI-based Lime Explainer, a machine learning algorithm, to analyze patient data to predict whether a person is likely to be diagnosed with diabetes. It then provides a recommendation system for patients with diabetes to help them manage their disease. The system uses several features such as age, gender, height, and blood sugar levels to predict the risk of diabetes. The XAI-based Lime Explainer then uses these features to identify the most important factors that influence the likelihood of a patient being diagnosed with diabetes. It also provides recommendations to patients on how they can modify their lifestyle to reduce their risk of diabetes or manage their illness. The results of the system show that it can accurately predict the risk of diabetes, while also providing explanations of why certain factors are important.

Nagaraj et al. [19] focus on the sentiment analysis of diabetes diagnosis health care as it is a major health issue in the world today. To this end, they used a machine learning technique called support vector machine (SVM) to classify tweets into two classes: positive and negative. The dataset used for this study consisted of tweets related to diabetes diagnosis health care, which were manually labeled as either positive or negative. The authors then used the SVM to classify the tweets into two classes. The results showed that the SVM was able to classify the tweets with an accuracy of 77%. The authors concluded that the SVM was effective in classifying tweets related to diabetes diagnosis and health care and could be used to improve the accuracy of sentiment analysis in this field.

Nagaraj et al. [20] proposed the system has two main components: a grid search and a random forest. The grid search algorithm is used to identify the optimal combination of model parameters, and the random forest algorithm is used to build the prediction model based on the identified optimal parameters. The system is tested on a real-world dataset of diabetes patients and is shown to have high accuracy and precision. The system is also compared to existing medical expert systems and is found to be more accurate and precise than existing systems. The chapter concludes by highlighting the potential value of the proposed system for improving the accuracy of DM prediction in medical settings.

Deny et al. [21] proposed a model-based control system for glucose regulation, which uses blood glucose readings, carbohydrate intake, and insulin dosage to adjust glucose levels. The proposed system uses a model predictive control (MPC) algorithm to estimate the optimal insulin dosage for each patient, which is then used to adjust the dosage as needed. The authors first present a model of glucose-insulin dynamics and discuss the parameters used in the model. They then describe the MPC algorithm and its implementation, which is based on a genetic algorithm. Finally, they present the results of their model-based control system on a real-life patient dataset. The results show that the proposed model-based control system was able to maintain stable glucose levels over the course of two weeks. Overall, this chapter provides a promising approach to glucose regulation for type 2 DM. The proposed model-based control system showed significant improvements in glucose control compared to manual adjustment of insulin dosage. The results suggest that this system could be used to improve glucose control in type 2 DM patients.

Brintha et al. [22] proposed a system designed to provide personalized food recommendations to diabetic patients, with the goal of helping them better manage their condition. The system uses ANN and CNN techniques to predict the diabetic patient's future food preferences and make personalized food recommendations accordingly. The authors also proposed a novel approach to help diabetic patients to make better decisions regarding their food choices. The system collects data from a variety of sources, including the patient's medical history, lifestyle, and dietary habits. It then uses ANN and CNN techniques to predict the patient's future food preferences. The authors tested the system using a dataset of diabetic patients and found that it was effective in predicting patients' food preferences and providing personalized food recommendations.

Revathi et al. [23] proposed a network that uses a PSO-based feature selection algorithm to select the most relevant features from the input images. The features are then used to construct a deep CNN, which is trained and tested on a large dataset of DR images. The results show that the proposed approach outperforms existing methods in terms of accuracy and specificity and can achieve a sensitivity of 95.41%. Furthermore, the proposed approach is computationally efficient and can be used to detect DR in a shorter time frame.

To achieve this, data mining is crucial in the creation of such diagnostic and prognostic tools for diabetes [24–42].

13.4 MATERIALS AND METHODS

13.4.1 DATA SOURCE

In this chapter, two different datasets were utilized to train and test novel methods for predicting a diabetes diagnosis. The first dataset was extracted from a different set of questions raised by the different patents. The sample question and the respective response are given in Figure 13.1.

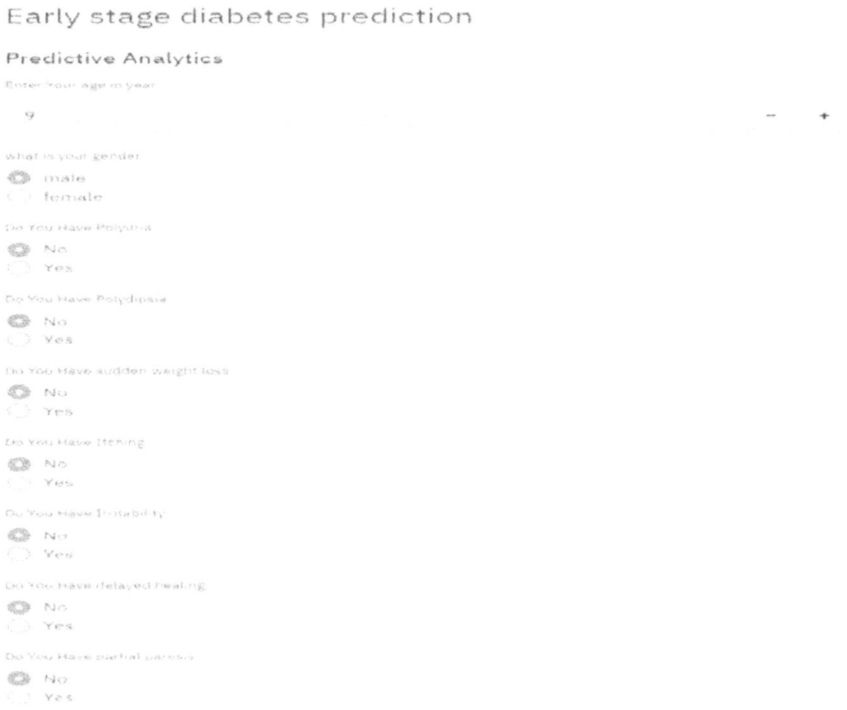

Early stage diabetes prediction

Predictive Analytics

Enter Your age in year

9   −   +

What is your gender
● male
○ female

Do You Have Polyuria
● No
○ Yes

Do You Have Polydipsia
● No
○ Yes

Do You Have sudden weight loss
● No
○ Yes

Do You Have itching
● No
○ Yes

Do You Have Irritability
● No
○ Yes

Do You have delayed healing
● No
○ Yes

Do You Have partial paresis
● No
○ Yes

FIGURE 13.1   Patients details collection from survival questions and response.

The second dataset, which was taken from the UCI machine learning repository, is frequently used to make predictions about the development of diabetes. This dataset is frequently used by machine learning researchers. The National Institute of Diabetes and Digestive and Kidney Diseases provided these statistics. The goal of the dataset is to ascertain whether a patient has diabetes using the diagnostic metrics in the collection. These cases were chosen from a larger database under several constraints. Women of Pima Indian descent who are at least 21 years old make up the entirety of the clinic's patrons. The dataset has 768 rows and 8 columns, as well as some medical indexes, and the purpose is to do exploratory data analysis on the state of diabetes. The dataset features are described in Figure 13.2.

13.4.2   PROPOSED METHOD

The analytical system is built from the data collection unit as the foundation cluster, and datasets containing the history of pharmaceutical data of a patient are important for forecasting autoimmune illnesses. Datasets like these can be found in databases like Kaggle. PIMA Indian Dataset for Diabetes is one such dataset that might be useful, and any additional relevant datasets can be collected and combined to produce the final dataset. The final dataset can now be uploaded to the cloud workspace that is hosting a machine learning instance. The machine

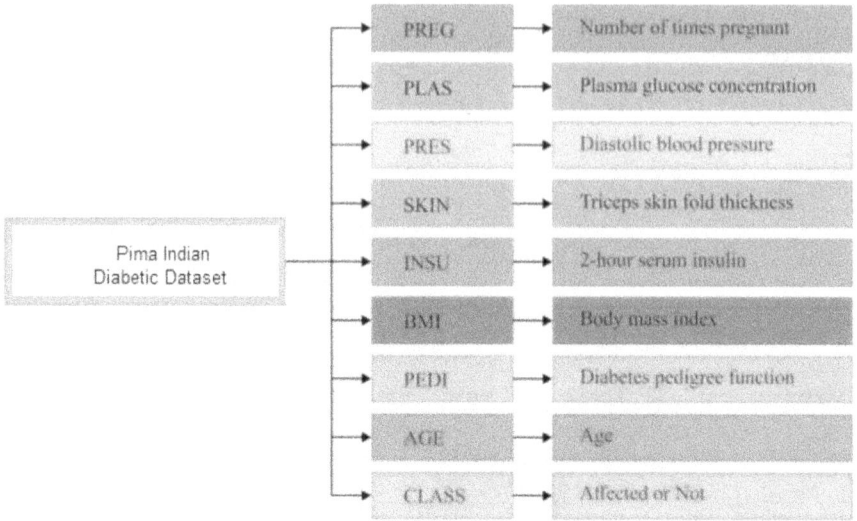

FIGURE 13.2   PIDD features.

learning instance examines the data and extracts the dataset's unique fields. Feature extraction is the term for this process. Furthermore, the extracted structures would now be configurable by the user. The user can now choose which fields should be studied with a prognostic algorithm and which fields should be the possible outcomes of the analyzed fields. Any augmentations can also be planned. This is the stage where you choose whatever features you want to use. The LGBM algorithm is utilized to train and test the dataset because it provides the highest level of accuracy for the dataset under consideration. Once the algorithm has been chosen, the dataset can be separated into two halves for training and testing.

The usual methods are used to calculate data in datasets that need to be used for training and testing. This algorithm will utilize the data in the dataset to train itself based on the outcome field existing in the dataset, and it will use the remaining split to test the accuracy of prediction once the training and testing splits have been selected by the user.

The model is ready to use once the "training and testing" is completed. When a similar dataset with suitable input fields is loaded, this prediction model running the LGBM algorithm will be ready to forecast the chance of persistent autoimmune disease. The user must ensure that all patient information is collected by the dataset used to train and test the model, or else the prediction conclusion will be wrong, as the model is not 100% accurate in prediction. After the analysis is completed with the analytical model, the estimated findings can be seen and retrieved in a variety of formats, including XML, CSV, spreadsheet, and Word document, depending on the user's preference. The accuracy of such enrichments can be pre-determined in the training and testing stages, and the results can be fine-tuned by running the algorithm with any available improvements. The flow

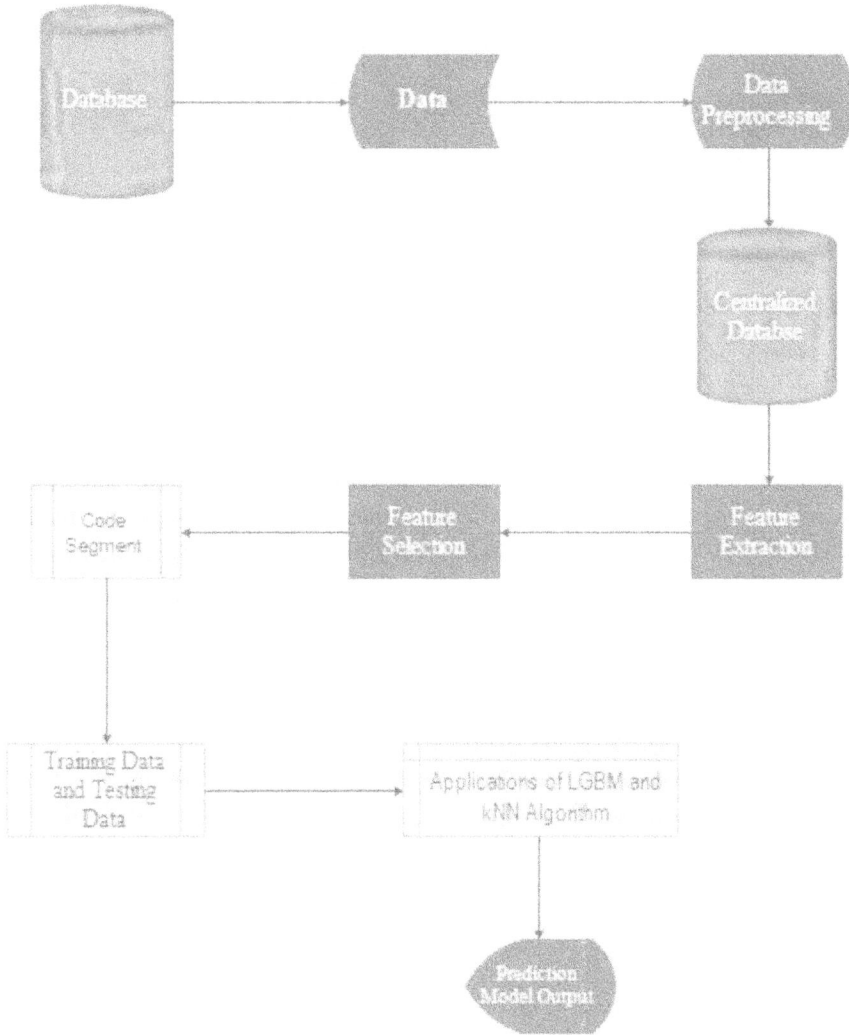

FIGURE 13.3   Proposed system architecture.

of the proposed model is illustrated in Figure 13.3. The most effective way to prevent overfitting using regularization is to add a penalty term to the cost function that penalizes overly complex models. This penalty term is typically a function of the weights and biases of the model and can take the form of a Y or Z regularization. Y regularization adds a penalty proportional to the sum of the absolute value of the weights, while Z regularization adds a penalty proportional to the sum of the squares of the weights. The penalty term encourages the model to use only the most important features, which helps to reduce overfitting. Additionally, techniques such as early stopping and dropout can be used to further reduce the chances of overfitting.

13.5 RESULTS AND DISCUSSION

Two distinct datasets for DM and Python were used to demonstrate the proposed model validation (Python Software Foundation, Wilmington, DE, USA). A computer system with an Intel® Pentium® 1.9 GHz processor, a 64-bit operating system, Microsoft® Windows 10, 4 GB of RAM, and Java JDK 1.8 was used to put the suggested technique into practice. The outcome of the proposed model was examined by accuracy, precision, recall, F1 measures, and ROC.

13.5.1 EARLY-STAGE DIABETES DETECTION WITH QUESTIONER DATASET

Feature engineering and visualization of the data were done in the first stage. Then, we took the early-stage diabetes detection dataset and applied the simple classification algorithms to it. If the result is normal, the person is healthy and does not have any diabetes. If the model predicted positive, then the person had to use the model that was trained on PIDD for more accurate results. Figure 13.4 depicts the correlation between different questions with features. The data transformation for the PIMA dataset includes feature selection, outlier detection, and imputation (Table 13.1).

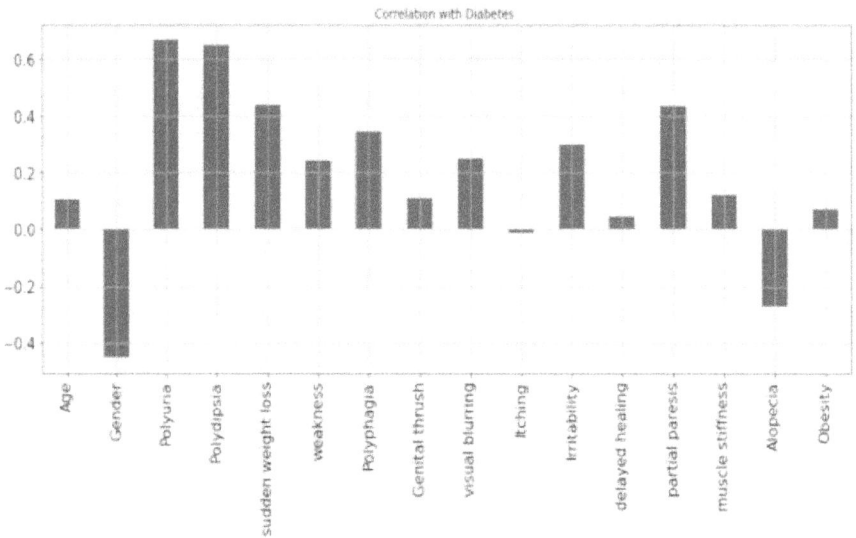

FIGURE 13.4   Correlation with features and target column in early-stage diabetes dataset.

TABLE 13.1
Early-stage Diabetes Prediction Model Results

Early-Stage Diabetes Diagnosis				
Algorithms	Accuracy	Precision	Recall	F1	ROC
Logistic regression	0.94	1	0.91	0.95	0.95
Random forest	**0.97**	**1**	**0.93**	**0.96**	**0.96**

13.5.2 Early-Stage Diabetes Detection with PIDD Dataset

Table 13.2 and Figures 13.5 to 13.10 show the results from the proposed model from the electronic health records. The user interface is shown in Figure 13.11. The parameters taken into account for each of the generated models in the ensemble are learning rate and activation functions.

TABLE 13.2
PIDD Dataset Result

PIDD Dataset	
Algorithms	**Accuracy**
Logistic regression	0.82
Gaussian naïve Bayes	0.68
K-neighbors classifier	0.81
XG BOOST	0.86
LightGBM	0.90
LightGBM +KNN	**0.91**

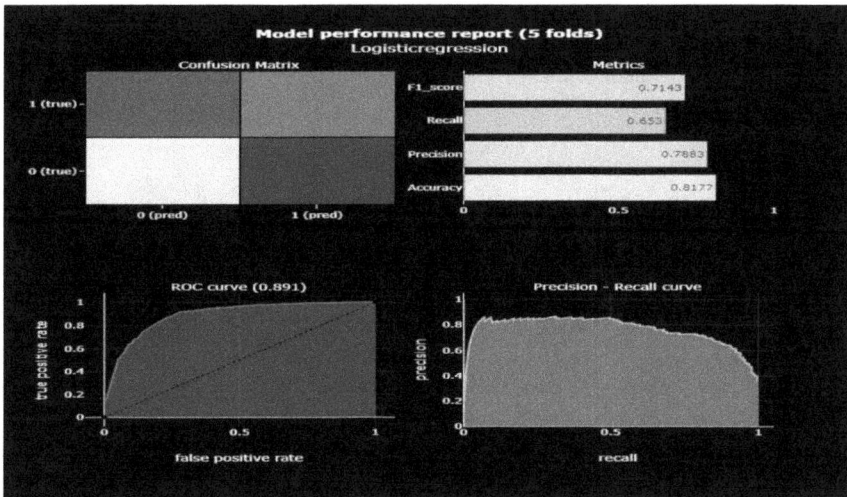

FIGURE 13.5 Logistics regression model.

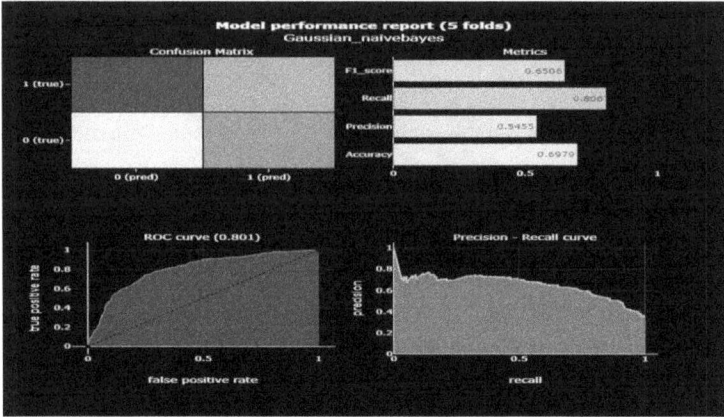

FIGURE 13.6   Gaussian naïve Bayes model.

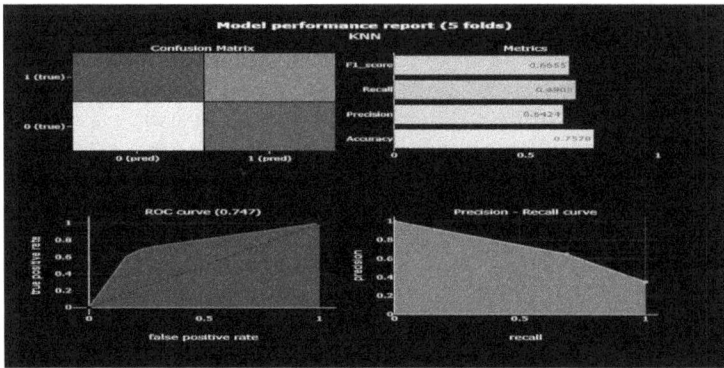

FIGURE 13.7   KNeighbors classifier model.

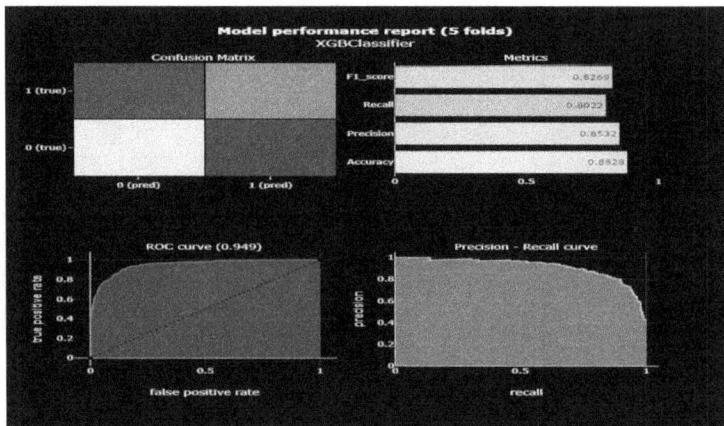

FIGURE 13.8   XGBoost model.

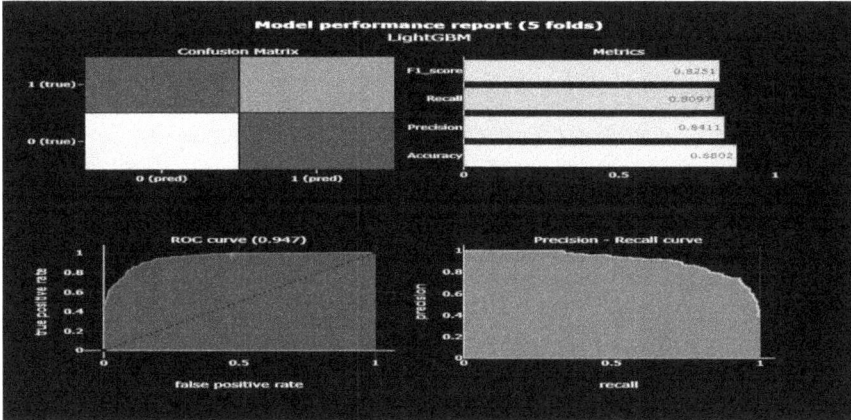

FIGURE 13.9   Light GBM model.

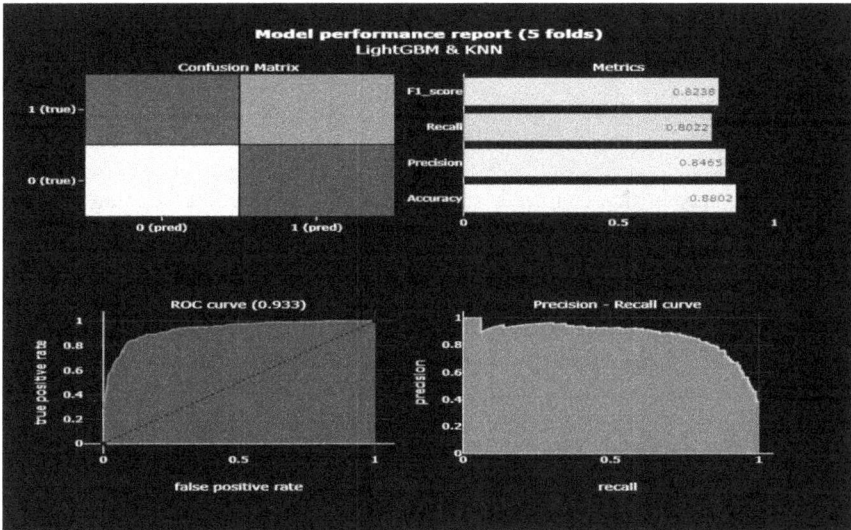

FIGURE 13.10   Light GBM + KNN model.

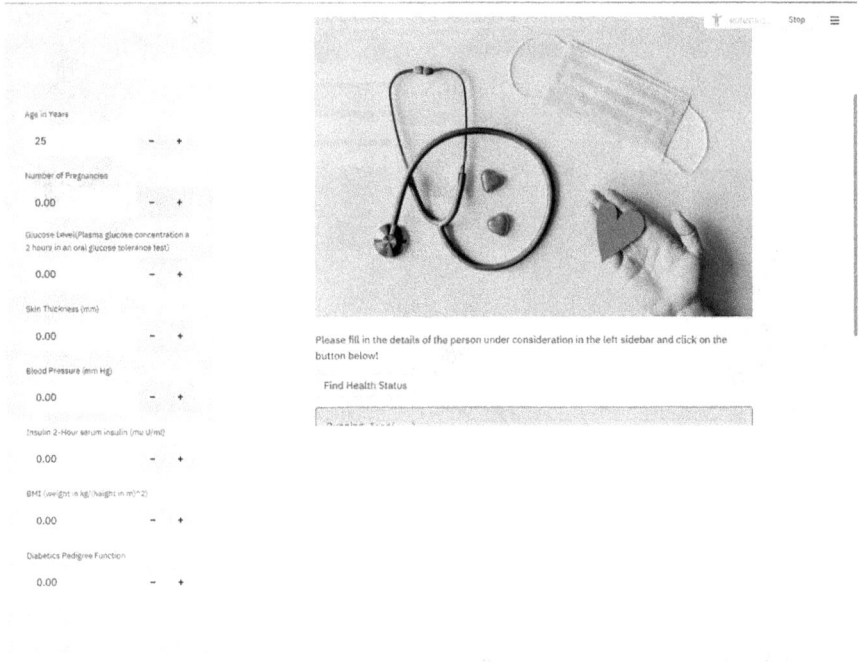

FIGURE 13.11 User interface for PIDD (LightGBM+KNN MODEL).

13.6 CONCLUSION

The overall study in this chapter is to improve diabetes prediction using machine learning techniques. Initially, we did a literature survey on various research papers about diabetic prediction using machine learning. We tried to detect diabetes at an early stage using a questionnaire dataset that does not involve any medical diagnosis. The highest accuracy is obtained for the random forest algorithm (0.97). We then tried to predict diabetes based on PIDD (Pima Indian Diabetic Dataset), which contains the various features and the target column. We classified the target column as binary (diabetic or non-diabetic). Various classification and ensemble algorithms were applied. Finally, the hybrid algorithm LightGBM+KNN (0.91) gave the highest accuracy. For both models, we created a user interface using the Streamlit library in Python.

REFERENCES

1. Mishra, P., Sharma, A., & Badholia, A. (2021). Predictive modeling and analytics for diabetes using a machine learning approach. Information Technology in Industry, 9(1), 215–223.
2. Rey, J. B., & Hawks, M. (2022). Prevention or delay of Type 2 diabetes mellitus: Recommendations from the American Diabetes Association. American Family Physician, 105(4), 438–439.
3. http://diabetesindia.com/

4. Itrat, M., & Akhlaq, S. (2022). Prevalence, pattern and perceived benefits of unani medicines usage in diabetes: A patient-based survey at a Primary Health Centre of Bengaluru, India. Journal of Herbal Medicine, 35, 100591.

5. https://my.clevelandclinic.org/health/diseases/7104-diabetes-mellitus-an-overview/

6. https://www.diabetes.co.uk/diabetes_care/blood-sugar-level-ranges.html

7. Joshi, R., & Alehegn, M. (2017). Analysis and prediction of diabetes diseases using machine learning algorithm: Ensemble approach. International Research Journal of Engineering and Technology, 4(10), 426–435.

8. Eswari, T., Sampath, P., & Lavanya, S. J. P. C. S. (2015). Predictive methodology for diabetic data analysis in big data. Procedia Computer Science, 50, 203–208.

9. Iyer, A., Jeyalatha, S., & Sumbaly, R. (2015). Diagnosis of diabetes using classification mining techniques. arXiv preprint arXiv:1502.03774.

10. Rajesh, K., & Sangeetha, V. (2012). Application of data mining methods and techniques for diabetes diagnosis. International Journal of Engineering and Innovative Technology (IJEIT), 2(3), 224–229.

11. Kahramanli, H., & Allahverdi, N. (2008). Design of a hybrid system for the diabetes and heart diseases. Expert Systems with Applications, 35(1-2), 82–89.

12. Patil, B. M., Joshi, R. C., & Toshniwal, D. (2010, February). Association rule for classification of type-2 diabetic patients. In 2010 second international conference on machine learning and computing (pp. 330–334). IEEE.

13. Nagaraj, P., Deepalakshmi, P., Mansour, R. F., & Almazroa, A. (2021). Artificial flora algorithm-based feature selection with gradient boosted tree model for diabetes classification. Diabetes, Metabolic Syndrome and Obesity: Targets and Therapy, 14, 2789.

14. Nagaraj, P., & Deepalakshmi, P. (2022). An intelligent fuzzy inference rule-based expert recommendation system for predictive diabetes diagnosis. International Journal of Imaging Systems and Technology, 32(4), 1373–1396.

15. Nagaraj, P., & Deepalakshmi, P. (2021). Diabetes Prediction Using Enhanced SVM and Deep Neural Network Learning Techniques: An Algorithmic Approach for Early Screening of Diabetes. International Journal of Healthcare Information Systems and Informatics (IJHISI), 16(4), 1–20.

16. Nagaraj, P., Deepalakshmi, P., & Ijaz, M. F. (2022). Optimized Adaptive Tree Seed Kalman Filter for a Diabetes Recommendation System—Bilevel Performance Improvement Strategy for Healthcare Applications. In Cognitive and Soft Computing Techniques for the Analysis of Healthcare Data (pp. 191–202). Academic Press.

17. Nagaraj, P., Muneeswaran, V., Sabik Ali, R., Sangeeth Kumar, T., Someshwara, A. L., & Pranav, J. (2021). Flexible Bolus Insulin Intelligent Recommender System for Diabetes Mellitus Using Mutated Kalman Filtering Techniques. In Congress on Intelligent Systems: Proceedings of CIS 2020, Volume 2 (pp. 565–574). Springer Singapore.

18. Nagaraj, P., Muneeswaran, V., Dharanidharan, A., Balananthanan, K., Arunkumar, M., & Rajkumar, C. (2022, April). A Prediction and Recommendation System for Diabetes Mellitus using XAI-based Lime Explainer. In 2022 International Conference on Sustainable Computing and Data Communication Systems (ICSCDS) (pp. 1472–1478). IEEE.

19. Nagaraj, P., Deepalakshmi, P., Muneeswaran, V., & Muthamil Sudar, K. (2022, July). Sentiment Analysis on Diabetes Diagnosis Health Care Using Machine Learning Technique. In Congress on Intelligent Systems: Proceedings of CIS 2021, Volume 1 (pp. 491–502). Singapore: Springer Nature Singapore.

20. Nagaraj, P., Muneeswaran, V., & Deshik, G. (2022, August). Ensemble Machine Learning (Grid Search & Random Forest) based Enhanced Medical Expert Recommendation System for Diabetes Mellitus Prediction. In 2022 3rd International Conference on Electronics and Sustainable Communication Systems (ICESC) (pp. 757–765). IEEE.

21. Deny, J., Rajalakshmi, P., Muneeswaran, V., Sudharsan, R. R., & Nagaraj, P. (2022, August). Automation of Glucose Control for Type-2 Diabetes Mellitus. In 2022 3rd International Conference on Electronics and Sustainable Communication Systems (ICESC) (pp. 79–83). IEEE.

22. Brintha, N. C., Nagaraj, P., Tejasri, A., Durga, B. V., Teja, M. T., & Kumar, M. N. V. P. (2022, June). A Food Recommendation System for Predictive Diabetic Patients using ANN and CNN. In 2022 7th International Conference on Communication and Electronics Systems (ICCES) (pp. 1364–1371). IEEE.

23. Revathi, B., Elizabeth, S. K., Nagaraj, P., Birunda, S. S., & Nithya, D. (2023, February). Particle Swarm Optimization based Detection of Diabetic Retinopathy using a Novel Deep CNN. In 2023 Third International Conference on Artificial Intelligence and Smart Energy (ICAIS) (pp. 998–1003). IEEE.

24. https://www.kaggle.com/uciml/pima-indians-diabetes-database/

25. Varma, C. G., Nagaraj, P., Muneeswaran, V., Mokshagni, M., & Jaswanth, M. (2021, May). Astute Segmentation and Classification of Leucocytes in Blood Microscopic Smear Images Using Titivated K-means Clustering and Robust SVM Techniques. In 2021 5th International Conference on Intelligent Computing and Control Systems (ICICCS) (pp. 818–824). IEEE.

26. Sharan, E. S., Kumar, K. S., & Madhuri, G. (2021, July). Conceal Face Mask Recognition using Convolutional Neural Networks. In 2021 6th International Conference on Communication and Electronics Systems (ICCES) (pp. 1787–1793). IEEE.

27. Nagaraj, P., Muneeswaran, V., Reddy, L. V., Upendra, P., & Reddy, M. V. V. (2020, May). Programmed Multi-classification of Brain Tumor Images Using Deep Neural Network. In 2020 4th international conference on intelligent computing and control systems (ICICCS) (pp. 865–870). IEEE.

28. Nagaraj, P., & Deepalakshmi, P. (2020). A framework for e-healthcare management service using recommender system. Electronic Government, an International Journal, 16(1-2), 84–100.

29. Harinath Reddy, C., Koushik Kumar, B. V., Sai Teja Varma, N., Vidya, S., Nagaraj, P., & Muthamil Sudar, K. (2021, May). Risk Prediction of Lung Disease Using Deep Learning Approach. In International Conference on Image Processing and Capsule Networks (pp. 462–471). Cham: Springer.

30. Muneeswaran, V., Nagaraj, P., Rajasekaran, M. P., Kumar, K. V., Kumar, C., & Reddy, Y. (2022). Programmed Identification of Glaucoma Using Tree Seed Optimized Histogram Manipulation. In Artificial Intelligence and Evolutionary Computations in Engineering Systems (pp. 355–365). Singapore: Springer.

31. Alagarsamy, S., & Nagaraj, P. (2022, January). Detection of Tumor Region in MRI Images Using Kernel Fuzzy C Means with PSO. In 2022 International Conference on Computer Communication and Informatics (ICCCI) (pp. 1–6). IEEE.

32. Nagaraj, P., Muneeswaran, V., Sabik Ali, R., Sangeeth Kumar, T., Someshwara, A. L., & Pranav, J. (2020, September). Flexible Bolus Insulin Intelligent Recommender System for Diabetes Mellitus Using Mutated Kalman Filtering Techniques. In Congress on Intelligent Systems (pp. 565–574). Singapore: Springer.

33. Muneeswaran, V., Nagaraj, P., & Ijaz, M. F. (2022). An Articulated Learning Method Based on Optimization Approach for Gallbladder Segmentation from MRCP Images and an Effective IoT Based Recommendation Framework. In Connected e-Health (pp. 165–179). Cham: Springer.

34. Sudar, K. M., Nagaraj, P., Yeshwanth, K. V., Kumar, Y. D., Kumar, V. S. J., & Reddy, V. N. S. (2022, May). Recognitionof Diseases in Paddy Using Deep Learning. In 2022 6th International Conference on Intelligent Computing and Control Systems (ICICCS) (pp. 1458–1463). IEEE.

35. Sudar, K. M., Nagaraj, P., Prakash, B., Reddy, M. M., Naidu, M. M., & Kumar, H. (2022, May). Development of Tomato Leaf Disease Prediction System to the Farmers by using Artificial Intelligent Network. In 2022 6th International Conference on Intelligent Computing and Control Systems (ICICCS) (pp. 955–961). IEEE.

36. Kumar, B. M., Rao, K. R. K., Nagaraj, P., Sudar, K. M., & Muneeswaran, V. (2022, April). Tobacco Plant Disease Detection and Classification using Deep Convolutional Neural Networks. In 2022 International Conference on Sustainable Computing and Data Communication Systems (ICSCDS) (pp. 490–495). IEEE.

37. Sudar, K. M., Nagaraj, P., Jeereddy, H. R., & Dasi, L. R. (2022, April). Convolutional Neural Network based Alzheimer's Disease Prediction in MRI Images. In 2022 International Conference on Sustainable Computing and Data Communication Systems (ICSCDS) (pp. 452–457). IEEE.

38. Birunda, S. S., Nagaraj, P., Narayanan, S. K., Sudar, K. M., Muneeswaran, V., & Ramana, R. (2022, January). Fake Image Detection in Twitter using Flood Fill Algorithm and Deep Neural Networks. In 2022 12th International Conference on Cloud Computing, Data Science & Engineering (Confluence) (pp. 285–290). IEEE.

39. Vb, S. K. (2020). Perceptual image super resolution using deep learning and super resolution convolution neural networks (SRCNN). Intelligent Systems and Computer. Technology, 37(3), 3–8.

40. Nagaraj, P., Rao, J. S., Muneeswaran, V., & Kumar, A. S. (2020, May). Competent Ultra Data Compression by Enhanced Features Excerption Using Deep Learning Techniques. In 2020 4th International Conference on Intelligent Computing and Control Systems (ICICCS) (pp. 1061–1066). IEEE.

41. Muneeswaran, V., BenSujitha, B., Sujin, B., & Nagaraj, P. (2020). A compendious study on security challenges in big data and approaches of feature selection. International Journal of Control and Automation, 13(3), 23–31.

42. Sathiyamoorthi, V., Ilavarasi, A.K., Murugeswari, K., Ahmed, S. T., Devi, B. A., & Kalipindi, M. (2021). A deep convolutional neural network based computer aided diagnosis system for the prediction of Alzheimer's disease in MRI images. *Measurement*, 171, 108838, ISSN 0263-2241, 10.1016/j.measurement.2020.108838.

14 Deep Convolutional Neural Network Models for Early Detection of Breast Cancer from Digital Mammograms

A. Nithya and P. Shanmugavadivu
Department of Computer Science and Applications, The
Gandhigram Rural Institute (Deemed to be University),
Gandhigram, Dindigul, Tamil Nadu, India

14.1 INTRODUCTION

Cancer develops when abnormal body cells begin to rapidly split on a mass scale and then infect the normal cells and turn them into malignant cells. Breast cancer tops the list of claiming lives due to cancer. Invasive and non-invasive breast cancers are the two subtypes. The cancerous, or malignant, invasive cells spread rapidly to the neighboring organs. Precancerous, or non-invasive, type is benign in nature and remains in the identified location. It may or may not ultimately progress into an aggressive breast cancer. The glands and milk ducts that transport milk are the area of the body where breast cancer is generally spotted. Breast cancer frequently metastasizes to other organs, turning them malignant. Additionally, it spreads to other organs through the bloodstream. There are numerous forms of breast cancer, and each one spreads at a distinct rate. In 2018, 627000 women lost their lives to breast cancer, represented by the World Health Organization (WHO) [1]. The USA tops the list in the world of the victims of breast cancer. Breast cancer comes in four different forms. The first type of cancer is ductal carcinoma in situ, a form of early-stage breast cancer that is detected in the covering of breast milk ducts. Up to 70–80% of cases of another type of breast cancer are diagnosed. The third form of cancer is inflammatory breast cancer, in which the skin and lymphatic arteries of the breast are aggressively and swiftly penetrated by cancer cells. Breast cancer that has spread to other bodily areas is the fourth kind of breast cancer [2].

Numerous diagnostic procedures, including magnetic resonance imaging (MRI), ultrasound, mammography, and biopsies, provide images needed for classification. During mammography screening, X-rays are used to capture the breast image for

DOI: 10.1201/9781003469605-14

diagnosis. If any abnormal findings are seen, the doctor may advise a biopsy. Doctors recommend for ultrasound imaging, to be able to validate the presence/ absence of breast cancer. If tests conducted during a symptomatic examination are proved to be inconclusive, the doctor recommends breast MRI as it can provide the intrinsic details for easy diagnosis. The primary diagnostic tool for determining whether a suspected area is carcinogenic is a biopsy. About 80% of women who get a breast biopsy do not have a cancerous tumor [3,4].

The accurate classification of breast cancer used by popular machine learning (ML) techniques has triggered the interest of many researchers in recent years. ML includes the subfield of artificial intelligence (AI). Many researchers apply ML to retrain their models, which helps them perform better. When the amount of data is minimal, ML produces promising outcomes. But, when the amount of data is enormous, it is proved to be inappropriate. The ML model falls into one of three categories of ML: supervised, unsupervised, and reinforcement model. The supervised models learn from labeled datasets (containing both inputs and class values). The unsupervised ML models learn from unlabeled data. The reinforcement models get tuned based on rewards for accurate computation and penalties for inaccurate ones. These algorithms pull the most relevant data from prior knowledge for regression/classification [5].

Deep learning (DL) is an unsupervised method that accumulates knowledge from image datasets. The data could be unlabeled or unstructured. A deep neural network has more hidden layers rather than two. In essence, the input layer is the top layer and the output layer is the bottom layer. Neural network, the intermediate layer other than the input and output layers, is the hidden layer. Neurons refer to the node present in the layer. Convolution neural network (CNN) is vibrantly used to classify the breast images. The dataset of breast cancer image inputs is used for model training and testing. The images are provided to CNN as inputs along with the corresponding weights [6,7]. To reduce misclassification and improve performance of the models, the weights are updated. Conventionally the CNN models contain a convolution layer, an activation layer, a pooling layer, and a fully connected (FC) layer. By convolving the input image with reference to the filter or kernel, the convolution layer aims to extract the essential properties from the source image. This process greatly helps in dimensionality reduction. The activation function such as ReLu helps to confine the unbounded intermediate values into bounded values. The pooling layer extracts the prominent features in the form of classification, identification, detection, etc. The task of classification is carried out by the FC layers [8].

The use of ML models in image processing could be a useful tool for identification and diagnosis. Without human effort or assistance, DL models have a greater capacity to discover breast cancer at an earlier stage [9]. The design and performance of the DL models are problem specific; it is important to confirm the suitability of a DL by exploring the performance of selected models on breast cancer detection. This research work intends to analyze performance of the pre-trained models, namely VGG19, ResNet50V2, InceptionResNetV2, DenseNet201, and EfficientNetB6. These transfer learning models provide commendable solutions for image segmentation, classification, and analysis. The results of each DL model were comparatively analyzed. Every DL model offers ample scope for fine-tuning by adjusting its architecture, and optimizing the hyper-parameter values. The pre-trained DL models (i.e., transfer learning models) are proven to handle complex real-time problems better than the ML models. In this research, DenseNet201 model is vouched to be the best performing DL model. The quality metrics used for the quantitative performance analysis were accuracy, precision, recall, and F1-score.

This chapter's goal is to describe the processes for diagnosing breast cancer and determining whether it is benign or malignant. The DDSM and INbreast datasets were used in the experimental analysis. Each model is improved by retraining the final layer using our breast mammography dataset while freezing the pre-trained weights of the primary layers.

14.2 RELATED WORKS

The development of a computer system that can recognize breast tumors from mammograms has undergone a number of attempts. Numerous authors have used various ML approaches, such as feature extraction, feature selection, and image pre-processing, to decrease the amount of features, speed up computation, and enhance accuracy. The most efficient DL method currently applied in the medical field is CNN modeling, which has been shown to outperform more conventional methods [10–13].

There have been many attempts to create a computer system that can recognize breast cancers from mammograms. To decrease the amount of features, decrease computation time, and increase accuracy, some authors have used a variety of ML approaches, such as image pre-processing, feature extraction, feature selection, etc. The CNN models have been exposed to be more efficient than conventional techniques and are currently the most often utilized DL methodology in the medical field. Z. Hussain et al. [14] developed a transfer learning-based CNN model to detect the presence and absence of breast abnormalities in DDSM mammograms dataset and classify the tumors as benign or malignant. They combined transfer learning-based VGG-16 with a data augmentation method to enhance the instances of the training data. Their techniques obtained 88% accuracy.

M. Alkhaleefah et al. created a double shot transfer learning (DSTL)-based model that may be utilized for both classification and augmentation. A huge dataset that was roughly comparable to the target dataset was used for DSTL in addition to fine-tune the parameters of the pre-trained network. The networks were modified using the target dataset [15].

A. Perre et al. proposed three different networks based on transfer learning techniques, namely VGG-m, Caffe, and VGG-f. These pre-trained CNN models' output was inspected twice, once with and once without image normalization, throughout the fine-tuning process to look for any mammography anomalies. They evaluated the results of an SVM that had been given CNN-obtained features [16]. A mobile network, residual network, and modified VGG were created by A. Khamparial et al. [17]. According to research findings on the DDSM dataset, the proposed learning model produced 88.3% accuracy and attained 80.8% precision when the epoch is 15.

A hybrid model of VGG, ResNet, Xception, and ResNext was introduced by L. Falconi et al. Their CBIS-DDSM dataset trial, with fine-tuning, showed increased effectiveness in VGG16 with the value of AUC is 0.844. P. Kaur et al. experimented with a novel methodology using mini-MIAS dataset. K-mean convergence in an integrated feature extraction framework for speeding up reliable features (SURFs). The combination of multiclass SVM and deep neural network (DNN) received 70% training and 30% testing [18]. Using various datasets, namely DDSM, MIAS, LAPIMO, and BancoWeb, K. Shaikh et al. tested a CNN model utilizing accuracy, which was 87.5% [19]. In order to categorize mitoses, Wahab et al. utilized a transfer learning CNN and another CNN with the learned parameters. Precision, recall, and F-measure from their approach were 0.50, 0.80, and 0.621, respectively [20].

Without adjusting the source network layers, Cao et al. [21] combined the different feature groups using random forest dissimilarity (ResNet125). Using the dataset "ICIAR2018," classification accuracy increased to 82.90%. Using a 224×224 pixel input image and 14 layers, CNN was used to train by Charan et al. [22]. This network's accuracy on the MIAS database was 65%. This chapter proposes a pre-trained-based CNN model for classifying breast cancer in mammography images.

14.3 MATERIALS AND METHODS

14.3.1 MATERIALS

The experimental study of this chapter has been done on two digital breast X-ray databases, namely DDSM and INbreast.

14.3.1.1 DDSM

This dataset has over 2600 cases that are compiled based on the severity of the disease. In the DDSM, for each patient mammograms are taken in four views. The patient's age, the screening exam's date, and the breast density as determined by a professional radiologist utilizing the American College of Radiology reporting system [23]. Pixel-level ground truth anomaly indicators are used to identify cases with suspicious regions. In this research, 641 patients with benign and 688 patients with malignant, totaling 5316 images, were included in the subgroup of 1329 cases evaluated. This dataset has been shown to be pertinent to this investigation because it focuses specifically on classifying instances as benign or malignant.

14.3.1.2 INbreast

Digital mammogram images taken from the Portuguese University Hospital's Breast Center (Centro Hospitalar de S. Joao [CHSJ], Porto) were integrated into the INbreast database with the approval of the hospital's ethics committee and national data protection commission. The INbreast dataset contains 115 patients' images in both breast perspectives (MLO and CC). Each of the 90 women who impacted both breasts underwent four mammograms, while only two mammograms were conducted on the 25 patients who underwent mastectomy (i.e., 50 mammograms). Hence, 115 patients' MLO and CC pictures were used to create 410 mammograms altogether. This covers both benign and cancerous instances [24].

14.3.2 CONVOLUTIONAL NEURAL NETWORKS

In this subsection, the fundamental element of each CNN architecture is described. CNN is a subset of deep neural network, and it is predominantly employed for image

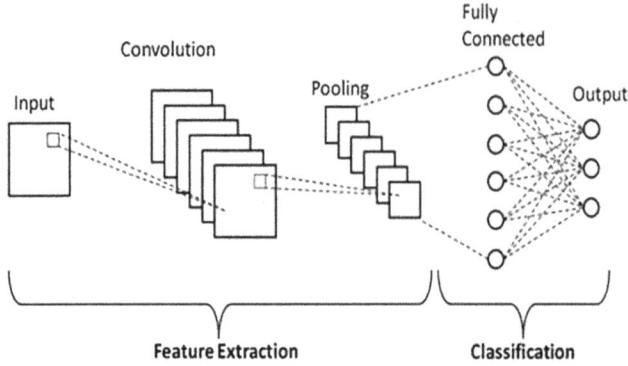

FIGURE 14.1 CNN architecture.

recognition and classification. CNNs have recently emerged as a turn-key technique in image processing, particularly for face detection, text processing, and medical imaging [25,26]. Since their creation in 1989, CNNs have been effectively utilized for image classification, segmentation, and many more applications. The visual processes of the human brain are designed to be similar to those of the CNNs. Neurons in the brain are related to one another in their immediate surroundings. Convolutional, pooling, and FC layers collaborate to generate the image used for feature extraction. The CNN extracts the topological features of an image, which are not spatially correlated. A fundamental CNN architecture is shown in Figure 14.1.

14.3.2.1   Convolutional Layers

The CNN layers are organized in accordance with the local connection and weight distribution idea to produce feature maps with input items assigned to all neurons. Above mentioned, both metrics use the densely populated local pixel neighborhood to decrease the number of input parameters while preserving the location independence of local pixel attributes. In CNN, the convolution layer performs convolution operation on the input pixels and a convolution mask (i.e., filter or kernel). The unbounded values computed by convolution are treated by an appropriate activation function such as ReLu and softmax and are transformed into bounded values, to ensure clarity of learning. The order of selection of input image pixels for convolution is decided by the size of the convolution filter.

14.3.2.2   Pooling Layer

Convolution is the first layer, followed by a pooling layer and uses a subsampling technique to extract the vital information from the output of convolutional layers. This layer's main objective is to highlight an image's features as well as to shrink and achieve dimensionality reduction on the feature map. Max pooling and min pooling are two prominent types of operations carried out on this layer [27].

14.3.2.3   Fully Connected Layer

The last layer of the CNN is the classifier, which establishes the class of the input data based on the feature map produced from the input data. The number of output classes is equal to the number of FC layer units [28].

TABLE 14.1

Description of Hyperparameter

Name of the Hyperparameter	Description
Learning rate	The preliminary learning rate for the CNN architecture is the most important hyperparameter that has a large impact on how well a model works. The model requires additional iterations because the initial learning rate was low.
Hidden layer	Although adding more hidden layer units could improve the model, doing so would decrease computational efficiency.
Dropout rate	Dropout rates are a regularization strategy that decreases overfitting by fostering the validity accuracy and, thus, the generalizing power.
Batch size	To update the parameters, the network receives the quantity of sub-samples.
Activation function	DL approaches are able to learn nonlinear prediction limits due to activation functions.
Number of epoch	The number of training iterations the entire training dataset has undergone.

The CNN model's performance is dependent on the values assumed by the hyperparameters, which in turn decides the accuracy. Some researchers attempt to fine-tune the hyperparameters in order to attain better results. Table 14.1 provides the hyperparameters for the CNN architecture along with a description of each one.

Several convolutional layers are present in deep CNN architectures. The AlexNet is a CNN architecture that differs from Basic CNN in that it has five convolutional layers. VGGNet replicates AlexNet in many ways. In order to extract more complicated characteristics, it employs 3×3 convolutions as well as numerous smaller-sized filters. The number of layers in various versions of VGGNet varies, including VGGNet16 (16 layers) and VGGNet19 (19 levels). The VGGNet's regular architecture makes it appealing. Unfortunately, because of its depth, it takes a time-consuming process for trains to compute, which causes the issue of disappearing gradients. ZF-Net is an architecture of Alex-Net that has been slightly altered, as shown by their feature maps of convolutional networks. With 22 layers, the GoogLeNet architecture is thought to be more intricate and deeper. This design uses the CNN's inception module and focuses on different convolutional layers [29].

In this chapter, the performance analysis of fine-tuned VGG19, ResNet50V2, InceptionResNetV2, DenseNet201, and EfficientNetB6 on the DDSM and INbreast datasets are documented.

14.3.3 PRE-TRAINED DCNN MODELS

14.3.3.1 VGG 19

The VGG19, which contains 19 layers, uses 16 convolutional layers and 3 fully connected layers to classify the images into 1000 object categories. The ImageNet database, which has one million images in 1000 classes, was used to train this algorithm. Convolutional layers are particularly popular for picture classification because each one employs multiple 3×3 filters. This model creates the label for the object in the given image after receiving a 224×224 image.

14.3.3.2   ResNet50V2

A massive architecture called ResNet50V2 was derived from ResNet50 and got improved in the later years to perform better than the earlier versions of architectures like ResNet101. The ResNet is a modern CNN that uses the remaining blocks in the design to solve vanishing gradients. Multiple residual blocks are placed on top of one another in a residual network. Each residual block is made up of connections that take shortcuts by skipping one or more layers. The pre-activation of weight layers is used by ResNet50V2. On the datasets, ResNet50V2 produces precise predictions.

14.3.3.3   InceptionResNetV2

This network blends a specific ResNet design with an Inception-v3 network architecture. The batch normalization is used as the standard layers. The networks' depth and the number of inception blocks are increased using the leftover modules. The Inception-ResNet-v2 architecture consists of one stem block and three different sets of inception blocks. The first block consists of five inception modules with seven convolution blocks each. Ten inception modules with five convolution blocks each are found in the first block, and five inception modules with four convolution blocks each are found in the third and final block. Both of these blocks contain two depletion blocks with numerous convolutional layers, average pooling, and fully connected layers. The Softmax activation function is used at the output layer.

14.3.3.4   DenseNet201

Each layer in DenseNet receives additional inputs from all the preceding layers in addition to its own feature maps. Due to getting the feature map of all prior layers, the network has fewer channels, 3×3 convolution with the growth rate k as an additional number of channels for each layer, along with batch normalization (BN) and ReLU.

The neural network's total number of layers is indicated by the 201 in DenseNet-201. The combination of various layers is a common DenseNet201 construction. It consists of two dense blocks (1×1 and 3×3 convolutions), five convolutions and pooling layers, three transition layers, one classification layer, and three transition layers.

14.3.3.5   EfficientNetB6

In 2019, EfficientNet was developed. Despite its disadvantage of having a somewhat slower learning rate than ResNet, it is believed to have adequate computing speed and accuracy for our application. CNNs are typically enhanced through the use of model extensions. The performance improves with network depth. The number of nodes can be increased or decreased to develop effective models as needed. However, these adjustments need to be made manually, and after multiple attempts, a superior CNN can be built utilizing hyperparameters.

14.4 METHODOLOGY

In a neural network, the neurons and synapses link to a mathematical model to simulate the human brain. In essence, DL trains the model using the CNN layer. Five different DL models' abilities to discriminate between typical and abnormal mammography pictures were analyzed. The proposed study compares the performance of five various models, including VGG19, ResNet50V2, InceptionResNetV2, DenseNet201, and EfficientNetB6, and it is implemented in the following steps.

Phase I: Data pre-processing
Phase II: Training the five different types of models (VGG19, ResNet50V2, InceptionResNetV2, DenseNet201, EfficientNetB6) with transfer learning using DDSM and INbreast datasets
Phase III: Test and predict benign or malignant images
Phase IV: Compare the performance of these five models with standard metrics

14.4.1 PHASE I: DATA PRE-PROCESSING

The mammography images in the database include a variety of undesirable visual features, noise, and artefacts, making them low-quality images that are certain to reduce classification accuracy. To get accurate results out of the DL models, the input images in the dataset are pre-processed with artefact removal, image resizing, and data augmentation. In this research work the artefacts are removed using the thresholding technique [30] and the original images are scaled down to 224×224 pixels.

The essential element of data classification, and the most significant aspect of ML and DL models, is feature extraction. Features describe many patterns relating to various diseases. During the training phase of DL/ML models, these feature extraction components are crucial in determining the class labels of data samples. Therefore, for precise prediction, the training dataset should contain a substantial number of datasets representing both benign and malignant mammogram detection. The total number of images with and without data augmentation is shown in Table 14.2. For all experiments, traditional data augmentation is done by rescaling, shear range, zoom range, validation split, and horizontal flip. Data augmentation is used to improve the performance of models during training and testing datasets. Also, DL models need a lot of information in order to attain a better understanding during training and testing.

14.4.2 PHASE II: TRAIN THE FIVE DIFFERENT TYPES OF TRANSFER LEARNING MODELS

This phase targets to train the conventional pre-trained models, namely, VGG19, ResNet50V2, InceptionResNetV2, DenseNet201, and EfficientNetB6, using transfer

TABLE 14.2
Number of Original and Augmented Images

Datasets	Total Number of Images (Original)			Total Number of Images (Augmented)		
	Benign	Malignant	Total	Benign	Malignant	Total
DDSM	2600	2716	5316	5970	7161	13131
INbreast	36	76	112	5112	2520	7632

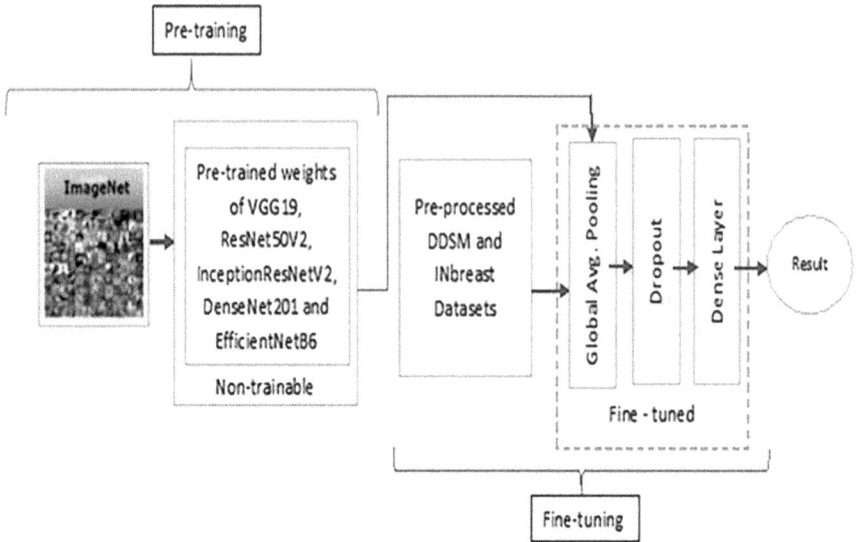

FIGURE 14.2   The proposed approach for selected model.

learning and global average pooling layer. An activation function used in an AI model is the powerhouse of a neural network. This research work has explored two activation functions, namely ReLu in the convolution layer and Softmax in the fully connected layers. Dropout (0.2) is used before the fully connected layer to eliminate the insignificant nodes for regularizing the network. Adam optimizer is used during the compilation of the developed model. Figure 14.2 shows the fine-tuned approach of selected models.

14.4.3   PHASE III: TEST AND PREDICT BENIGN OR MALIGNANT IMAGES

Once the proposed models were trained, the models were tested to predict the benign or malignant mammogram images using the test dataset. The results of models' testing depict that among those five models, the DenseNet201 almost reached the highest prediction.

14.4.4   PHASE IV: PERFORMANCE ANALYSIS

The standard performance parameters were used to examine and compare the experimental results of the five models.

These measurement parameters are defined as follows:

$$\text{Accuracy} = \frac{TP + TN}{TP + TN + FP + FN} \times 100 \qquad (14.1)$$

$$\text{Precision} = \frac{TP}{TP + FP} \qquad (14.2)$$

$$\text{Recall} = \frac{TP}{TP + FN} \times 100 \tag{14.3}$$

$$\text{F1} - \text{Score} = 2 \times \frac{precion * recall}{precion + recall} \tag{14.4}$$

Here, the number of correctly identified malignant samples is indicated by true positive (TP), whereas the number of correctly identified benign samples is shown by true negative (TN). As a result, the wrongly identified samples are represented as benign and malignant, respectively, by the abbreviations false negative (FN) and false positive (FP). The proposed fine-tuned CNN models were trained using the Adam optimizer with a learning rate of 0.01 and a loss function of binary cross-entropy across 50 epochs with a batch size of 32.

14.5 RESULTS AND DISCUSSION

The models were executed on Google colaboratory (Colab) using Lenovo with 8 GB RAM. Colab notebook is based on the Jupyter notebook, and it works on the Google docs objects. The notebooks are configured with the necessary DL and ML library files such as Tensorflow, Keras, matplotlib, and NumPy. The model's efficiency is also experimented by fine-tuning the hyperparameters suitable for normal and abnormal detection in mammogram images.

The developed model was trained by the Adam optimizer. For the DDSM and INbreast datasets, fixed batch size of 32 was chosen. The batch size taken into consideration here was reduced since it improves the model's test accuracy and speeds up network learning. Adam's optimization with learning rate is 0.01. The model is trained using Adam, which iteratively adjusts the network's weight based on the training dataset. From adaptive moment estimation, Adam is derived. There are training and testing subsets of the dataset.

The output from each of the five models for the DDSM dataset is shown in Table 14.3. With a testing loss of 0.1089 and a superior testing accuracy of 97.60%, the DenseNet201 model can be seen to perform better. Moreover, DenseNet201 has a maximum training accuracy of 98.17% while retaining a training loss of 0.0722. The output from each of the five models for the INbreast dataset is shown in Table 14.4. As can be observed, both models perform better on tests, with the DenseNet201 model providing a test accuracy of 96.74% and a test loss of 0.1956. Moreover, DenseNet201 has a maximum training accuracy of 95.89% while retaining a training loss of 0.2084.

Table 14.5 presents the results from all five models for the DDSM dataset with the following parameters, namely precision, recall, and F1-score for the type of benign and malignant. The DenseNet201 model produced good results for precision, recall, and F1-score for benign type as 0.97, 0.96, and 0.95. Malignant type recorded as follows: 0.96, 0.97, and 0.96. Table 14.6 presents the results from all five models for INbreast dataset with the same parameters for both benign type and malignant type. The DenseNet201 model also produced good results for precision, recall, and F1-score for benign type as 0.97, 0.96, and 0.96. The results for malignant type were recorded as follows 0.95, 0.96, and 0.97. The DenseNet201 model is

TABLE 14.3
Accuracy and Loss of Models on DDSM Dataset

Fine-Tuned Models	Value of Training Accuracy	Value of Training Loss	Value of Testing Accuracy	Value of Testing Loss
VGG19	94.62	0.1423	93.91	0.1626
ResNet50V2	95.38	0.257	95.32	0.497
InceptionResNetV2	86.07	2.0805	87.56	2.2543
EfficientNetB6	90.65	0.2412	90.03	0.2372
DenseNet201	**98.17**	**0.0722**	**97.60**	**0.1089**

TABLE 14.4
Accuracy and Loss of Models on INbreast Dataset

Fine-Tuned Models	Value of Training Accuracy	Value of Training Loss	Value of Testing Accuracy	Value of Testing Loss
VGG19	93.26	0.2143	92.78	0.2675
ResNet50V2	95.83	0.3489	94.65	0.2098
InceptionResNetV2	88.52	0.8052	87.95	0.8543
EfficientNetB6	94.52	0.2412	95.46	0.2372
DenseNet201	**96.74**	**0.1956**	**95.89**	**0.2084**

TABLE 14.5
Performance Analysis of Models on DDSM Dataset

Fine-Tuned Models	Class Type	Value of Precision	Value of Recall	Value of F1-score
VGG19	B	0.95	0.92	0.93
	M	0.94	0.96	0.93
ResNet50V2	B	0.95	0.90	0.92
	M	0.92	0.95	0.90
InceptionResNetV2	B	0.83	0.87	0.84
	M	0.85	0.86	0.83
EfficientNetB6	B	0.93	0.94	0.93
	M	0.96	0.95	0.94
DenseNet201	**B**	**0.97**	**0.96**	**0.95**
	M	**0.96**	**0.97**	**0.96**

performed well in both datasets as well as both benign (B) type and malignant (M) type detection and classification based on the performance metrics.

In Figures 14.3(a)-(e), the number of epochs considered for the experiment is shown on the X axis, while the accuracy and loss of the VGG19, ResNet50V2, InceptionResNetV2, DenseNet201, and EfficientNetB6 models relative to the DDSM

TABLE 14.6

Performance Analysis of Models on INbreast Dataset

Fine-Tuned Models	Class type	Value of Precision	Value of Recall	Value of F1-score
VGG19	B	0.94	0.92	0.93
	M	0.93	0.94	0.91
ResNet50V2	B	0.89	0.90	0.90
	M	0.88	0.89	0.91
InceptionResNetV2	B	0.79	0.80	0.78
	M	0.78	0.77	0.79
EfficientNetB6	B	0.96	0.94	0.95
	M	0.95	0.95	0.96
DenseNet201	B	0.97	0.96	0.96
	M	0.95	0.96	0.97

dataset are shown on the Y axis, respectively. Figures 14.4(a) to (e) show the loss and accuracy values of VGG19, ResNet50V2, InceptionResNetV2, DenseNet201, and EfficientNetB6 with respect to the INbreast dataset.

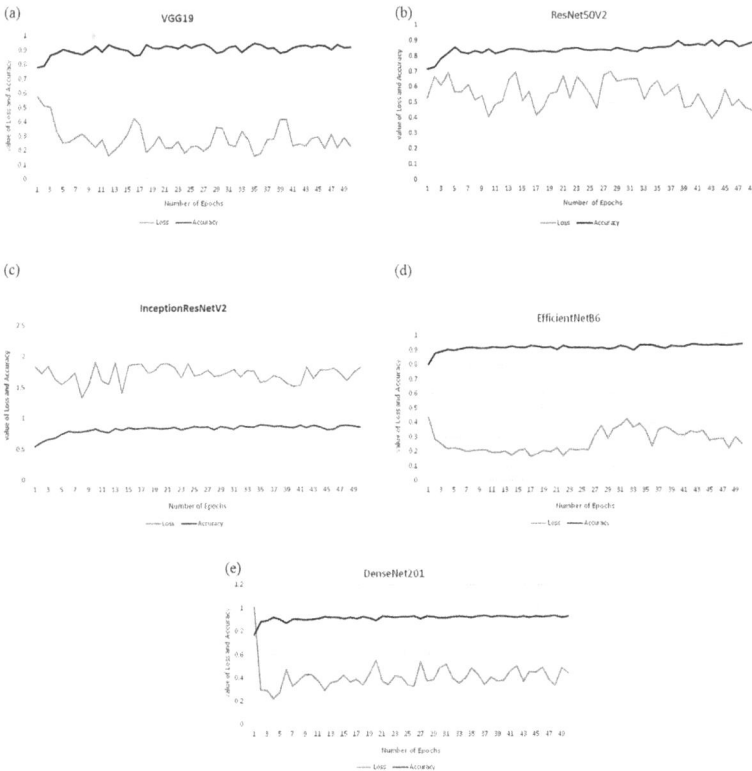

FIGURE 14.3 Accuracy and loss of models on DDSM datasets for (a) VGG19, (b) ResNet50V2, (c) InceptionResNetV2, (d) DenseNet201, and (e) EfficientNetB6.

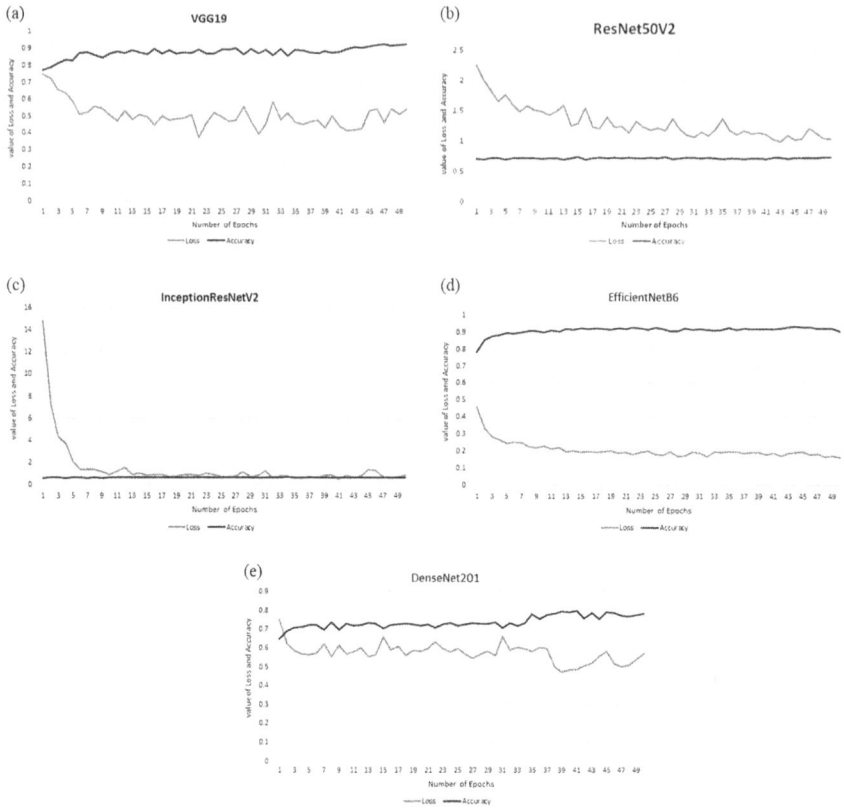

FIGURE 14.4 Value loss and value accuracy of INbreast datasets for (a) VGG19, (b) ResNet50V2, (c) InceptionResNetV2, (d) DenseNet201, and (e) EfficientNetB6.

14.6 CONCLUSION

The accurate classification of mammogram images into benign or malignant remains a challenge for radiologists while diagnosing breast cancer. In recent years, automated classification of mammogram images using transfer learning-based models for breast cancer diagnosis is a boon to radiologists to validate their medical inferences. This chapter has delineated the behavior of transfer learning-based neural network models viz., VGG19, ResNet50V2, InceptionResNetV2, DenseNet201, and EfficientNetB6 used in benign and malignant detection and classification. These five pre-trained and fine-tuned DCNN models were explored to discover the best-fit model delivering the most accuracy. This performance of the DenseNet201 model has yielded the maximum accuracy in both DDSM and INbreast datasets. This proposed model DenseNet201 has offered the maximum accuracy and in terms of precision, recall, and F1-score for benign and malignant type detection and classification.

REFERENCES

1. Breast Cancer. 2021. Available online: https://www.who.int/news-room/fact-sheets/detail/breast-cancer (accessed on 19 July 2021).
2. Sung, H.; Ferlay, J.; Siegel, R.L.; Laversanne, M.; Soerjomataram, I.; Jemal, A.; Bray, F. Global cancer statistics 2020: GLOBOCAN estimates of incidence and mortality worldwide for 36 cancers in 185 countries. CA Cancer J. Clin. 2021, 71, 209–249.
3. Lauby-Secretan, B.; Scoccianti, C.; Loomis, D.; Benbrahim-Tallaa, L.; Bouvard, V.; Bianchini, F.; Straif, K. Breast-cancer screening viewpoint of the IARC Working Group. N. Engl. J. Med. 2015, 372, 2353–2358.
4. Zahoor, S.; Lali, I.U.; Khan, M.A.; Javed, K.; Mehmood, W. Breast cancer detection and classification using traditional computer vision techniques: A comprehensive review. Curr. Med. Imaging 2020, 16, 1187–1200.
5. Xie, J.; Liu, R.; Luttrell IV, J.; Zhang, C. Deep learning based analysis of histopathological images of breast cancer. Front. Genet. 2019, 10, 80.
6. Lehman, C.D.; Yala, A.; Schuster, T.; Dontchos, B.; Bahl, M.; Swanson, K.; Barzilay, R. Mammographic breast density assessment using deep learning: Clinical implementation. Radiology 2019, 290, 52–58.
7. Le, H.; Gupta, R.; Hou, L.; Abousamra, S.; Fassler, D.; Torre-Healy, L.; Moffitt, R.A.; Kurc, T.; Samaras, D.; Batiste, R.; et al. Utilizing automated breast cancer detection to identify spatial distributions of tumor infiltrating lymphocytes in invasive breast Cancer. Am. J. Pathol. 2020, 190, 1491–1504.
8. Huang, D.; Bai, H.;Wang, L.; Hou, Y.; Li, L.; Xia, Y.; Yan, Z.; Chen,W.; Chang, L.; Li,W. The application and development of deep learning in radiotherapy: A systematic review. Technol. Cancer Res. Treat. 2021, 20, 15330338211016386.
9. Burt, J.R.; Torosdagli, N.; Khosravan, N.; Raviprakash, H.; Mortazi, A.; Tissavirasingham, F.; Hussein, S.; Bagci, U. Deep learning beyond cats and dogs: Recent advances in diagnosing breast cancer with deep neural networks. Br. J. Radiol. 2018, 91, 20170545.
10. Chatfield, K.; Simonyan, K.; Vedaldi, A.; Zisserman, A. Return of the devil in the details: Delving deep into convolutional nets. arXiv 2014, arXiv:1405.3531.
11. Simonyan, K.; Zisserman, A. Very deep convolutional networks for large-scale image recognition. arXiv 2014, arXiv:1409.1556.
12. Shen, D.; Wu, G.; Suk, H.-I. Deep learning in medical image analysis. Med. Image Anal. 2017, 19, 221–248.
13. Litjens, G.; Kooi, T.; Bejnordi, B.E.; Setio, A.A.A.; Ciompi, F.; Ghafoorian, M.; van der Laak, J.A.; van Ginneken, B.; Sánchez, C.I. A survey on deep learning in medical image analysis. Med. Image Anal. 2017, 42, 60–88. [CrossRef] [PubMed].
14. Hussain, Z.; Gimenez, F.; Yi, D.; Rubin, D. Differential data augmentation techniques for medical imaging classification tasks. AMIA Annu. Symp. Proc. Arch. 2017, 2017, 979–984.
15. Alkhaleefah, M.; Ma, S.-C.; Chang, Y.-L.; Huang, B.; Chittem, P.K.; Achhannagari, V.P. Double-shot transfer learning for breast cancer classification from X-ray images. Appl. Sci. 2020, 10, 3999.
16. Perre, A.C.; Alexandre, L.; Freire, L.C. Lesion classification in mammograms using convolutional neural networks and transfer learning. Comput. Methods Biomech. Biomed. Eng. Imaging Vis. 2018, 7, 550–556.
17. Khamparia, A.; Bharati, S.; Podder, P.; Gupta, D.; Khanna, A.; Phung, T.K.; Thanh, D.N.H. Diagnosis of breast cancer based on modern mammography using hybrid transfer learning. Multidimens. Syst. Signal Process. 2021, 32, 747–765.

18. Kaur, P.; Singh, G.; Kaur, P. Intellectual detection and validation of automated mammogram breast cancer images by multi-class SVM using deep learning classification. Inform. Med. Unlocked 2019, 16, 100151.

19. Shaikh, K.; Krishnan, S.; Thanki, R. Deep Learning Model for Classification of Breast Cancer, in Artificial Intelligence in Breast Cancer Early Detection and Diagnosis; Springer: Berlin/Heidelberg, Germany, 2021; pp. 93–100.

20. Wahab, N.; Khan, A.; Lee, Y.S. Transfer learning based deep CNN for segmentation and detection of mitoses in breast cancer histopathological images. Microscopy 2019, 68, 216–233.

21. Cao, H.; Bernard, S.; Heutte, L.; Sabourin, R. Improve the performance of transfer learning without fine-tuning using dissimilarity based multi-view learning for breast cancer histology images. In Proceedings of the 15th International Conference, ICIAR 2018, Póvoa de Varzim, Portugal, 27–29 June 2018; Springer: Berlin/Heidelberg, Germany, 2018.

22. Charan, S.; Khan, M.J.; Khurshid, K. Breast cancer detection in mammograms using convolutional neural network. In Proceedings of the 2018 International Conference on Computing, Mathematics and Engineering Technologies (iCoMET), Wuhan, China, 7–8 February 2018; IEEE: New York, NY, USA, 2018.

23. Heath, M.; Bowyer, K.; Kopans, D.; Moore, R.; Kegelmeyer, W.P. The digital database for screening mammography. In Proceedings of the 5th International Workshop on Digital Mammography, Toronto, ON, Canada, 11–14 June 2000; pp. 212–218.

24. Moreira, I.C.; Amaral, I.; Domingues, I.; Cardoso, A.; Cardoso, M.J.; Cardoso, J.S. INbreast: Toward a full-field digital mammographic database. Acad. Radiol. 2012, 19, 236–248.

25. Houssein, E.H; Emam, M.M; Ali, A.A; Suganthan, P.N. Deep and machine learning techniques for medical imaging-based breast cancer: A comprehensive review. Expert SystAppl 2020, 167, 114161.

26. Yap, M.H.; Pons, G.; Martí, J.; Ganau, S., Sentís, M., Zwiggelaar, R., Davison, A.K., Martí, R. Automated breast ultrasound lesions detection using convolutional neural networks. IEEE J Biomed Health Inform 2017, 22(4):1218–1226.

27. Lumini, A; Nanni, L. Deep learning and transfer learning features for plankton classification. Ecol Inform 2019, 51, 33–43.

28. Gaspar, A; Oliva, D.; Cuevas, E., Zaldívar, D., Pérez, M.; Pajares, G. Hyperparameter optimization in a convolutional neural network using metaheuristic algorithms. In Metaheuristics in Machine Learning: Theory and Applications. Springer, 2021, pp. 37–59.

29. Sathiyamoorthi, V.; Ilavarasi, A.K.; Murugeswari, K.; Thouheed Ahmed, S.; Aruna Devi, B.; Kalipindi, M. A deep convolutional neural network based computer aided diagnosis system for the prediction of Alzheimer's disease in MRI images. Measurement 2021, 171, 108838, ISSN 0263-2241, 10.1016/j.measurement.2020.108838.

30. Nithya, A. and Shanmugavadivu, P., An Introspective Performance Analysis of Threshold-based Segmentation Techniques on Digital Mammograms, International Journal of YMER, 20(11), 176–195.

15 Case Study

Deep Learning-Based Approach for Detection and Treatment of Retinopathy of Prematurity

S. Karkuzhali
Department of Computer Science and Engineering, Mepco
Schlenk Engineering College, Sivakasi, Tamil Nadu, India

K. Murugeswari
School of Computing Science and Engineering,
VIT Bhopal University, Madhya Pradesh, India

Thendral Puyalnithi
Department of Artificial Intelligence & Data Science, Mepco
Schlenk Engineering College, Sivakasi, Tamil Nadu, India

S. Senthilkumar
Department of Chemistry, Ayya Nadar Janaki Ammal
College, Sivakasi, Tamil Nadu, India

G. Ganesan
School of Computing Science and Engineering,
VIT Bhopal University, Madhya Pradesh, India

15.1 INTRODUCTION

Retinopathy of prematurity (ROP) is an eye condition that primarily affects young infants' fundus vasculature. The disease's effects can be slight, leaving no obvious abnormalities, or they can be severe, resulting in neovascularization, retinal detachment, and perhaps even childhood blindness. Plus, the condition, which is clinically identified by spotting specific morphological alterations to the blood vessels present in the retina of premature newborns, is an essential indicator for starting therapy for ROP. Around the world, ROP is a major factor in preventable

DOI: 10.1201/9781003469605-15

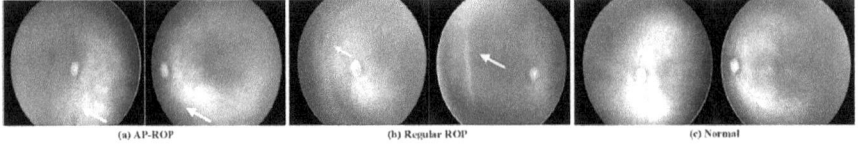

(a) AP-ROP   (b) Regular ROP   (c) Normal

FIGURE 15.1   A schematic diagram of various fundus images of an eye.

childhood blindness. If the illness is not identified and adequately treated in its early stages, it could result in irreversible blindness. ROP frequently occurs in conjunction with Plus disease, a retinal illness marked by aberrant blood vessel dilatation and tortuosity [1].

"Childhood blindness refers to a collection of disorders and conditions beginning in childhood or early adolescence, which if left untreated, culminates in blindness or severe visual impairment that are likely to be untreatable later in life," according to WHO. One of the main causes of irreversible but preventable childhood blindness is ROP, a retinal illness that affects the undeveloped retina of preterm infants. Over 3.5 million preterm babies are born each year in India, and as economic conditions and standards of life have improved, so too has the infant survival rate. Despite this, because of the high birth rate, improved survival of low birth weight children, and a lack of effective operational standards for mandated ROP screening, the vulnerability of infants in rural regions to visually impaired diseases like ROP is increasing. More than 60,000 infants in India are said to require (treatment-grade) ROP each year, according to reports. However, ROP-related blindness is largely avoidable if diagnosed and treated in a timely manner [2].

ROP is one of the most frequent causes of childhood blindness in premature infants, and aggressive posterior retinopathy of prematurity (AP-ROP) is a special type of ROP that, if not recognized and treated early, will advance quickly into the fifth stage of ROP and even blindness. APROP is uncommon and has few symptoms, which makes it simple for mistakes to occur. Using computer-assisted methods, clinicians can accurately diagnose AP-ROP early on [3]. Figure 15.1 shows the schematic diagram of various fundus images of an eye.

15.2   LITERATURE SURVEY

Wang et al. [1] demonstrated that deep neural networks (DNNs) can be trained using sizable datasets to automatically detect ROP in pictures of the retinal fundus with good sensitivity and accuracy without the need for expert feature specification. The generated DNNs achieved equivalent performance and produced the detection prediction extremely well when compared with human experts with sufficient clinical knowledge in ROP diagnosis. Additionally, it consistently makes the same diagnosis on a given image, which is challenging for a human ophthalmologist. To imitate the advice of various experts, multiple DNN models can be trained and combined. We shall put this to the test in subsequent work. Additionally, compared to the method in the literature, the proposed method in this study is more appropriate for use in an automated ROP screening system.

The test conducted in a clinical environment demonstrated the Deep ROP platform's outstanding performance. According to the findings, whereas ROP detection performed admirably prospectively, ROP grading did not. There could be two causes. One is that compared to characteristics between "normal" cases and "ROP" cases, those between "mild ROP" cases and "severe ROP" patients are harder to differentiate. The second is that the Gr-generalization Net's performance is worse than the Id because Net's fewer cases were used to construct it than were used to develop the Id-Net. For a number of reasons, the clinical setting test is a crucial step in telemedicine ROP screening programs and multihospital collaboration. In non-specialized hospitals, it permits ROP pre-screening and evaluation of patients.

Second, it speeds up the process of gathering a sizable dataset for fine-grained ROP grading and removes the data usage bottleneck caused by the isolation of data in separate hospitals. Third, the cloud-based platform can gather fresh information, expanding the area covered by ROP features and enhancing the ROP detection algorithm. For instance, in the study's web-based test, 4908 photos of 944 incidents involving 404 infants were gathered over the course of 10 months. These data items were greater in size than published datasets [4]. Figure 15.2 shows the Flow diagram of ROP diagnosis using ResNET. Figure 15.3 shows the A cloud-based DNN model for diagnosis of ROP.

Bao et al. (2021) reviewed telemedicine as a technique for remote image interpretation that can deliver medical care to isolated areas, but it still needs local workers to be trained. Computer-based image analytical systems for ROP were subsequently developed using the data gathered from telemedicine image collections. The aforementioned systems have so far primarily been created through the use of multiple machine learning, deep learning (DL), and classic machine learning. Various computer-aided ROP systems based on traditional machine learning have become available over the past 20 years and have attained satisfactory performance, including RISA, ROPtool, and CAIER. Additionally, highly accurate automated ROP diagnosis tools based on DL are being created for clinical applications. Figures 15.4 and 15.5 show the image labeling process and architecture diagram of DNN [5]. Figure 15.6 shows the flowchart for database search and study selection.

Chang et al. looked for randomized controlled trials and nonrandomized comparative studies that had been published as of March 2022 in the CENTRAL, Embase, MEDLINE, and CINAHL databases. Studies with comparable populations and treatment standards that used bevacizumab, ranibizumab, aflibercept, or laser for ROP were considered. The Grading of Recommendations, Assessment, Development and Evaluation methodology was used to analyze studies, and those that had biased case selection, nonrandomized case-control, or no control group were disqualified. The absolute primary retreatment rate for each modality was calculated using frequentist meta-analyses of proportions, and Bayesian network meta-analyses compared pairs of treatments for type 1 and Zone I ROP [6].

Su et al. (2022) describe the therapeutic antagonists of three different types, including peptides, nonpeptides, and monoclonal antibodies, which effectively inhibit pathological apelin/APJ signaling activation and have been used to treat a variety of diseases and conditions, including hypertension, renal ischemia, pulmonary disorders,

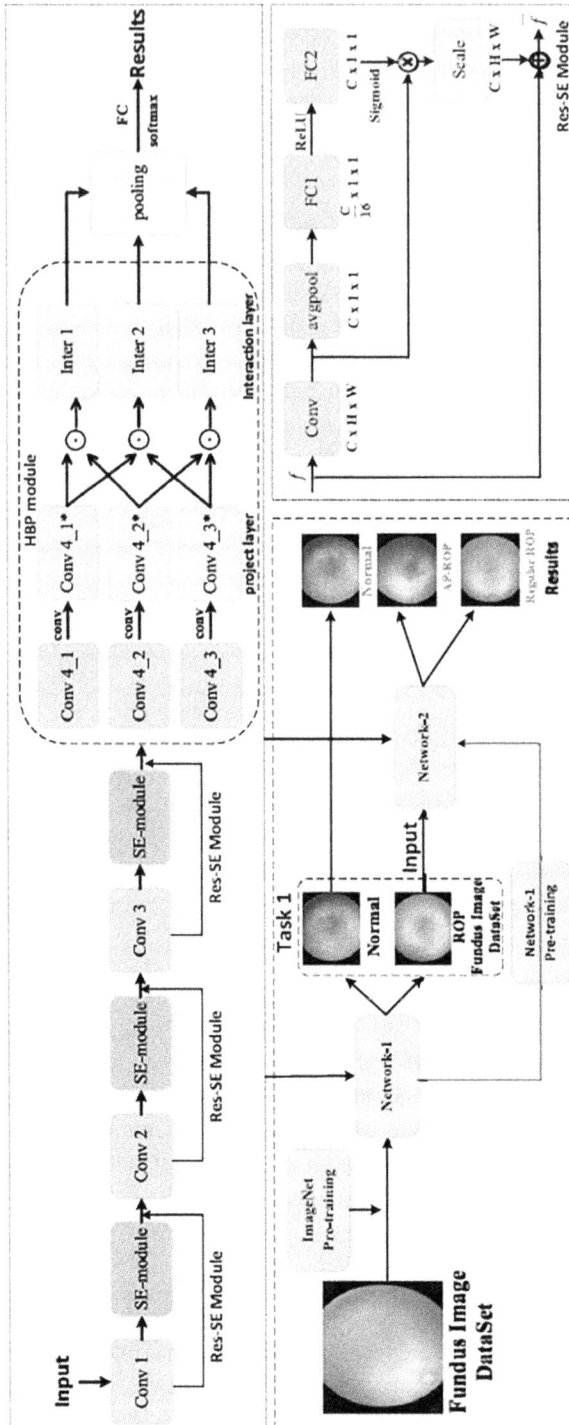

FIGURE 15.2 Flow diagram of ROP diagnosis using ResNET.

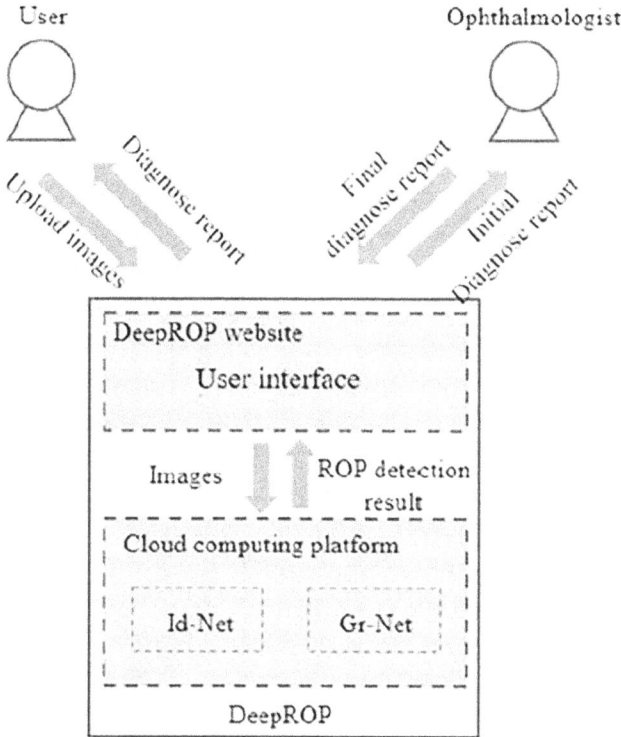

FIGURE 15.3 A cloud-based DNN model for diagnosis of ROP.

polycystic ovary syndrome, endothelial dysfunction, cardiac hypertrophy, chronic heart failure, tumor metastasis, harmful virus infiltration at the central nervous system, and pathological retinal ROP, a prominent retinal condition that frequently results in childhood blindness, primarily involves abnormal apelin/APJ signaling. As a result, we speculate that all three types of antagonists that are specific to apelin peptides and the APJ receptor and have been reviewed in this study may be clinically useful in reducing the abnormal retinal vasculature associated with ROP. These therapeutic antagonists that target the pathogenic apelin/APJ signaling activity must undergo clinical trials to prove their effectiveness [7].

Park et al. (2021) found that therapeutic antagonists of three different types, including peptides, nonpeptides, and monoclonal antibodies, effectively inhibit pathological apelin/APJ signaling activation and have been used to treat a variety of diseases and conditions, including hypertension, renal ischemia, pulmonary disorders, polycystic ovary syndrome, endothelial dysfunction, cardiac hypertrophy, chronic heart failure, tumor metastasis, harmful virus infiltration at the central nervous system, and pathological retinal. Eighty-five singleton preterm newborns (24.5 weeks gestational age [GA] at delivery–30 weeks) with either preterm labor with intact membranes (PTL) or preterm premature rupture of membranes

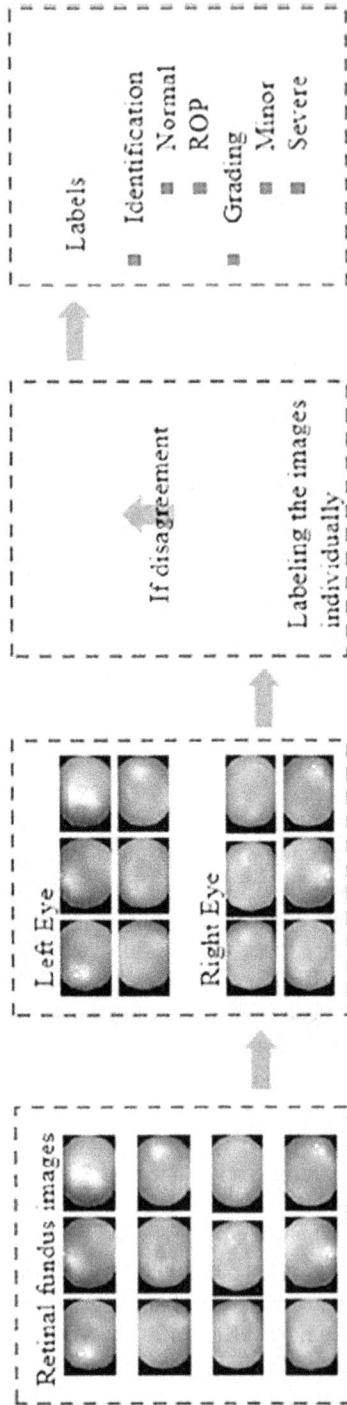

FIGURE 15.4 Image labeling process.

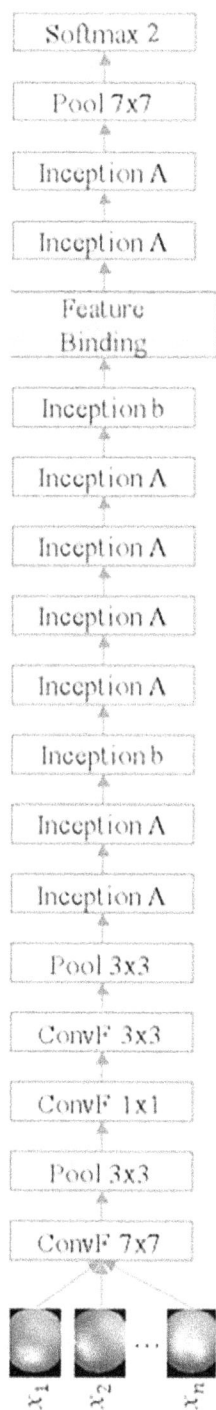

FIGURE 15.5 Architecture diagram of DNN.

```
┌─────────────────────────────────────┐
│ 800 records identified from MEDLINE, │
│ EMBASE, Cochrane Library,            │
│ ClinicalTrials.gov, and other reviews│
└─────────────────────────────────────┘
                  │
                  ▼
┌─────────────────────────────────────┐
│ 539 records after duplicates removed │
└─────────────────────────────────────┘
                  │
                  ▼
┌─────────────────────────────────────┐
│ 539 records included on title and    │
│ abstract review                      │
└─────────────────────────────────────┘
                  │                    ┌────────────────────────────┐
                  ├───────────────────▶│ 444 excluded as irrelevant  │
                  │                    │ to our subject              │
                  ▼                    └────────────────────────────┘
┌─────────────────────────────────────┐
│ 95 full-text articles assessed for   │
│ eligibility                          │
└─────────────────────────────────────┘
                  │                    ┌──────────────────────────────────────────────┐
                  │                    │ 65 excluded:                                   │
                  │                    │ 38 Intervention or outcome not of interest     │
                  ├───────────────────▶│ 8 Non-comparative study                        │
                  │                    │ 17 Follow up studies of included studies       │
                  │                    │ 1 Non-conventional follow up                   │
                  │                    │ 1 Conference abstract (non-peer reviewed)      │
                  ▼                    └──────────────────────────────────────────────┘
┌─────────────────────────────────────┐
│ 30 studies included in meta-analysis │
│ 11 Bevacizumab vs Laser              │
│ 6 Ranibizumab vs Laser               │
│ 5 Bevacizumab vs Ranibizumab         │
│ 3 Bevacizumab vs Ranibizumab vs Laser│
│ 2 Aflibercept vs Laser               │
│ 1 Ranibizumab vs Aflibercept         │
│ 1 Bevacizumab vs Aflibercept         │
│ 1 Bevacizumab vs Ranibizumab vs Aflibercept │
└─────────────────────────────────────┘
```

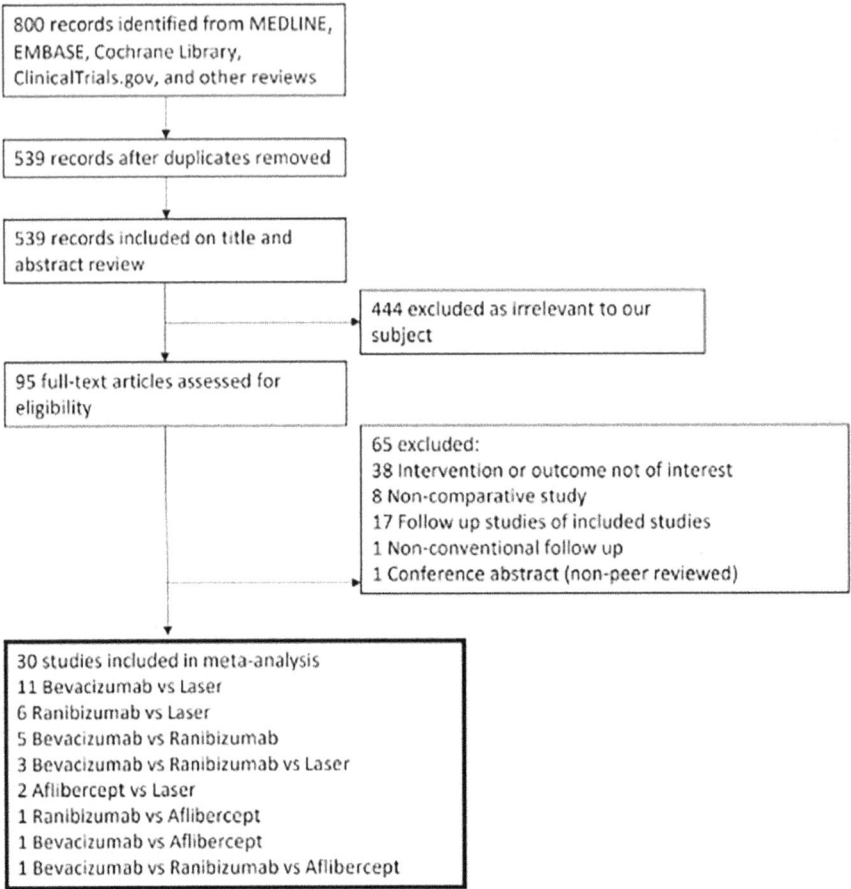

FIGURE 15.6 Flowchart for database search and study selection.

were studied for the prevalence of ROP without FGR (birth weight 5th percentile for GA), preterm-PROM membranes. The advancement of inflammation in the extra-placental membranes (EPM), chorionic vessels (CV), and umbilical cord were used to categorize the patients (UC) [8]. Figure 15.7 shows the architecture diagram for ROP diagnostic method employing U-COSFIRE filters. Figure 15.8 shows the flow diagram for blood vessel segmentation using the adaptive method. Figure 15.9 shows the right and left eyes in a schematic with zone borders.

Chiang et al. (2021) created a consensus agreement called the International Categorization of Retinopathy of Preterm, which establishes a uniform terminology for ROP classification. It was first released in 1984, then it was enlarged, then it was republished in 2005. This article introduces a third revision, the International Classification of Retinopathy of Prematurity, Third Edition (ICROP3), which is now

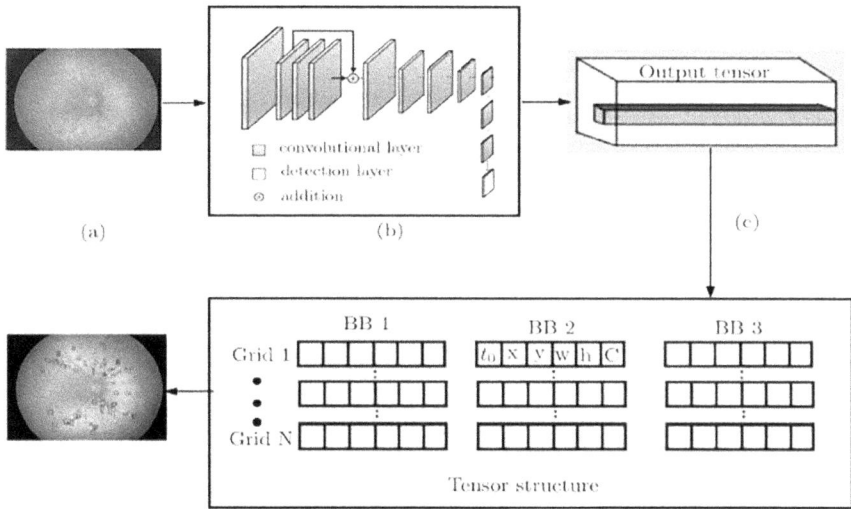

FIGURE 15.7 The architecture diagram for ROP diagnostic method employing U-COSFIRE filters.

necessary due to issues like: (1) worries about subjectivity in crucial disease classification components; (2) advancements in ophthalmic imaging; and (3) novel pharmacologic therapies (such as anti-vascular endothelial growth factor agents) with distinct regression and reactivation features after treatment compared with existing standards [9].

Campbell et al. (2022) are members of the ICROP3 committee who labeled two distinct datasets of 30 fundus pictures each for stage (0e5) and disease (plus, preplus, neither) using an open-source platform. A continuous label for plus (1e9) and stage (1e3) for each image was created by averaging these results. Additionally, experts were asked to assess the relative severity of the plus disease in each image. Additionally, the Imaging and Informatics in ROP DL system assigned each image a vascular severity score, which was correlated with each grader's diagnostic labeling and the stage of the disease determined by ophthalmoscopic examination [10]. Figure 15.10 shows the example images for determination of plus disease and stage by members of the International Classification of Retinopathy of Prematurity (ICROP) committee. Figure 15.11 shows the spectrum of disease severity for plus and stage in ROP.

Iwahashi et al. (2021) gathered the following information from the patient's medical records: gender, gestational age at birth, birth weight, ROP stage, postmenstrual age (PMA) at LSV, surgical technique, preoperative injection of anti-VEGF medicines, additional retinal operations, and lensectomy during follow-up [11].

Coyner et al. (2022) discussed how a large amount of diverse, carefully picked data are needed to develop powerful artificial intelligence (AI) models for analyzing medical images; however, gathering this data might be difficult due to privacy issues, the rarity of some diseases, or the accuracy of the diagnostic labels. Gathering data for

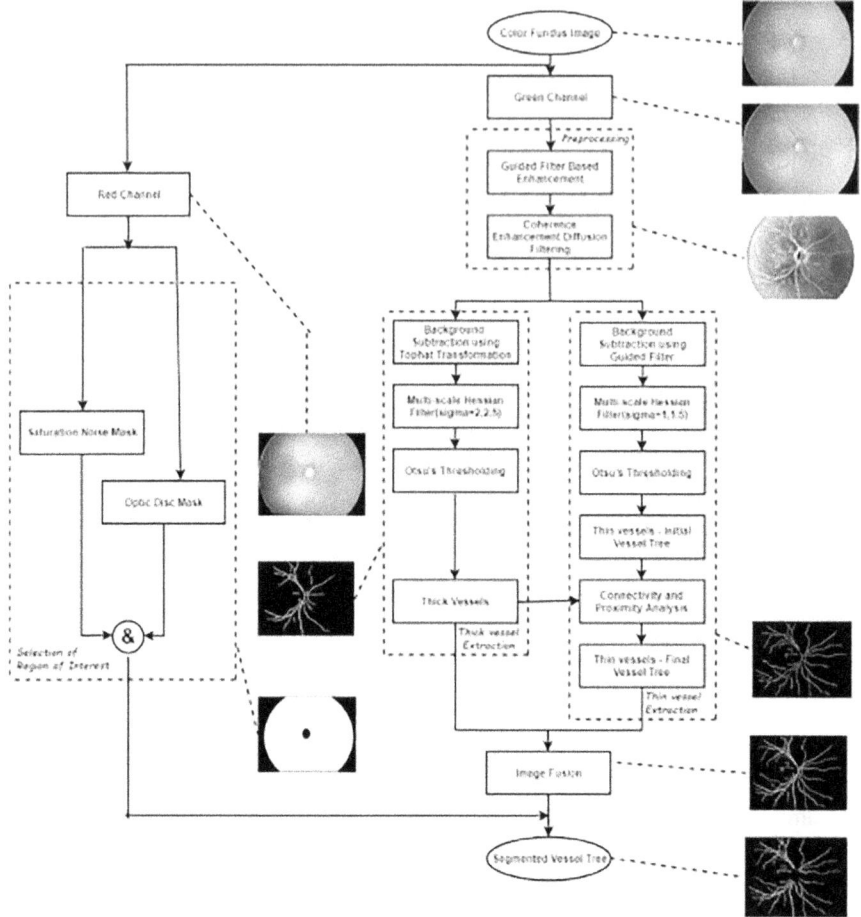

FIGURE 15.8   Flow diagram for blood vessel segmentation using adaptive method.

ROP, the disease that could cause blindness, experiences these difficulties. Because they can create extremely realistic images, progressive growing generative adversarial networks (PGANs) may be helpful in expanding the number and diversity of medical datasets [12].

Podraza et al. (2020) discovered that the condition comprises two distinct postnatal phases, the first of which is thought to be brought on by hyperoxia. Blood transfusions, which introduce "non-physiological" adult hemoglobin (HbA) into the newborn circulation instead of the physiological fetal hemoglobin, are one of the most significant risk factors for ROP in standard clinical practice (HbF). Since HbA and HbF have differing affinity for oxygen, HbA will release more oxygen into the retina than HbF. Instead of adult blood, it is hypothesized that this significantly larger input of oxygen from HbA may be seen as hyperoxia by the pertinent retinal

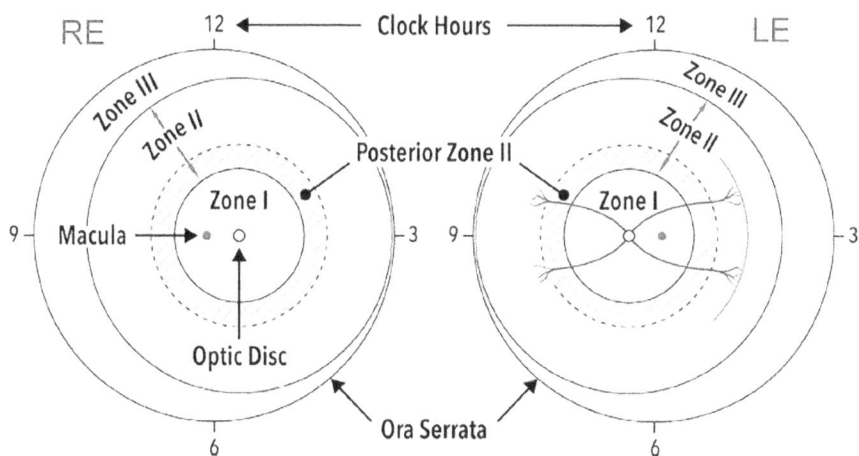

FIGURE 15.9 Right and left eyes are shown in a schematic with zone borders and clock hour sectors to indicate where vascularization is present and how much retinopathy there is.

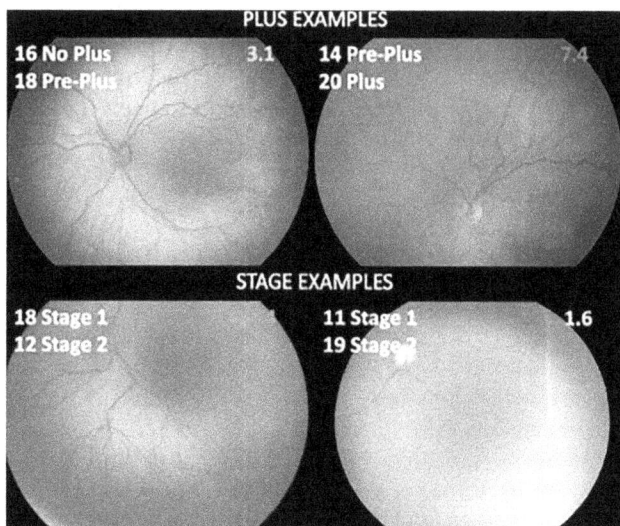

FIGURE 15.10 Example images for determination of plus disease and stage by members of the International Classification of Retinopathy of Prematurity (ICROP) committee.

receptors. In light of the aforementioned factors, I contend that the genesis and progression of ROP is significantly influenced by the introduction of non-physiological HbA from adult donors during blood transfusion for anemia. According to this theory, there is a threshold for HbA at which the chain of events outlined in the pathogenesis of ROP is set off. I suggest beginning a new branch of medicine called neonatal transfusion medicine in order to prevent ROP. Instead of

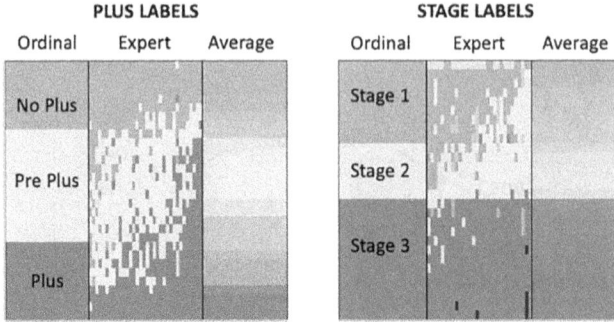

FIGURE 15.11   Spectrum of disease severity for plus and stage in ROP.

using adult blood to treat premature newborns (who are at risk for ROP), this technology would collect and prepare umbilical cord blood from the placenta of healthy newborns, which contains about 100% HbF [13].

Al Amro et al. (2018) briefed that blindness can be avoided with early detection and proper treatment. The basis in the care of this condition is an effective and timely screening examination of the retina by an experienced ophthalmologist who treats premature newborns with ROP. This timing should also be known by all neonatologists and pediatricians who treat these preterm infants who are at danger. This useful guideline aims to instruct ophthalmologists, neonatologists, and other healthcare professionals in Saudi Arabia on the most recent indications for ROP screening and management in order to avoid or reduce difficulties down the road. This useful recommendation was developed by the Ministry of Health's National Eye Health Program (NEHP) and Neonatology Services Improvement Program. It also received support from the Saudi Ophthalmological Society (SOS) [14].

Tu et al. (2020) discussed in this retrospective investigation, data on preterm infants who were less than 1500 g at birth and who received total parenteral nutrition (TPN) for at least seven days between January 2009 and November 2017. By employing various lipid emulsions during two different epochs— epoch 1 (soybean-based lipid emulsions, January 2009–February 2014) and epoch 2 (fish oil–containing lipid emulsions, January 2015–November 2017)—we compared clinical results. The incidence of ROP and the number of ROP cases necessitating bevacizumab therapy were the main outcomes assessed [15].

Tao et al. (2020) examined 75 newborns who were born within 28 weeks of their first period (PMA) were included in the study. The goal variable was evaluated as being the quantity of PC procedures for ROP [16].

Desideri et al. (2022) discussed how the role of AI and DL models in the field of ophthalmology has recently attracted growing interest on a global scale. DL models are regarded as the cutting-edge AI technology at the moment. In fact, DL systems are able to identify, characterize, and quantify abnormal clinical characteristics.

Several retinal illnesses, including glaucoma, are currently being studied in relation to the importance for early diagnosis and management. The early diagnosis of diabetic retinopathy (DR), wet age-related macular degeneration (w-AMD), ROP, and glaucoma has shown encouraging results when the DL model is applied to fundus pictures, visual fields, and optical coherence tomography (OCT) imaging. Without ignoring the current limitations and difficulties in adopting AI and DL models, we analyze the available evidence of AI applied to ocular illnesses in this study. We also consider potential future advances and therapeutic implications [17].

An observational, retrospective research by Chaves-Samaniego et al. (2020) included 233 preterm infants who were evaluated between 1999 and 2019. For postnatal weight gain in the first four weeks of life, birth weight, gestational age, mechanical ventilation, transfusion, the presence of sepsis, persistence of arterial ductus, necrotizing enterocolitis, intraventricular hemorrhage, or periventricular leukomalacia, it was discovered that there were significant differences between the ROP groups. While the ROP group that did require therapy experienced a mean postnatal weight increase of 9.50 5.45 g/day, the ROP group that did not require therapy experienced a mean postnatal weight gain of 12.75 5.99 g/day [18].

Navarro-Blanco et al. (2020) discussed the lack of ophthalmologists who specialize in the treatment of preterm infants in every hospital that provides neonatal care in Europe, and in Spain, in particular, which is a worry when it comes to ROP screening. A total of 99 public and private hospitals that cared for newborns with birth weights ≤ 1500 g underwent an analysis of ROP screening in neonatal units by Moral Pumarega et al. Only 39% of the hospitals surveyed had pediatric ophthalmologists on staff, whereas the other centers allowed any of the on-staff ophthalmologists to do examinations, according to their findings [19].

Khurram et al. (2021) found that a hyperpigmented torpedo maculopathy lesion was discovered in one of the eyes of a prematurely born newborn with bilateral ROP (one eye cured), while the other eye had microphthalmia, a congenital cataract, and non-specific pigmentary retinopathy. Laboratory tests later revealed elevated plasma IgG and IgM for toxoplasmosis following negative TORCH screening [20].

All analyses in the study by Fleck et al. (2022) were done by eye, not by subject. Only data from the 24-week core study were used to determine how long it took for disease, stage 3 ROP, and AP-ROP to regress. The first observation of a certain trait ceasing to exist was used to characterize the regression of plus illness or other ROP symptoms. Mild, moderate, or severe disease was classified as occurring in at least two quadrants. If an additional therapy was administered, an undesirable retinal structure emerged, the newborn died, or the trial was discontinued, the eyes were censored (no longer counted) [21].

Zhou et al. (2022) found that the retina and its vasculature are further harmed by the progression of ROP. The disease's long-term effects, like choroidal thinning and foveal dysplasia, were sustained by teenagers who contracted ROP as infants, according to newly available research. These results may be related to the electroretinogram's substantial photoreceptor malfunction. Since the 1980s, there has been a noticeable increase in neonatal care, and now, more prematurely born babies survive and grow up. There is currently little research on the visual abilities and ocular structure of preterm adults. This study's main objective was to describe the visual abilities of a group of young adults who were prematurely born. We also sought to determine whether ROP could predispose the adults born preterm to longer-term visual dysfunctions, taking into consideration the sneaky character of ROP. All participants gave their informed consent. The ethics committee and institutional review board gave their approval. We classified data according to better BCVA (strong eyes) and poorer BCVA (weak eyes) while examining best-corrected visual acuity (BCVA), refractive errors, and contrast sensitivities (CSs), as previously described [22].

In a study by Chen et al. (2021), each infant's oxygen saturations and percentage of inspired oxygen (FiO2) were manually retrieved from the EHR (PMA) up until 31 weeks' postmenstrual age. Weekly calculations of FiO2 and cumulative minimum, maximum, and mean oxygen saturation were made. To identify infants that had TR-ROP, random forest models were trained with five-fold cross-validation using gestational age (GA) and cumulative minimum FiO2 at 30 weeks PMA. Due to the small number of newborns, a secondary receiver operating characteristic (ROC) curve analysis without cross-validation was out [23].

Scruggs et al. (2022) found that to evaluate early vitreoretinal pathologic features objectively, en face and B-scan imaging of the peripheral retina should be acquired. These features include the distinction between anterior avascular and vascularized retina, the presence of early ridge formation, and tiny neovascular tufts [24].

As part of the Imaging and Informatics in ROP (i-ROP) cohort study, Hanif et al. (2022) used wide-angle retinal pictures from patients having diagnostic ROP exams to train DL neural networks. In ROP retinal fundus images from two datasets, neural networks were trained with either class or comparative labels representing disease severity. All networks were tested using a different test dataset after training and validation in one of two binary classification tasks: normal vs aberrant or plus versus nonplus [25].

In Nepal and Mongolia, Cole et al. (2022) used the Forus 3nethra Neo (Forus Health) and RetCam Portable (Natus Medical, Inc.) to capture fundus images. The International Classification of ROP was used to analyze the medical record and assess the overall severity of ROP (ICROP). Using a reference standard diagnostic, the presence of plus illness was identified separately in each image. On pictures from the RetCam, the i-ROP DL algorithm was trained to identify the disease and assign a vascular severity score (VSS) ranging from 1 to 9 [26,27]. Figure 15.12 shows the comparison of the preterm without ROP versus the preterm group with ROP in terms of best-corrected visual acuity (BCVA), sphere refraction, cylinder refraction, and contrast sensitivity (CS) between the preterm (A, C, E, and H) and term groups (B, D, F, and J).

Lower contrast sensitivity in young adults who had ROP

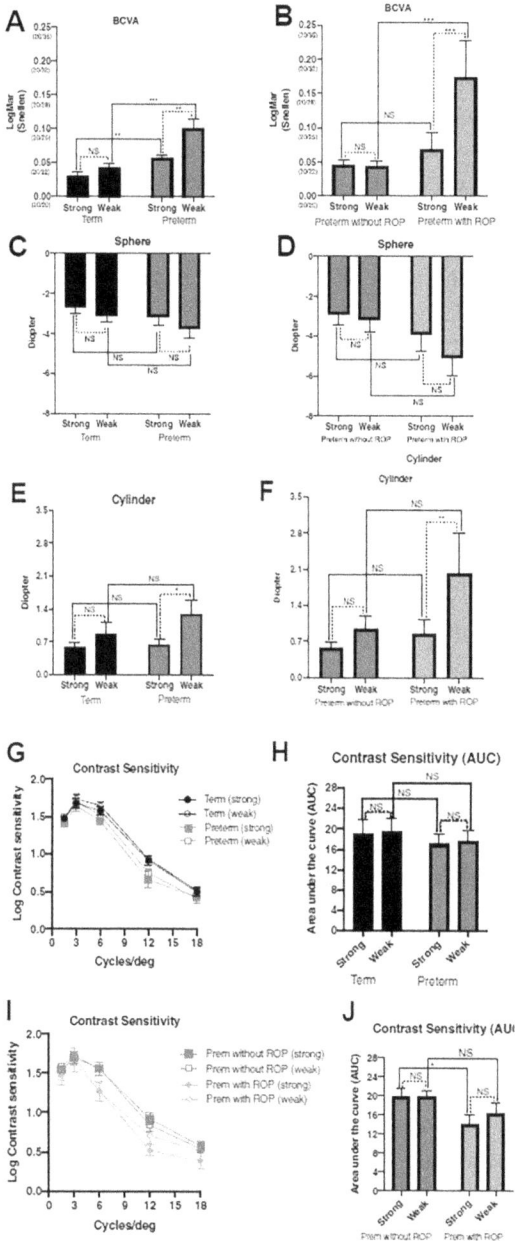

FIGURE 15.12 Comparison of the preterm without retinopathy of prematurity (ROP) versus the preterm group with ROP in terms of best-corrected visual acuity (BCVA), sphere refraction, cylinder refraction, and contrast sensitivity (CS) between the preterm (A, C, E, G and I) and term groups (B, D, F, H and J).

15.3 CONCLUSION

A vasoproliferative retinal condition called ROP mostly affects newborn preterm infants. It can be avoided as a contributor to childhood blindness. ROP has risen to the top of the list of preventable childhood blindness around the world since preterm newborns are now living longer. This avoidable blindness can be avoided with a quick screening exam performed by an ophthalmologist within a few weeks of birth. Although screening techniques and recommendations are closely followed in affluent countries, they are not in place in emerging economies like China and India, which have the highest rate of preterm births worldwide. If prompt action is not taken to address the issue, the burden of this blindness in these countries is expected to rise significantly in the future. When ROP initially appeared, it was known as retrolental fibroplasia. Since then, a great deal of research has been conducted on this illness, which has been the subject of numerous epidemics that have occurred and continue to occur in various parts of the world. However, only a small number of thorough reviews that address all facets of ROP have been published to date. This overview emphasizes the illness management tactics used in the past, present, and future. The pediatricians' expertise of ROP could use some updating.

15.4 FUTURE DIRECTION

15.4.1 Newer ROP Predictor

Early detection of ROP is essential for better results and early therapy. Only the two most significant risk factors—gestational age and birth weight—are used in the current screening recommendations; postnatal factors are not. However, only around 10% of the premature infants tested require medical attention. In an effort to predict ROP, several neonatal scoring systems, including the Clinical Risk Index for Babies, the Scores for Neonatal Acute Physiology (SNAP), and the SNAP-Perinatal Extension-II, have been developed. However, none of these systems demonstrated sufficient predictive ability for severe ROP. In order to decrease the number of ROP screening exams, it is necessary to improve the present screening protocols by creating new, better predictors.

15.4.2 Low Weight Growth Percentage

Currently, it is recognized as a risk factor for ROP to have low weight gain by six weeks following premature birth. The weight at six weeks of life less the birth weight divided by the birth weight is the proportion of the weight gain. Birth weight and gestational age alone are not believed to be as accurate indicators of severe ROP as low weight gain proportion, or weight increase less than 50% of birth weight in the first six weeks of life. Binenbaum et al. discovered that a birth weight-gestational age-weight increase model might decrease the requirement for tests by 30% in a high-risk cohort while still identifying all newborns needing an examination.

A surveillance algorithm is the WINROP algorithm. Researchers created WINROP to identify newborns at risk for severe ROP. From birth to 36 weeks after conception, serum IGF-1 levels and body weight are measured monthly for WINROP.

The WINROP algorithm was able to identify every preterm newborn later diagnosed with severe ROP in their initial prospective research, which involved 50 preterm infants. Since then, the WINROP method has been verified in numerous cohorts across a wide range of nations. According to this research, the WINROP algorithm is a reliable ROP screening tool that can be used to target care for people who are most at risk for ROP. WINROP is currently being evaluated in a significant multi-center international trial to confirm its efficacy.

15.4.3 TELE SCREENING

The gold standard for ROP screening is prompt referral by pediatricians and comprehensive evaluation by a skilled ophthalmologist. The use of digital retinal imaging is becoming more and more crucial for ROP screening. These digital imaging tools are being used efficiently by non-ophthalmologists who are being trained, such as newborn nurses and technicians. By electronically transferring the photos that these paramedical staff members take, pediatric ophthalmologists' services can be made available in remote areas. According to researchers, remote examination of the trained technicians' digital retinal images collected by them can lower referral-warranted ROP. According to the findings of these research, tele screening offers potential approaches for outreach ROP screening and will enable access to diagnostic expertise in underserved regions of both developed and developing nations.

15.4.4 OCT

The imaging technique known as optical coherence tomography, which provides cross-sectional images of the retina, has been widely applied to adult patients. Despite not being widely used in ROP, this technology is already shedding fresh light on the normal development of the retina, the acute ROP process, and its long-term aftereffects at the cellular and subcellular level.

Delivery weight, gestational age, weight increase, blood transfusions from the time of birth to the sixth week of life, and oxygen usage all factor into the ROPScore. After doing a linear regression analysis on 16 variables, researchers created this score. The study included 474 individuals, and the scores' respective areas under the receiver operating characteristic curve for predicting any stage and severe ROP were 0.77 and 0.88. They came to the conclusion that ROPScore is a promising technique that may be more accurate at predicting ROP in extremely low birth weight preterm infants than birth weight and gestational age. Additionally, the score is simple enough for ophthalmologists or the nursing staff to utilize it regularly while screening for ROP.

15.5 LIMITATIONS

First off, there are not enough "severe ROP" instances to guarantee the clinical test's generalization performance. Second, the technology that has been created can only assess the severity of ROP. In our upcoming research, we want to gather more information and score ROP in more precise categories like "plus-disease," "stage," and "zone." Third, whether the cloud platform's predictions will affect ophthalmologists' diagnoses in comparison to clinical testing without the platform is an unanswered question. Future testing of the platform should pay more attention to detail.

REFERENCES

1. Wang, J., Ju, R., Chen, Y., Zhang, L., Hu, J., Wu, Y., Dong, W., Zhong, J. and Yi, Z., 2018. Automated retinopathy of prematurity screening using deep neural networks. EBioMedicine, *35*, pp. 361–368.
2. Al Amro, S.A., Al Aql, F., Al Hajar, S., Al Dhibi, H., Al Nemri, A., Mousa, A. and Ahmad, J., 2018. Practical guidelines for screening and treatment of retinopathy of prematurity in Saudi Arabia. Saudi Journal of Ophthalmology, *32*(3), pp. 222–226.
3. Nisha, K.L., Sreelekha, G., Sathidevi, P.S., Mohanachandran, P. and Vinekar, A., 2019. A computer-aided diagnosis system for plus disease in retinopathy of prematurity with structure adaptive segmentation and vessel based features. Computerized Medical Imaging and Graphics, *74*, pp. 72–94.
4. Podraza, W., 2020. A new approach to neonatal medical management that could transform the prevention of retinopathy of prematurity: Theoretical considerations. Medical Hypotheses, *137*, p. 109541.
5. Tu, C.F., Lee, C.H., Chen, H.N., Tsao, L.Y., Chen, J.Y. and Hsiao, C.C., 2020. Effects of fish oil-containing lipid emulsions on retinopathy of prematurity in very low birth weight infants. Pediatrics & Neonatology, *61*(2), pp. 224–230.
6. Navarro-Blanco, C., Pastora-Salvador, N., Sánchez-Ramos, C. and Peralta-Calvo, J., 2020, December. Assessment of non-expert ophthalmologists in the analysis of retinopathy of prematurity. In Anales de pediatria (pp. S1695–S4033).
7. Ramachandran, S., Niyas, P., Vinekar, A. and John, R., 2021. A deep learning framework for the detection of Plus disease in retinal fundus images of preterm infants. Biocybernetics and Biomedical Engineering, *41*(2), pp. 362–375.
8. Bao, Y., Ming, W.K., Mou, Z.W., Kong, Q.H., Li, A., Yuan, T.F. and Mi, X.S., 2021. Current application of digital diagnosing systems for retinopathy of prematurity. Computer Methods and Programs in Biomedicine, *200*, p. 105871.
9. Park, J.Y., Park, C.W., Moon, K.C., Park, J.S., Jun, J.K., Lee, S.J. and Kim, J.H., 2021. Retinopathy of prematurity in infants without fetal growth restriction is decreased with the progression of acute histologic chorioamnionitis: New observation as a protective factor against retinopathy of prematurity. Placenta, *104*, pp. 161–167.
10. Chiang, M.F., Quinn, G.E., Fielder, A.R., Ostmo, S.R., Chan, R.P., Berrocal, A., Binenbaum, G., Blair, M., Campbell, J.P., Capone Jr, A. and Chen, Y., 2021. International classification of retinopathy of prematurity. Ophthalmology, *128*(10), pp. e51–e68.
11. Iwahashi, C., Tachibana, K., Oga, T., Kondo, C., Kuniyoshi, K. and Kusaka, S., 2021. Incidence and factors of postoperative lens opacity after lens-sparing vitrectomy for retinopathy of prematurity. Ophthalmology Retina, *5*(11), pp. 1139–1145.
12. Chaves-Samaniego, M.J., Chaves-Samaniego, M.C., Hoyos, A.M. and Serrano, J.L.G., 2021. New evidence on the protector effect of weight gain in retinopathy of prematurity. Anales de Pediatría (English Edition), *95*(2), pp. 78–85.
13. Khurram, D., Ali, S.M., Nguyen, Q.D. and Kozak, I., 2021. Congenital ocular toxoplasmosis with torpedo maculopathy and retinopathy of prematurity in a premature baby. American Journal of Ophthalmology Case Reports, *23*, p. 101121.

14. Chen, J.S., Anderson, J.E., Coyner, A.S., Ostmo, S., Sonmez, K., Erdogmus, D., Jordan, B.K., McEvoy, C.T., Dukhovny, D., Schelonka, R.L. and Chan, R.P., 2021. Quantification of early neonatal oxygen exposure as a risk factor for retinopathy of prematurity requiring treatment. Ophthalmology Science, 1(4), p. 100070.

15. Zhang, R., Zhao, J., Xie, H., Wang, T., Chen, G., Zhang, G. and Lei, B., 2022. Automatic diagnosis for aggressive posterior retinopathy of prematurity via deep attentive convolutional neural network. Expert Systems with Applications, 187, p. 115843.

16. Chang, E.T., Josan, A.S., Purohit, R., Patel, C.K. and Xue, K., 2022. A network meta-analysis of retreatment rates following Bevacizumab, Ranibizumab, Aflibercept and laser for retinopathy of prematurity. Ophthalmology.

17. Su, J., Zhang, Y., Kumar, S.A., Sun, M., Yao, Y. and Duan, Y., 2022. APJ/apelin: A promising target for the treatment of retinopathy of prematurity. Drug Discovery Today.

18. Campbell, J.P., Chiang, M.F., Chen, J.S., Moshfeghi, D.M., Nudleman, E., Ruambivoonsuk, P., Cherwek, H., Cheung, C.Y., Singh, P., Kalpathy-Cramer, J. and Ostmo, S., 2022. Artificial intelligence for retinopathy of prematurity: Validation of a vascular severity scale against international expert diagnosis. Ophthalmology, 129(7), pp. e69–e76.

19. Coyner, A.S., Chen, J.S., Chang, K., Singh, P., Ostmo, S., Chan, R.P., Chiang, M.F., Kalpathy-Cramer, J., Campbell, J.P. and Imaging and Informatics in Retinopathy of Prematurity Consortium, 2022. Synthetic medical images for robust, privacy-preserving training of artificial intelligence: Application to retinopathy of prematurity diagnosis. Ophthalmology Science, 2(2), p. 100126.

20. Tao, K., 2022. Postnatal administration of systemic steroids increases severity of retinopathy in premature infants. Pediatrics & Neonatology, 63(3), pp. 220–226.

21. Desideri, L.F., Rutigliani, C., Corazza, P., Nastasi, A., Roda, M., Nicolo, M., Traverso, C.E. and Vagge, A., 2022. The upcoming role of Artificial Intelligence (AI) for retinal and glaucomatous diseases. Journal of Optometry.

22. Fleck, B.W., Reynolds, J.D., Zhu, Q., Lepore, D., Marlow, N., Stahl, A., Li, J., Weisberger, A., Fielder, A.R. and RAINBOW Investigator Group, 2022. Time course of retinopathy of prematurity regression and reactivation after treatment with ranibi-zumab or laser in the RAINBOW trial. Ophthalmology Retina, 6(7), pp. 628–637.

23. Zhou, T.E., Kassis, P.O., Qian, C., Bérubé-Thevenet, R., Chappaz, A., Hamel, P., Chemtob, S., Nuyt, A.M. and Luu, T.M., 2022. Reduced contrast sensitivity in young adults who had retinopathy of prematurity. Ophthalmology Retina, 6(8), pp. 744–746.

24. Scruggs, B.A., Ni, S., Nguyen, T.T.P., Ostmo, S., Chiang, M.F., Jia, Y., Huang, D., Jian, Y. and Campbell, J.P., 2022. Peripheral OCT assisted by scleral depression in retinopathy of prematurity. Ophthalmology Science, 2(1), p. 100094.

25. Hanif, A., Yıldız, İ., Tian, P., Kalkanlı, B., Erdoğmuş, D., Ioannidis, S., Dy, J., Kalpathy-Cramer, J., Ostmo, S., Jonas, K. and Chan, R.P., 2022. Improved training efficiency for retinopathy of prematurity deep learning models using comparison versus class labels. Ophthalmology Science, 2(2), p. 100122.

26. Cole, E., Valikodath, N.G., Al-Khaled, T., Bajimaya, S., Sagun, K.C., Chuluunbat, T., Munkhuu, B., Jonas, K.E., Chuluunkhuu, C., MacKeen, L.D. and Yap, V., 2022. Evaluation of an artificial intelligence system for retinopathy of prematurity screening in Nepal and Mongolia. Ophthalmology Science, 2(4), p. 100165.

27. Sathiyamoorthi, V., Ilavarasi, A.K., Murugeswari, K., Ahmed, S. T., Devi, B. A. and Kalipindi, M., 2021. A deep convolutional neural network based computer aided diagnosis system for the prediction of Alzheimer's disease in MRI images. Measurement, 171, p. 108838, ISSN 0263-2241, 10.1016/j.measurement.2020.108838.

Index

For Product Safety Concerns and Information please contact our EU
representative GPSR@taylorandfrancis.com
Taylor & Francis Verlag GmbH, Kaufingerstraße 24, 80331 München, Germany

www.ingramcontent.com/pod-product-compliance
Lightning Source LLC
Chambersburg PA
CBHW060337220326
41598CB00023B/2732